Oxford Cases in Medicine and Surgery

Oxford Cases in
Medicine and Surgery

Hugo Farne
Junior Doctor; St Mary's Hospital,
Paddington, London, UK

Edward Norris-Cervetto
Junior Doctor; Royal Berkshire Hospital,
Reading, UK

James Warbrick-Smith
Junior Doctor; Gloucestershire Royal Hospital, UK

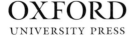
OXFORD
UNIVERSITY PRESS

OXFORD

UNIVERSITY PRESS

Great Clarendon Street, Oxford OX2 6DP

Oxford University Press is a department of the University of Oxford.
It furthers the University's objective of excellence in research, scholarship,
and education by publishing worldwide in

Oxford New York

Auckland Cape Town Dar es Salaam Hong Kong Karachi
Kuala Lumpur Madrid Melbourne Mexico City Nairobi
New Delhi Shanghai Taipei Toronto

With offices in

Argentina Austria Brazil Chile Czech Republic France Greece
Guatemala Hungary Italy Japan Poland Portugal Singapore
South Korea Switzerland Thailand Turkey Ukraine Vietnam

Oxford is a registered trade mark of Oxford University Press
in the UK and in certain other countries

Published in the United States
by Oxford University Press Inc., New York

British Library Cataloguing in Publication Data

Data available

Library of Congress Cataloging in Publication Data

Data available

Typeset by MPS Limited, A Macmillan Company
Printed in Italy
on acid-free paper by LEGO SpA-Lavis, TN

ISBN 978–0–19–956052–3

10 9 8 7 6 5 4 3 2 1

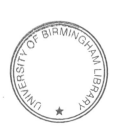

Foreword

There is an abundance of excellent medical and surgical textbooks, written in both traditional and more novel formats. However, in a climate in which the content and mode of delivery of medical education remain in constant flux there remains a need for new resources that stimulate interest in the reader as well as providing the important and relevant facts. *Oxford Cases in Medicine and Surgery* fulfils this need. This book's uniqueness – and its educational value – stems from the way that the authors have approached the learning aspect from direct clinical symptoms, highlighting the most important differential diagnoses but also explaining how to differentiate them. This approach represents the book's real strength, mirroring as it does the integrated systems-based approach that is commonly used by many medical schools.

In my experience as a clinical teacher, course organiser, and examiner over the past decade, this is the first book that has attempted to bring together, and explain from a basic science concept, the reasons for the clinical picture or condition. This will help readers enormously, whether they are under-graduate or post-graduate medical, dental, or nursing students. It is an important book for those who wish to understand the reasons for clinical presentations and their differing management.

Mr Christopher LH Chan
Senior Lecturer/Honorary Consultant Surgeon
Barts and The London School of Medicine and Dentistry

Introduction

Why we wrote this book

The inspiration for this book comes from our time as medical students. The problem we found with existing textbooks was twofold.

Firstly, most books are organized by pathology. For example, they may have chapters on 'cardiology' that then discuss specific conditions, like 'myocardial infarction', in detail. But patients do not present with ready-made diagnoses like 'myocardial infarction'. They present with symptoms, such as 'chest pain', which could be a myocardial infarction – but could also be anything from reflux oesophagitis to aortic dissection.

Secondly, there are also textbooks based around cases rather than pathologies. Our experience is that these tend to skip over the diagnostic approach too quickly, in order to move on to a discussion of the underlying disease. Many give the reader so much information in the initial case presentation that the diagnosis is virtually made for you. For example, a '62-year-old diabetic male with sudden onset, crushing chest pain; tachycardia on examination; ST elevation on his ECG, plus raised troponins' has a myocardial infarction. But by giving so much information upfront, these books neglect to address what many students find most challenging – how do you decide what information to collect in order to make a diagnosis? Patients present with symptoms such as 'chest pain' and it is your job to elicit the key clues on history and examination, and to arrange the key investigations that will confirm that this is a myocardial infarction and rule out other diagnoses.

Knowing what to do when faced simply with 'confusion' or 'abdominal pain' can be daunting and tricky – we know, and that is what motivated us to write this book.

We hope this book will help you start thinking like a diagnostician from your first day on the wards. Thus, we hope you will be able to work out why your patient is short of breath or has abdominal pain in a way that is safe and efficient, and avoids you missing important diagnoses. Even with detailed knowledge of anatomy, physiology, biochemistry, pathology, history-taking, examination skills, and data interpretation, it can be difficult to integrate everything when faced with acutely ill patients on the wards. We benefited greatly from case-based seminars that taught us a hypothesis-driven, logical, step-by-step approach to diagnosis. Our hope is that this book emulates the teaching that we found so beneficial.

Finally, we wanted to write a workbook that students will enjoy using and where even the simplest concepts are clearly explained.

The need for a logical diagnostic approach

Looks like an elephant. Sounds like an elephant. Smells like an elephant. Probably an elephant. Experienced clinicians often use pattern recognition to guide diagnosis. As a student, you will begin to do this rapidly for conditions that you will encounter frequently – chances are that, by now, you easily recognized that the 62-year-old diabetic male mentioned above was having a myocardial infarction.

Pattern recognition is useful and efficient, and we have tried to illustrate stereotypical presentations of some diseases in our short cases.

Looks like a crocodile. Sounds like a crocodile. Smells like a crocodile... but is actually an alligator. Pattern recognition is a problem when a disease presents in a way that mimics another disease. For example, patients with oesophageal spasm may describe the same pain as those with an acute coronary syndrome. Such diagnostic puzzles are the stuff that hospital grand rounds and television shows are made of. But misdiagnosis due to (incorrect) pattern recognition can have disastrous consequences – you could inadvertently thrombolyse a patient you thought was having a myocardial infarction but actually had an aortic dissection. This is one reason why it is important to always follow a logical diagnostic approach.

Looks like an elephant. Sounds like a lion. Not sure what it smells like. Must be a...? You cannot recognize a pattern you have never seen before, an especially big problem for the inexperienced medical student starting their clinical placements. On other occasions, the symptoms may not fit any known pattern, and even experienced clinicians may struggle initially with the diagnosis. This is another reason for having a logical diagnostic approach.

A logical approach to diagnosis

Below is an outline of the diagnostic strategy we have used throughout this book. We recognize that, over time, everyone develops their own diagnostic strategy and that tutors may teach you differing approaches. This is simply one that has worked for us.

'*50-year-old male with chest pain*'. It is tempting to assume that he is having a myocardial infarction, like the 62-year-old diabetic male mentioned above. However,...

- **Step 1:** Think of all the things that could cause this presentation. Use anatomy, a surgical sieve (e.g. INVITED MD), etc. to come up with as long a list as possible.

- **Step 2:** Highlight from your list the most common causes. For example, acute coronary syndrome is a common cause of chest pain, viral costochondritis is not. Mark the ones that you *must* exclude because they are lethal. In the case of chest pain, Boerhaave's perforation of the oesophagus is important as, if untreated, it carries a 100% mortality.

- **Step 3:** Think of key clues in the patient history for each of the diagnoses. For example, patients with Boerhaave's perforation of the oesophagus invariably give a history of vomiting immediately before onset of the pain. Now take a history that deliberately tries to pick up these clues, rather than just going through a set of 'standard' questions which may miss things. Also consider the patient themselves (e.g. their age, occupation, etc.) and how this affects the relative likelihoods of your differential diagnoses. *Has the patient's history or epidemiological factors made any diagnoses more/less likely?*

- **Step 4:** Think of key clues on examination for your diagnoses. For example, patients with a pneumothorax will have an area of the chest that is hyperexpanded, hyper-resonant to percussion, with absent breath sounds. Perform a thorough examination looking for these clues. *Have your examination findings made any diagnoses more/less likely?*

Step 1: What could it be?	Step 2: What is most likely? What must I exclude (*)?	Step 3: Key clues on history?	Step 4: Key clues on examination?	Step 5: Key clues on basic investigations?	Step 6: Patient improving with management?
Acute coronary syndrome Pneumothorax Aortic dissection Boerhaave's perforation Peptic ulcer disease Stable angina Musculoskeletal Oesophagitis (e.g. due to reflux) Oesophageal spasm Pulmonary embolism Pleurisy (secondary to infection) Anxiety Myopericarditis Aortic aneurysm Coronary spasm Cholecystitis Pancreatitis	**Acute coronary syndrome*** Pneumothorax* Aortic dissection* Boerhaave's perforation* Peptic ulcer disease **Stable angina*** **Musculoskeletal** Oesophagitis Oesophageal spasm **Pulmonary embolism*** Pleurisy **Anxiety** Myopericarditis Aortic aneurysm Coronary spasm Cholecystitis Pancreatitis	Acute coronary syndrome* Pneumothorax* Aortic dissection* Boerhaave's perforation* Peptic ulcer disease Stable angina* Musculoskeletal Oesophagitis Oesophageal spasm **Pulmonary embolism*** Pleurisy Anxiety Myopericarditis Aortic aneurysm Coronary spasm Cholecystitis Pancreatitis	Acute coronary syndrome* **Pneumothorax*** Aortic dissection* Boerhaave's perforation* Peptic ulcer disease Stable angina* Musculoskeletal Oesophagitis Oesophageal spasm Pulmonary embolism* Pleurisy Anxiety Myopericarditis Aortic aneurysm Coronary spasm Cholecystitis Pancreatitis	Acute coronary syndrome* **Pneumothorax*** Aortic dissection* Boerhaave's perforation* Peptic ulcer disease Stable angina* Musculoskeletal Oesophagitis Oesophageal spasm Pulmonary embolism* Pleurisy Anxiety Myopericarditis Aortic aneurysm Coronary spasm Cholecystitis Pancreatitis	Acute coronary syndrome* **Pneumothorax*** Aortic dissection* Boerhaave's perforation* Peptic ulcer disease Stable angina* Musculoskeletal Oesophagitis Oesophageal spasm Pulmonary embolism* Pleurisy Anxiety Myopericarditis Aortic aneurysm Coronary spasm Cholecystitis Pancreatitis
50-year-old male with chest pain	50-year-old male with chest pain	50-year-old male with sharp, left-sided chest pain, came on suddenly whilst watching TV. Smoker with known COPD. No risk factors for venous thrombosis.	Upper left zone of chest is hyper-resonant with reduced air entry and reduced vocal resonance. Chest not tender to palpation. No signs of DVT in calves.	Chest radiograph shows air in pleural space on left, with lung collapsing away from the upper left apex.	Patient improves after insertion of a chest drain for pneumothorax. Chest pain resolves completely.

- **Step 5:** Don't order a set of 'standard' investigations. Think about those investigations that will help confirm or dismiss each diagnosis. Also include those that are relevant for management. Thus urea and electrolytes are necessary if a patient is put nil by mouth and on intravenous fluids, or started on drugs that are renally excreted or potentially nephrotoxic. Try to prioritize investigations into those that are more readily available (e.g. an MRI head scan is not a viable option for everyone who presents with a fall). Also think about which investigations are safe for this patient – is radiation exposure necessary, is the woman pregnant, do they have contraindications to MRI? *Then ask yourself, have your investigation results made any diagnoses more/less likely?*
- **Step 6:** Always try to confirm your diagnosis. *Is the patient getting better with your management for your proposed diagnosis? If not, why not?*

What this book *is* about

✓**Common acute presentations**: We cover 29 of the most common patient presentations in acute general medicine (internal medicine for our American readers) and general surgery. These reflect both the general medical and surgical syllabus at UK medical schools and those presentations that you are most likely to encounter during clinical attachments.

✓**Diagnostic strategy**: This book is primarily a diagnostic manual. It should equip the student with a framework for thinking about the most common general medical and surgical presentations.

✓**Pattern recognition**: The cases are loosely based on real clinical scenarios, although any likeness to a particular patient or individual is unintended. Some cases represent stereotypical presentations of diseases, from which the student may begin to pick up pattern recognition skills. Others illustrate more unusual presentations, and are designed to keep readers on their toes and remind them to keep an open mind at all times.

✓**Basic management**: For completeness, we include a discussion of the basic management for many of the diseases featured in the cases. Points on management cover the core knowledge expected of a medical student but are necessarily brief. We have tried to highlight areas of contention, and to refer to landmark trials and guidelines where relevant. Some of this is covered under our 'viva questions'.

What this book is *not* about

✗**Every possible diagnosis**: It is not logistically possible to condense the entirety of the medical and surgical syllabus into a book of this style – indeed such an attempt would run counter to the aims of this book. Our aim is to cover the most *common* presentations, and in so doing we also cover the most common diagnoses. We are fully aware that many diagnoses are not covered. But our hope is that we have provided a framework that will enable the reader to exclude the more common conditions, and be able to deal intelligently with clinical conundrums. The reader should be equipped to recognize the salient features of the case in question, and know when to ask for specialist help.

A case-based book which attempted to cover all possible diagnoses which may be encountered would not only be so long as to be unwieldy, but would also run the risk of suggesting that pattern recognition is a surrogate for a rational diagnostic strategy.

✗**Basic sciences and clinical skills**: This book does not aim to teach disease pathology or how to take a history, examine a patient, and how to interpret basic investigations (biochemistry, haematology, radiology). However, we believe that this book can be fruitfully read alongside books and teaching about basic science and clinical skills.

✗**Specialities**: It should also be noted that the cases covered reflect only a selection, albeit a broad one, of the diseases and presentations that a medical student needs to cover. The bulk of the omissions relate to the specialities (e.g. obstetrics and gynaecology, paediatrics, ear, nose, and throat, ophthalmology, etc.) and general practice (family medicine).

✗**Epidemiology**: This book does not contain detailed epidemiological data on the exact likelihood of diagnoses, because such data are rarely available and hardly memorable. Instead, we consider diagnoses to be either 'common', 'occasional', or 'very rare'. This is based on data, where available, or the cumulative experience of our senior reviewers (all of them consultants of many years' standing).

✗**Detailed management**: This book does not focus on drug doses, surgical techniques, or other details of management, because these can already be found in other textbooks.

How to use this book

A workbook, not a reference text: This is intended to be an exercise text where you 'learn by doing'. Try to cover up the answers and work through the text (without cheating!) to get the most out of it.

Find a presentation: We have structured this book by presenting complaint, rather than pathology, because patients present with 'chest pain' rather than 'aortic dissection'. For ease of reference there is also an index by disease. Each chapter can be read individually, so the student can read those that relate to the presentation they last encountered or that was most recently discussed. Every chapter contains a core case, short cases, and viva questions, in that order.

Core case: Each core case is a clinical problem that walks you through the diagnostic approach. The information the clerking doctor might receive is provided in an initial box, followed by a question. The answer follows, with another section with clinical information and another question, and so on.

Short cases: The short case 'vignettes' are designed to highlight some of the other conditions that can present in a similar manner (indeed, with the same symptom). They will help develop your 'pattern recognition' of some diseases, but also remind you that pathologies can masquerade as one another, hence the need for a logical approach.

Viva questions: These questions are designed to test aspects of anatomy, pharmacology, physiology, etc. related to the cases. We hope they will prepare the reader for the inevitable quizzing that occurs on teaching ward rounds or in theatres/operating rooms.

Graphical features: Questions are on a red background. Font sizes in a differential diagnosis illustrate how likely a diagnosis **is** (or isn't). Important points are in **red** or **bold** text.

Acknowledgements

Miss P. J. Clarke, Dr J. Dwight, Mr A. Handa, Dr T. Lancaster, and Dr T. Littlewood: thank you for sharing your invaluable clinical and educational experience with us, and for tirelessly reviewing all of the chapters over the past 2 years.

Dr P. Dennis and Dr T. Lancaster: thank you for your case-based seminars, which inspired this book. We hope to have captured the essence of what you taught us as medical students.

Dr C. Conlon, Professor T. Hope, Dr N. Meston, Mr R. Mihai, Dr A. Slater, Professor C. Tapper, Dr W. Thevathasan, Dr C. M. Norris, and Dr T. Walker: thank you for specialist advice when we were out of our depth.

Dr R. Graham and Dr J. Teh: thank you for helping us obtain elusive images.

Miss C. Connelly, Miss H. Edmundson, and the staff from OUP: thank you for believing in our project, encouraging us, and mentoring us as first time authors.

Emily: thank you for being so patient and discreet.

Rachel: thank you for cooking your boys endless amounts of brain food.

Editorial advisors

Dr J Dwight MD FRCP
Consultant Cardiologist, Department of Cardiology, John Radcliffe Hospital, Oxford

Dr T Lancaster MRCP MRCGP
General Practitioner and Director of Clinical Studies, John Radcliffe Hospital, Oxford

Dr T Littlewood MD FRCP FRCPath
Consultant Haematologist, Department of Haematology, John Radcliffe Hospital, Oxford

Mr A Handa MBBS FRCS
Clinicial Tutor & Consultant Vascular Surgeon, Nuffield Dept of Surgery, John Radcliffe Hospital, Oxford

Miss P J Clarke MD FRCS
Consultant Breast & General Surgeon, John Radcliffe Hospital, Oxford

Contents

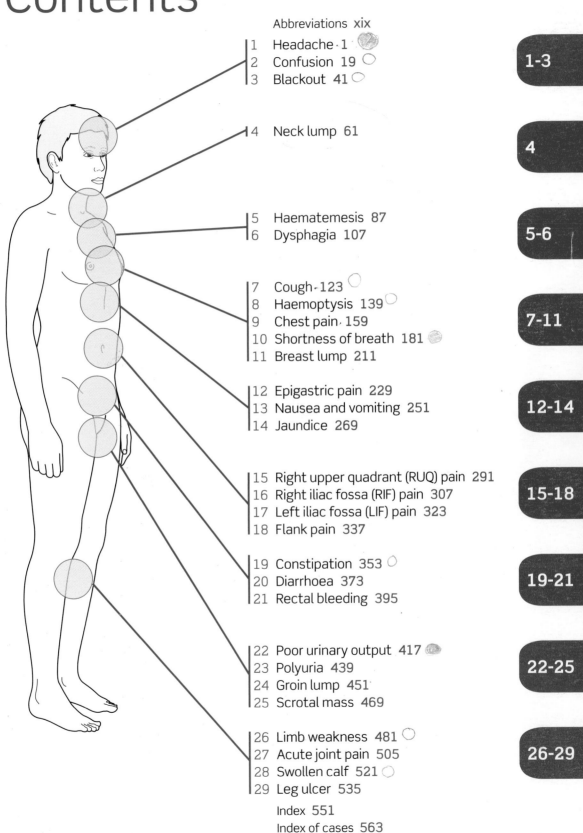

List of abbreviations

AAA	abdominal aortic aneurysm
ABC	airways, breathing, and circulation
ABG	arterial blood gas
ABPI	ankle–brachial pressure index
ACA	anterior cerebral artery
ACE	angiotensin-converting enzyme
ACEi	angiotensin-converting enzyme inhibitor
ACTH	adrenocorticotropic hormone
ADH	antidiuretic hormone
ADP	adenosine diphosphate
A&E	Accident and Emergency [Department]
AFP	alpha-fetoprotein
ALP	alkaline phosphatase
ALT	alanine aminotransferase
AMA	antimitochondrial antibodies
AMTS	Abbreviated Mental Test Score
ANA	antinuclear antibodies
APTT	activated partial thromboplastin time
ARBs	angiotensin II receptor blockers
ARDS	acute respiratory distress syndrome
ASIS	anterior superior iliac spine
ASMA	antismooth muscle antibodies
AST	aspartate aminotransferase
ATLS	advanced trauma life support
AV [node]	atrioventricular [node]
BCG	bacille Calmette–Guérin [vaccine against tuberculosis]
b.d.	twice a day [drug dosing]
BMI	body mass index
BNF	British National Formulary
BP	blood pressure
BPH	benign prostatic hyperplasia
bpm	beats per minute
BPPV	benign paroxysmal positional vertigo
BTS	British Thoracic Society
CABG	coronary artery bypass graft
cANCA	cytoplasmic-staining antineutrophil cytoplasmic antibodies
CBT	cognitive behavioural therapy
CCB	calcium-channel blocker
CCK	cholecystokinin
CCP	cyclic citrullinated peptide
CEA	carcinoembryonic antigen
CLO	columnar lined oesophagus
CMV	cytomegalovirus

CNS	central nervous system
COCP	combined oral contraceptive pill
COPD	chronic obstructive pulmonary disease
COX	cyclooxygenase
CRP	C-reactive protein
CSF	cerebrospinal fluid
CT	computed tomography
CT-KUB	CT of kidneys, ureters, and bladder
CTPA	CT pulmonary angiogram
CVP	central venous pressure
DCBE	double-contrast barium enema
DIC	disseminated intravascular coagulation
DSM-IV	Diagnostic and Statistical Manual of Mental Disorders, 4th edition
DVLA	Driver and Vehicle Licensing Agency
DVT	deep vein thrombosis
EBV	Epstein–Barr virus
ECG	electrocardiogram
EEG	electroencephalogram
eGFR	estimated glomerular filtration rate
ELISA	enzyme linked immunosorbent assay
ENT	ear, nose, and throat
ERCP	endoscopic retrograde cholangiopancreatography
ESR	erythrocyte sedimentation rate
ESWL	extracorporeal shock wave lithotripsy
EUS	endoscopic ultrasound
FAP	familial adenomatous polyposis
FATP1	fatty acid transporter protein 1
FBC	full blood count
FER	forced expiratory ratio
FEV_1	forced expiratory volume in 1 second
FiO_2	fraction of inspired oxygen
FMTC	familial medullary thyroid carcinoma
FNA	fine needle aspiration
FOBT	faecal occult blood test
FVC	forced vital capacity
G6PDH	glucose-6-phosphate dehydrogenase
GCA	giant cell arteritis
GCS	Glasgow Coma Scale
GGT	gamma-glutamyl transferase
GI	gastrointestinal
GORD	gastro-oesophageal reflux disease
GP	general practitioner
GTN	glyceryl trinitrate
GUM	genitourinary medicine
Hb	haemoglobin
HDL	high-density lipoprotein
β-HCG	β-human chorionic gonadotropin
HDU	high-dependency unit

HiB	*Haemophilus influenzae* B
HIT	heparin-induced thrombocytopenia
HNPCC	hereditary non-polyposis colorectal cancer
HOCM	hypertrophic obstructive cardiomyopathy
HONK	hyperosmotic non-ketotic [coma/acidosis]
HPOA	hypertrophic pulmonary osteoarthropathy
HR	heart rate
HRT	hormone replacement therapy
IBD	inflammatory bowel disease
IBS	irritable bowel syndrome
ICD-10	WHO International Statistical Classification of Diseases and Related Health Problems, 10th revision
ICDs	implantable cardioversion devices
Ig	immunoglobulin
IM	intramuscular
INO	internuclear ophthalmoplegia
INR	international normalized ratio
IPAA	ileal pouch–anal anastomosis
ITP	immune thrombocytopenic purpura
ITU	intensive therapy unit
IV	intravenous
IVC	inferior vena cava
IVF	*in vitro* fertilization
IVP	intravenous pyelogram/pyelography
IVU	intravenous urogram/urography
JVP	jugular venous pressure
LABA	long-acting β_2-agonist
LACA	long-acting anticholinergic
LAD	left anterior descending coronary artery
LDH	lactate dehydrogenase
LDL	low-density lipoprotein
LFTs	liver function tests
LHRH	luteinizing hormone-releasing hormone
LIF	left iliac fossa
LMN	lower motor neuron
LMWH	low-molecular weight heparin
LNG-IUD	levonorgestrel-releasing intrauterine device
LP	lumbar puncture
LPL	lipoprotein lipase
LUQ	left upper quadrant
LUTS	lower urinary tract symptoms
MCA	middle cerebral artery
MC&S	microscopy, culture, and sensitivities
MCPJs	metacarpophalangeal joints
MCV	mean corpuscular volume
MDT	multidisciplinary team
MEN	multiple endocrine neoplasia
MI	myocardial infarction
MMSE	Mini Mental State Exam

MRCP	magnetic resonance cholangiopancreatography
MRI	magnetic resonance imaging
MRU	magnetic resonance urogram
MSU	mid-stream urine
MTC	medullary thyroid carcinoma
NBM	nil by mouth
NG	nasogastric [tube]
NICE	National Institute for Health and Clinical Excellence
NIV	non-invasive ventilation
NSAID	non-steroidal anti-inflammatory drug
NSCLC	non-small cell lung cancer
NSTEMI	non-ST elevation myocardial infarction
NUD	non-ulcer dyspepsia
NYHA	New York Heart Association
o.d.	once a day [drug dosing]
OGD	oesophagogastroduodenoscopy
OSCE	Objective Structured Clinical Examination
P_aCO_2	arterial partial pressure of carbon dioxide
P_aO_2	arterial partial pressure of oxygen
pANCA	perinuclear-staining antineutrophil cytoplasmic autoantibodies
PBC	primary biliary cirrhosis
PCA	posterior cerebral artery
PCD	primary ciliary dyskinesia
PCNL	percutaneous nephrolithotomy
PCOM	posterior communicating artery
PE	pulmonary embolism
PEF	peak expiratory flow
PEFR	peak expiratory flow rate
PET	positron emission tomography
P_i	inorganic phosphate
PK	pyruvate kinase
PMN	polymorphonuclear leucocyte
PPAR	peroxisome proliferator-activated receptor
PPI	proton-pump inhibitor
PSA	prostate-specific antigen
PSC	primary sclerosing cholangitis
PT	prothrombin time
PTH	parathyroid hormone
PTHrP	parathyroid hormone-related peptide
PUJ	pelvi-ureteric junction
q.d.s.	four times a day [drug dosing]
RAPD	relative afferent papillary defect
RBC	red blood cell [count]
RCA	right coronary artery
RIF	right iliac fossa
RLN	recurrent laryngeal nerve
RUQ	right upper quadrant
SACD	subacute combined degeneration of the cord
SAH	subarachnoid haemorrhage

SALT	speech and language therapist
SC	subcutaneous
SCLC	small cell lung cancer
SIADH	syndrome of inappropriate ADH secretion
SLE	systemic lupus erythematosus
SOL	space-occupying lesion
SSRV	small structured round virus
STEMI	ST elevation myocardial infarct
SVC	superior vena cava
T_3	tri-iodothyronine
T_4	thyroxine
TB	tuberculosis
t.d.s.	three times a day [drug dosing]
TFTs	thyroid function tests
TG	thyroglobulin
TIA	transient ischaemic attack
TIBC	total iron-binding capacity
TIPS/TIPSS	transjugular intrahepatic portosystemic shunt
TMJ	temporomandibular joint
TNF	tumour necrosis factor
tPA	tissue plasminogen activator
TPN	total parenteral nutrition
TRAM	tranverse rectus abdominis myocutaneous [flap]
TSH	thyroid-stimulating hormone
TTG	tissue transglutaminase
TURP	transurethral resection of the prostate
TWOC	trial without catheter
UC	ulcerative colitis
U&Es	urea and electrolytes
UMN	upper motor neuron
UTI	urinary tract infection
VTE	venous thromboembolism
WCC	white cell count
WLE	wide local excision

Headache

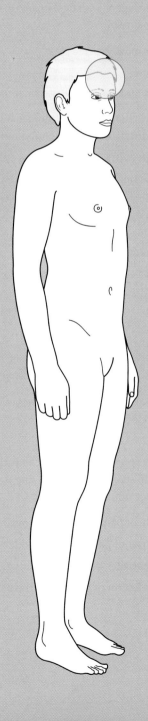

Core cases

> ! *Read through the sections in red, covering up the sections in white that follow so that you don't see the answer. At the end of each red section, try to answer the question before reading on.*

Core case

Mr Lennon is a 74-year-old gentleman referred to the hospital by his general practitioner (GP) because of a severe headache.

Headache is a common symptom with many causes. It is essential to rule out the sinister causes first, i.e. those that require urgent investigation and management because if left untreated they cause lasting damage and/or mortality.

What sinister causes must you rule out?

The sinister causes can be remembered using the mnemonic VIVID:

Vascular: subarachnoid haemorrhage (SAH), haematoma (subdural or extra-dural), cerebral venous sinus thrombosis, cerebellar infarct

Infection: meningitis, encephalitis

Vision-threatening: temporal arteritis[†], acute glaucoma, pituitary apoplexy, posterior leucoencephalopathy, cavernous sinus thrombosis

Intracranial pressure (raised): space-occupying lesion (SOL; e.g. tumour, abscess, cyst), cerebral oedema (e.g. trauma, altitude), hydrocephalus, malignant hypertension

Dissection: carotid dissection

[†] Note that temporal arteritis is another name for giant cell arteritis, a systemic vasculitis. The term temporal arteritis is more common when headache is the presenting symptom.

Taking a good history is key to any diagnosis, but particularly so when tackling headache as the symptom is so subjective and examination findings are often unhelpful.

With a mental list of the sinister causes, what questions will you ask first in the history? What 'red flags' will help you exclude the sinister causes?

The approach to headache is the same as that to pain anywhere in the body: you need to start by characterizing the pain. One useful way of doing this is by following another mnemonic, SOCRATES:

Site of pain, and has it moved since it began?

Onset of pain – was it sudden or gradual, and did something trigger it?

Character of pain – stabbing, dull, deep, superficial, gripping, tearing, burning?

Radiation of pain – has the pain spread?

Attenuating factors – does anything make the pain better (position? medications?)

Timing of pain – how long has it gone on for, has it been constant or coming and going?

Exacerbating factors – does anything make the pain worse (moving? breathing?)

Severity – on a scale of 0 to 10, where 10 is the worst pain ever (e.g. childbirth).

In addition, you should enquire about the presence or absence of the following 'red flags':

- **Decreased level of consciousness.** This is a worrying feature of any medical presentation. Combined with headache, SAH needs exclusion. If there is a history of **head injury**, it could suggest a subdural haematoma (fluctuating consciousness) or extradural haematoma (altered consciousness following a lucid interval). Meningitis and encephalitis can also affect consciousness.

- **Sudden onset, worst headache ever.** Suggests SAH, with blood in the cerebrospinal fluid (CSF) irritating the meninges. It can be informative to ask the patient whether they remember the *exact* moment when the headache started – a very severe headache of almost instantaneous onset is characteristic of SAH. Patients describe it like, for example, 'being hit on the head with a baseball bat'.

- **Seizure(s) or focal neurological deficit** (e.g. limb weakness, speech difficulties). Suggests intracranial pathology.

- **Absence of previous episodes.** Recurrent episodes are usually less sinister. A new onset of headache suggests a new pathology. In someone over 50 years old, a new onset headache should raise your suspicions of temporal arteritis until proven otherwise.

- **Reduced visual acuity.** Temporal arteritis is common in older patients. Transient blindness (amaurosis fugax) is usually due to a transient ischaemic attack (TIA), but these rarely produce a headache. In the context of headaches, loss of vision can be due to temporal arteritis, carotid artery dissection causing decreased blood flow to the retina, or acute glaucoma.

- **Persistent headache, worse when lying down,** and coupled with **early morning nausea.** Suggests raised intracranial pressure. This is worse when lying flat for prolonged times (e.g. overnight) due to the effect of gravity, but can even occur when the patient is bending over. Headaches that are worse when standing up suggested *reduced* intracranial pressure and are common after a lumbar puncture (LP), but these are *not* sinister and resolve with hydration and lying down for several hours.

- **Progressive, persistent headache.** This could be an expanding SOL (e.g. tumour, abscess, cyst, haematoma).

- **Constitutional symptoms.** Weight loss, night sweats, and/or fever may suggest malignancy, chronic infection (e.g. tuberculosis), or chronic inflammation (e.g. temporal arteritis).

You start by characterizing Mr Lennon's headache. He tells you the pain is on the right side of his head and hasn't ever moved. It started 4 days ago, since when it has been getting worse. He can only characterize it as intense. He has tried over-the-counter analgesics with no benefit, and when asked specifically, says there is no change with position or time of day.

He has had no changes in consciousness, nor seizures, that he is aware of. When asked about other symptoms, he tells you he has found it hard to eat and open his mouth properly since yesterday because of jaw pain. He has not noticed any constitutional symptoms, and he hasn't noticed any change in vision. He has never had anything like this before.

How does this information help focus the differential diagnosis and your approach?

Mr Lennon gives a good description of his headache. The gradual onset over 4 days makes a number of the more sinister causes less likely, specifically SAH. In addition, one of the red flags is present: a new onset headache in someone older than 50. In such presentations, particularly given suggestive symptoms like possible jaw claudication, your priority is to exclude temporal arteritis.

Whilst you have begun to narrow your diagnosis, you still want to exclude sinister causes with your examination and investigations.

What signs will you look for on clinical examination?

Basic observations

- **Altered consciousness.** Assess Mr Lennon's Glasgow Coma Scale (GCS) score, although it is likely to already be obvious from the history taking. The significance of altered consciousness is discussed above.
- **Blood pressure and pulse.** Check for malignant hypertension.
- **Temperature**. Fever and headache suggests meningitis or encephalitis.

Focal neurological signs

Note that the list below is not exhaustive.

- **Focal limb deficit.** Makes intracranial pathology more likely.
- **Third nerve palsy.** This consists of ptosis (droopy eyelid), mydriasis (dilated pupil), and an eye that is deviated down and out. One cause is an SAH due to a ruptured aneurysm of the posterior communicating artery (PCOM). PCOM aneurysms are a cause of headache.
- **Sixth nerve palsy.** Convergent squint and/or failure to abduct the eye laterally. This nerve can be compressed either directly by a mass or indirectly by raised intracranial pressure. Remember that the sixth nerve has the longest intracranial course and is therefore most likely to get compressed at some point.
- **Twelfth nerve palsy.** Look for tongue deviation. A twelfth nerve palsy can arise from a carotid artery dissection.

- **Horner's syndrome.** Triad of partial ptosis, miosis (constricted pupil), and anhydrosis (dry skin around the orbit). Results from interruption of the ipsilateral sympathetic pathway. In the context of our differential diagnosis, Horner's syndrome should raise suspicions of a carotid artery dissection (ask about neck pain) or cavernous sinus lesion.

Eye inspection

- **Exophthalmos?** This may indicate a retro-orbital process such as cavernous sinus thrombosis.
- **Cloudy cornea? Fixed, dilated/oval pupil?** This may suggest acute glaucoma.
- **Optic disc appearance on fundoscopy.** Look for papilloedema, indicating raised intracranial pressure.

Other

- **Reduced visual acuity.** This can suggest acute glaucoma or temporal arteritis for example.
- **Scalp tenderness.** Classically seen in temporal arteritis.
- **Meningism.** Check whether the patient has a stiff neck or photophobia, suggesting meningism due to infection or SAH.

On examination, Mr Lennon is not obviously photophobic as he is sitting in a well-lit environment. His heart rate is 84 beats/min (bpm), his blood pressure is 134/81 mmHg, and his temperature 36.5°C. Examination of his cranial nerves reveals reduced visual acuity in his right eye but not his left, which he previously hadn't noticed. Fundoscopy is normal. The rest of his cranial nerves are intact but you do notice that his right scalp is tender to light touch. There are no limb signs and no neck stiffness.

Mr Lennon is an elderly man with a 4-day history of new-onset right-sided temporal headache, possibly jaw claudication, a right-sided decrease in visual acuity, and a tender scalp.

What is the most likely diagnosis? What is the pathology, and why is it an emergency?

Mr Lennon's history and clinical features are highly suggestive of **temporal arteritis** (aka giant cell arteritis, GCA). This is a disease of unknown aetiology that typically appears in patients over 50 years of age. It is characterized by the formation of immune, inflammatory granulomas in the tunica media of medium/large-sized arteries. The inflammation (or thrombosis or spasm induced by it) can be sufficient to block the lumen of medium-sized arteries affected by this disease. Inflammation of the mandibular branch of the external carotid artery causes jaw claudication. Inflammation of the superficial temporal branch of the external carotid artery causes headache and scalp tenderness. Inflammation of the posterior ciliary arteries causes visual disturbances, due to ischaemia to either the retina (blurring, visual field loss) or the optic motor muscles (double vision = diplopia).

The reason to worry about this presentation is that with visual loss in one eye the other eye is at risk without prompt treatment. Temporal arteritis with visual disturbance is therefore an **ophthalmological emergency** and patients should be referred to the on-call ophthalmologist as soon as possible. Unfortunately, visual loss prior to arrival at hospital is unlikely to be reversed regardless of treatment.

1 | How will you proceed in light of your working diagnosis?

Having taken a full history and examined the patient, one should arrange only first-line investigations that are quick to do – such as blood tests to demonstrate an **elevated erythrocyte sedimentation rate (ESR) and C-reactive protein (CRP)** that would be consistent with a systemic inflammation such as temporal arteritis. Management should then aim to reduce the immune-mediated inflammation that is causing the ischaemia in Mr Lennon's arteries and the best way to do this is using **high-dose corticosteroids**.

Once initial treatment is under way, one can arrange for more time-consuming investigations to help confirm the diagnosis and rule out alternatives. In this case, a **temporal artery biopsy** should be arranged to help confirm the diagnosis (it will show granulomas in temporal arteritis). Note that the principal reason for urgent treatment of temporal arteritis is to protect the vision in the fellow, unaffected eye, rather than aiming to restore vision to the affected eye.

Mr Lennon's 40-year-old daughter has come to see her father. You have explained that you think he has temporal arteritis, an inflammation of some of the blood vessels supplying his head. Poor Miss Lennon is worried that she may have the same problem as she also frequently gets headaches.

You ask her to characterize the headache using **SOCRATES**. She tells you the headaches only affect the right side of her head. They come on over half an hour, and make her feel nauseated and sensitive to bright light and noise. She only finds relief by hiding in a dark room and getting some sleep. They last hours, but less than a day, and are relatively infrequent, occurring three or four times a year since her early twenties. You also ask about the red flags, none of which are present.

The lack of red flags makes a sinister cause of headache unlikely. But there are several non-sinister syndromes that cause headache. These syndromes are not 'benign' because they cause significant morbidity (in the form of pain). However, they are unlikely to cause lasting damage or mortality in the short term.

What different types of non-sinister headache are there?

Causes of non-sinister headache include:

Tension-type headache
Migraine
Sinusitis
Medication overuse headache
Temporomandibular joint (TMJ) dysfunction syndrome (TMJ syndrome)
Trigeminal neuralgia
Cluster headache

Some of these are 'primary headaches' because the symptom (headache) is primary, i.e. if the headaches were removed there would be no harmful pathology. This is in contrast to 'secondary headaches', where the headache is only one of many possible symptoms that result from pathology such as head trauma, intracranial lesion (e.g. tumour), vascular lesion (e.g. SAH), or infection. The following are secondary headaches: sinusitis, medication overuse headache, and TMJ syndrome. Sinusitis and TMJ syndrome cannot be diagnosed in the absence of additional symptoms. A diagnosis of medication overuse headache can only be made in patients using analgesic and/or migraine medication.

In addition to the pain history (e.g. SOCRATES), what questions should you ask to characterize non-sinister headaches?

- **Does the patient suffer from different types of headache?** If so, separate histories will be needed for each as they may reflect distinct syndromes. Thus patients with migraine are also vulnerable to medication overuse headaches from the treatment for their migraine.

- **Are there any predisposing (trigger) factors?** Factors such as stress and fatigue are known triggers for tension headaches and migraines. Some migraine sufferers point to certain foods as triggers (e.g. cheese, caffeine), and alcohol can trigger cluster headaches.

- **How disabling are the headaches?** Migraines render many sufferers incapable of performing even the activities of daily living for around a day. Cluster headaches are severely painful and disabling but often occur at night, allowing daytime duties to continue. Tension-type headaches usually allow normal activities to be continued.

- **Does the patient get an 'aura' before the headache?** Auras are usually visual phenomena, although focal neurological deficits (e.g. limb weakness) are sometimes present. About a third of migraine sufferers report auras as a feature of their migraines.

> Going back to the list of differential diagnoses above, what are the key features of each diagnosis in the history?

- **Tension-type headaches.** Very common. Often bifrontal pain. They are episodic, occurring with variable frequency. The pain is described as pressure or tightness around the head like a tightening band. Other than the headache there are no other features (e.g. no photophobia). The headaches last no more than a few hours and are not severely disabling. However, in rare cases they may occur almost daily, in which case they become disabling. Stress and fatigue are well-known trigger factors.

- **Migraine.** Common, although not as common as tension headaches, and twice as common in women than men. Migraines are stereotyped, i.e. attacks exhibit the same pattern of symptoms and become recognizable to patients. They are typically unilateral (migraine is a corruption of the Latin (*he*)*mi-cranium*). Associated with an aura in about a third of sufferers (**migraine with aura** or **classical migraine**, as opposed to **migraine without aura** or **common migraine**). The pain is described as throbbing or pulsatile. There is sensitivity to light, sound, and even smell, and nausea can also be a feature. Migraines last between 4 and 72 hours, unless successfully treated. Some patients suffer from **aura without migraine**. Such attacks are in the differential for TIAs (particularly in older patients) and epilepsy.

- **Sinusitis.** Patients usually report facial pain coming on over hours to days in conjunction with coryzal symptoms. The pain is tight, as in tension headaches, and is often exacerbated by movement. The headaches last several days, with a time course consistent with the infection. The headaches are moderately severe but not disabling. However, patients with chronic sinusitis may find the headaches frequent enough to interfere with their daily activities.

- **Medication overuse.** Surprisingly common, particularly in women (about five-fold the incidence in men). This is seen particularly with migraine medications and analgesics. The headaches experienced resemble either migraine or tension-type headaches. Most patients will be taking very large quantities of medication (on average 35 doses of six different agents a week). It is often difficult for patients to accept that the over-treatment of headache is actually the cause of their ongoing headaches. Treatment consists of withdrawal from analgesic use, which often results in a period of exacerbation before improvement occurs.

- **TMJ syndrome.** Most common in individuals aged 20–40, and four times more prevalent in women. As well as headache, patients get a dull ache in the muscles of mastication that may radiate to the jaw and/or ear. Patients also often report hearing a 'click' or grinding noise when they move their jaw.

- **Trigeminal neuralgia.** A rare condition, occurring more often in women, with a typical age of onset around 60–70 years. Patients complain of unilateral facial pain involving one or more of the divisions of the trigeminal nerve. The pain lasts only seconds, and can be triggered by eating, laughing, talking or touching the affected area. Although attacks last seconds, there may be several or even hundreds a day and patients can develop a longer-lasting background pain. Patients often avoid known triggers like shaving. Interestingly, attacks rarely occur during sleep, unlike migraine or cluster headaches.

- **Cluster headache.** Predominantly affects men. The headaches occur in 'clusters' for about 6–12 weeks every 1–2 years, hence the name. Attacks tend to occur at exactly the same time every day or night, like an alarm clock going off. The pain is focused over one eye. The pain is intense and causes the patient to wake up and can be so severe that suicide is contemplated, until the pain diminishes, around 20–30 minutes later. They will probably have a red, watery eye, rhinorrhoea, and Horner's syndrome, suggested by a history of ptosis. These headaches are very disabling.

> You ask the additional questions listed above. Miss Lennon tells you she sometimes gets 'normal' headaches, which respond to paracetamol, but it is these other headaches that she worries about. When you ask about any 'aura' or visual disturbance, she tells you they are often preceded by seeing a small black spot with bright, zig-zagging lines. When she has a headache, she has to stay in bed all day until it goes, but will be fit and well the day after.
>
> **What is the most likely diagnosis, given Miss Lennon's history?**

It may be tempting to dismiss Miss Lennon's headaches as tension headaches, which almost everyone experiences at some point. However, Miss Lennon describes a *unilateral* headache that makes her feel sick, photophobic, phonophobic, and is preceded by a visual phenomena (zig-zag lines). It is therefore very likely that Miss Lennon suffers from **migraine with aura**.

Migraine affects about 15% of the population, but many do not seek help as they think there is no treatment. This is not true, as acute abortive treatment including triptans ($5HT_1$-agonists such as sumatriptan), analgesics (aspirin, paracetamol), and anti-emetics (metoclopramide) have been shown to be highly effective if the patient takes them as soon as they feel a migraine coming on – something that most migraine sufferers recognize easily. Preventative treatments are only useful with high frequencies of attacks (e.g. fortnightly) and will usually only reduce migraine frequency by 50%.

> **Should you examine Miss Lennon and, if so, what would you look for? Should you order any investigations and, if so, which?**

All of the non-sinister causes of headache are diagnosed on history. However, you should conduct a physical examination, both to provide the patient with reassurance and to look for:

- **Blood pressure,** to exclude malignant hypertension.
- **Head and neck examination** for muscle tenderness, stiffness, or limited movement – which can occasionally mimic tension-type headaches. If present, such findings may need treatment in order to relieve the headache.
- **Focal neurological signs.** The presence of focal neurological signs in somebody with headache should alert you to intracranial pathology.
- **Fundoscopy,** to exclude raised intracranial pressure.

Investigations are only ever indicated where warranted by the history and examination and should not be ordered routinely.

Short cases

> Mrs Harrison is a 42-year-old who presents to accident and emergency (A&E) complaining of a severe headache and nausea. She has a history of migraine attacks but this time she says it is different – it came on suddenly after dinner, without warning, and felt as if someone had punched her in the back of the head. Her husband, annoyed at having to drive her to the hospital in the middle of the night, cynically thinks she is just having 'a bad migraine'.
>
> **What is the likely diagnosis? What key investigation should be requested?**

Patients know their disease better than any doctor, so if a patient tells you that something doesn't feel like what they normally have (e.g. migraines in this case), take them seriously. You should take a full history and examine the lady for key signs as discussed in the main case (e.g. neck stiffness suggesting meningism). But the history given is classic for an **SAH**, so you should arrange an urgent computed tomography **(CT) head scan**, looking for blood in the CSF (this appears bright on CT, for example in the Sylvian fissures). An LP looking for xanthochromia (yellow CSF due to bilirubin content) must be performed to exclude SAH if the CT is negative. Note that CT is only useful as an aid to diagnosis of SAH in the first days following a bleed – by approximately day 7 the scan will have ~50% sensitivity (i.e. you might as well flip a coin). LP should be delayed for 12 hours after the onset of the headache as false negative results can occur before that time. It remains reliable for up to 12 days (12 hour to 12 day rule).

If the CT confirms an SAH, Mrs Harrison will need urgent referral to a neurosurgical unit. Patients are initially managed with **nimodipine** (a calcium-channel blocker that reduces spasm of the ruptured cerebral artery, thus preventing ischaemia, i.e. a stroke) and bed rest.

If she survives and her symptoms improve, she should receive cerebral angiography to find the source of a bleed – usually a ruptured aneurysm. The neuroradiologist will usually be able to insert a platinum coil to cause the aneurysm to clot, scar, and heal. Coiling has been shown by the **ISAT Study**[1] to have fewer complications than surgically clipping the aneurysm via an open craniotomy. The family should be made aware that SAH carries a high risk of mortality and morbidity: 50% of patients die before arriving at hospital; a further 17% die in hospital; another 17% survive but with lasting neurological deficits; and only 17% survive without any sequelae.

[1] Molyneux AJ, Kerr RS, Yu LM, Clarke M, Sneade M, Yarnold JA, Sandercock P (2005). International subarachnoid aneurysm trial (ISAT) of neurosurgical clipping versus endovascular coiling in 2143 patients with ruptured intracranial aneurysms: a randomised comparison of effects on survival, dependency, seizures, rebleeding, subgroups, and aneurysm occlusion. *Lancet,* **366**: 809–817.

Mr McCartney is a 32-year-old salesman who is worried that he might be having repeated 'mini-strokes' (TIAs), like his father. He says that every couple of months he suffers from an attack where he sees a shimmering light in the corner of his eyes and gets a ringing in his ears. This usually occurs towards the end of the day, lasting half an hour. He is fully conscious throughout and never feels dazed or confused afterwards.

Could this gentleman be suffering from TIAs like his father?

TIAs and strokes are caused by areas of the brain ceasing to function due to a lack of blood (because of an embolism or haemorrhage) and are therefore characterized by 'negative', *loss of function*, symptoms and signs (loss of vision, numbness, loss of power in muscles). In contrast, epilepsy is caused by over-activation of areas of the brain and thus produces 'positive', *gain of function*, symptoms and signs (flashing lights, muscle convulsions, odd sensations in the skin). Migraine can produce both negative and positive symptoms. This gentleman describes clear gain of function symptoms (shimmering light, noises) that are more suggestive of epilepsy or migraine.

It could be epilepsy, but seizures tend to be followed by a post-ictal phase where the patient is exhausted and sometimes confused. It is therefore more likely to be a case of **migraine aura without headache**. A characteristic feature is a slow march of symptoms (e.g. visual disturbance affecting more and more of the visual field) then resolution in a similar fashion. Migraine without aura is an odd condition where patients experience the aura signs of typical migraine patients (e.g. shimmering lights with ziz-zagging edges, noises) but without the headache. One can reassure the patient that his symptoms are almost certainly not 'mini-strokes' but more likely due to a type of migraine without headaches. The patient may wish to have a trial of antimigraine medication as soon as one of these attacks starts (e.g. sumatriptan) or prophylactic medication to prevent it occurring (e.g. propanolol, pizitofen) and see if they help.

1

Ringo is a 16-year-old who presents with a runny nose and headache. He has been blowing out green mucus from his nose for a few days but has come to see you because the headache, which is located above his eyes, is now very bad. His nasal septum is slightly deviated and his forehead is indeed tender to gentle tapping.

Can we send this patient home on analgesia and rest?

It is possible that this young man simply has a viral rhinosinusitis, but the green mucus and the highly localized pain above his eyes suggest he may have developed an infection of his frontal sinuses.

Sinusitis usually affects the maxillary sinus and resolves spontaneously, occasionally needing a helping hand from antibiotics (e.g. amoxicillin) if it fails to resolve. However, **frontal sinusitis** can be particularly dangerous because it is possible for the bacteria to erode backwards into the brain, causing meningitis or a brain abscess. For this reason, a suspected case of frontal sinusitis should be taken seriously and referred to ear, nose, and throat (ENT) specialists who can arrange a CT head scan to check if either frontal sinus is affected. If it is, he will need antibiotics and draining of the frontal sinuses (antral lavage). It is possible that his deviated nasal septum is predisposing him to episodes of sinusitis and, if so, he could benefit from a re-arrangement of his nasal septum (septoplasty).

Short case

A 10-year-old girl is referred to the hospital by her GP for persistent headache in the occipital area that is worse in the morning. The parents have also noticed that she has become clumsy over the last few months. As part of your cranial nerve examination you perform fundoscopy, where you see the result shown in Fig. 1.1.

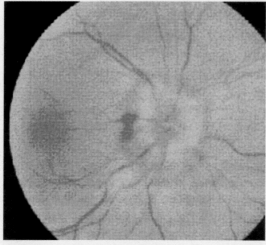

Figure 1.1 Fundoscopic view of the patient's retina. Both retinas had a similar appearance.
Reproduced from Fig. 1, p.449, in Oxford Handbook of Clinical Specialities, 7th edn, by Collier, Longmore, and Brinsden (2006). By permission of Oxford University Press.

What is your next step?

The appearance of the optic disc (poorly defined margins) is suggestive of **papill-oedema**, potentially due to raised intracranial pressure. This would be consistent with headaches which are worse in the morning. One cause of raised intracranial pressure is brain tumour, and in children most brain tumours are found in the posterior fossa that would explain the occipital headache. In addition, the most common type of tumour in children is a medulloblastoma in the cerebellum, which may explain her clumsiness. Thus you must rule out a **CNS tumour** as the problem in this child. An urgent **head magnetic resonance imaging (MRI) scan** should therefore be requested.

If a tumour is found, the neurosurgeon will use dexamethasone to reduce the brain inflammation (improving the headache) and discuss the surgical options to remove the tumour with the family.

Viva questions

What are the main causes of SAH?

The main causes of SAH are:

- **Rupture of an arterial aneurysm,** usually a 'berry aneurysm' at the junction between arteries of the circle of Willis (~45%)
- **Trauma** (~45%)
- **Arteriovenous malformations,** rupture of haemangiomas, rupture of cerebral vein around the brain-stem (~10%)

What is your differential diagnosis for intracranial tumours?

The list of possible intracranial tumours is very long but the most common are:

- **Secondary brain tumours (metastatic).** These are the *most common type of brain tumours* in adults, accounting for ~90% of all intracranial tumours. The five most common sources of primary cancer metastasizing to the brain are lung, kidney, breast, melanoma, and colon.
- **Primary brain tumours.** These can be divided into axial (within the brain parenchyma) and extra-axial:
  - **Axial** or **neuroepithelial tumours** (~50%). These are tumours of the brain matter itself. They include (the latter three are more common in children):
    Astrocytomas (glioblastoma multiforme is a grade 4 astrocytoma)
    Ependymomas
    Oligodendrogliomas
    Medulloblastomas
  - **Extra-axial**
    Meningioma (~15%). A slow-growing tumour of the meninges that compresses the brain. Often associated with neurofibromatosis type II (inherited predisposition to schwannomas and menin-giomas), these tumours can usually be surgically removed with good prognosis
    Vestibular schwannoma. Previously and incorrectly called an 'acoustic neuroma', this type of tumour is relatively common in young adults. It may compress cranial nerve VIII (hearing loss) and VII (facial palsy)
    Pituitary adenomas, prolactinomas, and craniopharyngiomas
    Other: choroid plexus papillomas, haemangiomas, pineal gland tumours, etc.

1

At what level of the spine should you insert a needle during an adult LP? What are the surface anatomy landmarks? What structures do you pass through as you perform an LP?

The spinal cord in adults ends at L1/L2, with peripheral nerves extending beyond that as a loose bundle of nerve fibres floating in CSF (the *cauda equina,* literally the 'horse's tail'). Modern studies have shown that in children the spinal cord ends only slightly lower (L2/L3) but certainly not as low as many older textbooks claim. A safe place to insert the needle is thus at or below L3/L4. This can be found by tracing a line between the posterior superior iliac crests (Tuffier's line), which marks the L4/L5 space.

The following structures are sequentially traversed as you perform an LP:

- Skin
- Subcutis
- Supraspinous ligament
- Interspinous ligament
- Ligamentum flavum (first 'give' as you push the needle)
- Dura mater (second 'give' as you push the needle)
- Arachnoid space – the destination

What are the indications, contraindications, and risks of an LP?

Indications

- **Diagnostic LP:** looking for oligoclonal bands (e.g. multiple sclerosis), high protein (Guillain–Barré syndrome), blood or bilirubin (e.g. SAH), pathogens (e.g. bacterial meningitis, viral encephalitis), malignant cells (e.g. CNS lymphoma), or a rapid improvement in gait and cognitive function after removal of 30 mL of CSF (e.g. normal pressure hydrocephalus).
- **Therapeutic LP:** intrathecal drug administration (e.g. haematological malignancy in children), temporary reduction in intracranial pressure (e.g. idiopathic intracranial hypertension).

Relative contraindications

- **Raised intracranial pressure** due to an SOL, as the sudden drop in pressure can cause the brainstem to cone through the foramen magnum. Suspect raised intracranial pressure in a history of early morning headaches, nausea, and vomiting that are made worse by lying down or straining; in anyone with impaired consciousness, papilloedema on fundoscopy, focal neurological signs (e.g. nerve VI palsy). If there is any doubt about an SOL then imaging should be performed prior to LP.
- **Increased bleeding tendency** (e.g. patient on warfarin, disseminated intravascular coagulation).
- **Infection at prospective site of puncture.**
- **Cardiorespiratory compromise.** Deal with this before doing any other procedure.

1

Risks

- **Headache.** About 30% of patients will get a headache due to the intracranial hypotension. This risk can be minimized by keeping the patient lying flat for at least 2 hours. Some needle types are less likely to cause headaches then others (smaller calibre is better).
- **Nerve root pain.** About 10% of patients will get pain in a lumbosacral nerve root distribution, due to irritation by the needle of one of the nerves that form the cauda equina. This can be minimized by inserting the needle slowly and withdrawing it from the cannula slowly. Provide analgesia and reassure the patient that the pain will gradually subside.
- Infection at the site of the puncture.

With regards to raised intracranial pressure, what are (1) its main symptoms and signs and (2) its main causes?

1) The main symptoms and signs of raised intracranial pressure are:
   Headache, often worse when lying down
   Nausea, usually first thing in the morning, after lying down all night
   Papilloedema, a swollen optic disc when visualized by fundoscopy
   Visual blurring
   Cushing's reflex, a paradoxical bradycardia and raised blood pressure, often with irregular breathing
   Cushing's peptic ulcer, causing epigastric pain

2) There are a variety of mechanisms that can lead to raised intracranial pressure:
   SOL, such as a tumour, haematoma, abscess, or cyst
   Cerebral oedema, secondary to trauma or some other lesion
   Increased blood pressure in the CNS, due to vasodilator drugs (glyceryl trinitrate (GTN) spray, Viagra), malignant hypertension, hypercapnic vasodilation, venous sinus thrombosis, or superior vena cava obstruction
   Increased volume of CSF (hydrocephalus), which can be due to obstruction of CSF drainage (e.g. by a tumour), dysfunction of the arachnoid granulations responsible for CSF reabsorption (e.g. SAH or meningitis irritating the granulations, idiopathic intracranial hypertension), or increased CSF production (by a choroid plexus papilloma)

For a range of Single Best Answer questions related to the topic of this chapter go to
www.oxfordtextbooks.co.uk/orc/ocms

Confusion

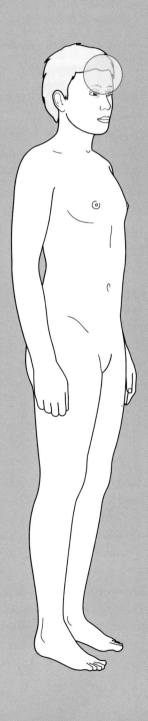

Core case

2

! *Read through the sections in red, covering up the sections in white that follow so that you don't see the answer. At the end of each red section, try to answer the question before reading on.*

Mrs Doolally is an 84-year-old woman who is referred by her general practitioner (GP) to her local hospital. She attends with her daughter, who reports that her mother is usually forgetful. However, when she visited that day she found that her mother was much worse than when she last saw her 3 days previously, as she was very '*confused*' and '*not herself*'.

'Confusion' is a very vague term that can refer to various medical syndromes, e.g. dementia, psychosis, etc.

What syndromes can cause a patient to appear 'confused'?

- **Delirium**: an acute impairment in cognitive ability together with impaired consciousness.
- **Dementia**: a chronic, progressive impairment in cognitive ability but with intact consciousness. Note that this is different from delirium and that you cannot diagnose dementia from a single mental status assessment.
- **Mental impairment**: a permanent impairment in cognitive ability.
- **Psychosis**: the patient may not be confused, but hallucinating or deluded due to a deranged personality and loss of contact with reality.
- **Receptive dysphasia**: the patient may have difficulties comprehending your questions (e.g. due to damage to Wernicke's area of the brain).
- **Expressive dysphasia**: the patient may be cognitively intact but have difficulties verbalizing an answer to your questions (e.g. due to damage to Broca's area of the brain).

It is often difficult to take a good history from a confused patient. However, you should nevertheless try to get some basic information from her.

What questions should you ask of all confused patients?

Remember to start by checking the patient's airway, breathing, and circulation (ABC) and whether they are in any pain that requires analgesia.

To work out what type of confusion this is, you should start by conducting a **quick screen of confusion** because if the patient does poorly in your screen, taking a conventional history may prove unhelpful. For this, you should ask all confused patients:

- **Are they oriented to time, place, and person? Can they tell you why they are here?** The Abbreviated Mental Test Score (AMTS) is a simple 10-question screening tool for assessing confusion where a score of less than 6/10 indicates cognitive impairment. An alternative is the 30-question Mini Mental

State Exam (MMSE), where a score of less than 26/30 indicates cognitive impairment.

* **Can they follow a three-step command?** This tests for receptive dysphasia.
* **Can they name three common objects?** This tests for expressive dysphasia.
* **Other symptoms?** Are they in pain? (even the most confused patient will complain of pain). You should also ask about breathlessness, cough, and urinary symptoms as a chest or urinary tract infection (UTI) is often the cause of confusion.

The Abbreviated Mental Test Score[†]

Remember this address: 33 Dorchester Street

Orientation in time

What time is it (nearest hour)?	1 point
What year are we in?	1 point
How old are you?	1 point

Orientation in space

What building are you in?	1 point

Orientation in person

Who am I? Who is that person (e.g. nurse)?	1 point

Long-term memory

What is your date of birth?	1 point
What year did the Second World War end (or alternative date, e.g. particular Olympic Games)?	1 point
Who is the current Prime Minister?	1 point

Short-term memory

Please count backwards from 20 to 1.	1 point
Can you remember the address I told you?	1 point

Score < 6 = dementia or delirium likely

[†] Based on Hodkinson HM (1972). Evaluation of a mental test score for assessment of mental impairment in the elderly. *Age and Ageing*, **1**: 233–238.

If they are accompanied, what information should you try to ascertain from their companion?

If they have been accompanied by someone who knows them, try to ascertain:

* **Their normal state.** It may be that they are behaving no differently from how they normally behave, but that it has been mistaken for confusion (e.g. if they have dementia, psychosis, mental impairment, etc.).

2

- The **time course** of their confusion. An acute onset argues against dementia and in favour of delirium.
- Their **drug history (including alcohol)**. Any number of drugs can cause confusion. Consider both the introduction and cessation of drugs.

This information is particularly important in elderly patients who may have dementia and/or be taking a number of medications which may or may not have changed recently. Remember that a history of dementia does not exclude an acute confusional state. On the contrary, such patients are at a greater risk of developing confusion in addition to their dementia.

If the patient has scored poorly on your quick screen of confusion and they are unaccompanied, you should move on quickly to the examination as conversation with the patient is unlikely to be productive.

Core case

Mrs Doolally is drowsy and confused with an AMTS of 5/10. She is able to follow a simple three-step command and correctly name three common objects. She reports that she fell over but otherwise is not sure why she has been brought in. She reports no other symptoms. Her daughter reports that her mother does not drink any alcohol. She takes a thiazide diuretic for hypertension, and is currently taking lactulose for constipation and clotrimazole for thrush.

Before you move on to examine Mrs Doolally, you should start formulating an idea as to what might be the cause of her acute confusion (delirium).

What causes of delirium can you think of?
The list is long and you may find using a surgical sieve is helpful.

Which of the diagnoses in your list are most likely in Mrs Doolally?

There are a number of different mnemonics for remembering a surgical sieve. The one used below is 'INVITED MD'. The diagnoses more likely in Mrs Doolally, given both what is most common and her age, are given in **bold type**.

Infectious (e.g. **chest**, **urinary**, encephalitis, brain abscess, sepsis)

Neoplastic (e.g. brain tumour)

Vascular (e.g. stroke, myocardial infarction causing hypoperfusion)

Immune (e.g. rare conditions such as neuropsychiatric lupus, Hashimoto's encephalopathy)

Trauma (e.g. **subdural haematoma**, extradural haematoma)

Endocrine (e.g. hypothyroidism, hyperthyroidism, diabetic ketoacidosis)

Drugs (e.g. intoxication or withdrawal of alcohol, opiates, or psychiatric medications; or **use of diuretics, digoxin, thyroid medication**). Drug toxicity accounts for 30% of delirium

Metabolic (e.g. hypoxia, hypercapnia, hypoglycaemia, **sodium or other electrolyte imbalances**, thiamine, folate, or vitamin B_{12} deficiencies)

Degenerative conditions. These will be chronic and will not cause the delirium, but they will predispose patients to becoming delirious

In elderly patients, don't forget that they may be hypothermic[†].

[†] While the surgical sieve approach is undoubtedly helpful for remembering a broad differential diagnosis, it is important to realize that some diagnoses do not 'pigeon-hole' precisely into categories. Hypothermia is a prime example.

Prior to taking a full history you should have checked Mrs Doolally's vital signs, to ensure that they are stable. These also provide some diagnostic information.

What vital signs would you be most interested in and why?

The vital signs of particular interest are:

* **Pulse and respiratory rate**: a tachycardia or tachypnoea could occur secondary to sepsis or haemorrhage.
* **Blood pressure**: hypoperfusion of the brain (due to systemic hypotension) decreases patient consciousness. Also consider the relationship between the pulse and blood pressure – is there hypertension and bradycardia? This is known as the Cushing response and is indicative of raised intracranial pressure.
* **Oxygen saturation**: hypoxia also affects consciousness and can be easily measured with a pulse oximeter.
* **Temperature**: fever may indicate an underlying infective process. Alternatively hypothermia also causes confusion and is not uncommon in the elderly.
* **Blood glucose**: hypoglycaemia or hyperglycaemia can depress consciousness. In patients with type 1 diabetes hyperglycaemia may be associated with ketoacidosis (which also affects the mental state). In type 2 diabetics, extreme hyperglycaemia may indicate a hyperosmolar non-ketotic (HONK) state. A BM (capillary glucose) is sufficient at this stage, although any abnormal result should be followed up with a venous blood sample.

Mrs Doolally's pulse is 108 bpm, her respiratory rate is 20/min, and her blood pressure 90/60 mmHg. Her oxygen saturation is 96% on room air, her temperature is 37.6°C and her blood glucose is 5.6 mM.

Confused patients may be inattentive, drowsy, and/or uncooperative, making a full examination difficult. Given this and the most likely diagnoses in your differential:

What are the most important signs to look for?

Even with patients who are difficult to examine, you should be able to do the following:

* **Consciousness**: assess this using the Glasgow Coma Scale (GCS). This was developed before head imaging modalities (computed tomography (CT) and magnetic resonance imaging (MRI)) where widely available and is a good prognostic indicator. It also enables you to track progression.

Glasgow Coma Scale

Best motor response

Moves arms in normal manner	6
Localizes hands to painful stimulus (e.g. push finger into angle of jaw)	5
Withdraws from painful stimulus (e.g. press hard on finger nails)	4
Flexes all limbs in response to pain	3
Extends all limbs in response to pain	2
No movement in response to pain	1

Glasgow Coma Scale (*Continued*)

Best verbal response

Talks fluently	5
Talks, but not fluently	4
Says words but sentences make no sense	3
Makes noise in response to painful stimulus	2
Silent despite painful stimulus	1

Best eye response

Eyes are spontaneously open and blinking naturally	4
Opens eyes in response to verbal command	3
Opens eyes in response to painful stimulus	2
Does not open eyes despite painful stimulus	1

GCS ≤8/15 = Patient cannot maintain own airway and will need a definitive airway i.e. intubation.

Based on: Teasdale G and Jennett B (1974). Assessment of coma and impaired consciousness: a practical scale. *Lancet*, **2**: 81–84.

- **Septic focus**: look for evidence of a septic focus such as:
  - **Chest**: look for signs of infection on percussion (dull) and auscultation (bronchial breathing, crackles).
  - **Urine**: check for suprapubic tenderness, and if there is a catheter bag check whether the urine is cloudy and send off a specimen for microscopy, culture, and sensitivities (MC&S).
  - **Cellulitis**: carefully inspect the skin. In diabetics pay particular attention to the feet, checking between the toes, as these are particularly vulnerable. Also check for any venous or arterial lines that may be a focus for infection.
  - **Meningitis**: check for neck stiffness and a purpuric rash suggestive of meningitis.
- **Pupils**: check these, looking for symmetry, size, and direct and consensual responses to light. You may find fixed dilated pupils (drug overdose, e.g. cocaine, tricyclic antidepressants; severe hypoxia; hypothermia; post-ictal), fixed pinpoint pupils (opiate or barbiturate overdose), or asymmetrical pupils suggestive of coning secondary to raised intracranial pressure or a third nerve palsy.
- **Focal neurological signs**: look for signs of focal neurological pathology (e.g. suggesting stroke or a space-occupying lesion): dysphasia, visual field defects, nystagmus, tone and reflex symmetry, plantar responses, focal weakness (moving all limbs if not cooperating), ataxia, and sensory or visual inattention.
- **Needle track marks**: suggests intravenous (IV) drug abuse.
- **Cherry red lips**: occurs in carbon monoxide poisoning …or lipstick.
- **Asterixis** (metabolic flap): suggests hypercapnia, hepatic encephalopathy, or uraemia as a cause.

- **Breath** for alcohol, fetor hepaticus (liver failure), uraemic fetor (renal failure), fruity (ketones in ketoacidosis).
- **Bitten tongue** and/or **posterior shoulder dislocation** suggests a convulsive seizure.

> You examine Mrs Doolally and find that she has a GCS of 12/15 (Eyes = 3, Verbal = 4, Motor = 5). Her lung fields are clear, her abdomen is soft and non-tender, there are no signs of cellulitis or meningism, and she does not have a catheter or any lines in place. There are no signs of focal neurology and her pupils are equal and reactive to light.
>
> **What investigations would you request?**

It can be difficult to discern the precise cause of delirium in many patients, even if the most common causes in a patient of this age are, statistically, infection or medications. Therefore, you should run a full 'confusion screen' consisting of:

- **Septic screen**: full blood count (FBC), C-reactive protein (CRP), blood cultures, urine dipstick and urine MC&S, chest radiography.
  - **FBC**: the white cell count (WCC) may be elevated if there is a systemic infection. Anaemia could contribute to hypoxia.
  - **CRP**: an elevated CRP points towards an inflammatory picture, although, as with the WCC, it is non-specific regarding the cause.
  - **Blood cultures**: these should be taken to look for infection and, if positive, to identify the organism and its sensitivity and resistance to various antibiotics. However, they take time to come back so are of more relevance in management than diagnosis.
  - **Urine analysis**: it is important that this is performed on a mid-stream urine (MSU) sample, in–out catheter sample, or suprapubic sample because the first part of a micturition stream will always be contaminated. Positive leucocyte esterase and nitrites indicate a UTI. A combination of positive glucose and ketones suggests diabetic ketoacidosis. A mid-stream sample can also be taken to look for specific bacteria.
  - **Urine microscopy, culture, and sensitivities (MC&S)**: as with the blood cultures, these should be taken to look for the offending organism if there are signs of infection on the urine dipstick.
  - **Chest radiograph**: consolidation is seen in a chest infection. An enlarged heart would be suggestive, although not diagnostic, of heart failure, which could be the cause of cerebral hypoperfusion.
- **Metabolic screen**: arterial blood gas (ABG), urea and electrolytes (U&Es), thyroid function, liver enzymes, thiamine, folate, vitamin B_{12}:
  - **ABG**: although you already have an idea of oxygen saturations from the pulse oximeter, this would provide further information about hypercapnia and acid–base balance. Uraemia, diabetic ketoacidosis, and some toxins can cause metabolic acidosis.
  - **U&Es**: a variety of different electrolyte imbalances can cause an acute confusional state, as can uraemia in renal failure.

2

- **Thyroid function tests (TFTs)**: if clinical signs or the history suggests hypo- or hyperthyroidism, you should investigate T3/T4 and TSH levels. In some hospitals this is routinely performed as a first-line investigation in confused patients.
- **Liver function tests (LFTs)**: liver failure can result in a hepatic encephalopathy and is suggested by deranged LFTs. Abnormal LFTs, in particular a disproportionately raised gamma-glutamyl transferase (GGT), may point to alcohol abuse.
- **Thiamine, folate, and vitamin B$_{12}$ levels**: if you suspect the patient is malnourished, e.g. a homeless patient, an alcohol or drug abuser, or an elderly patient living alone who appears cachexic (such patients may live on a minimal 'tea and toast' diet), then look for a deficiency in thiamine, folate, and vitamin B$_{12}$.

- **Toxicology screen**: before requesting a toxicology screen, think of which drugs the patient will realistically have consumed. This is a labour-intensive and expensive test, and thus the biochemistry department will not thank you for ordering it without good reason. In an elderly patient like Mrs Doolally, alcohol and prescription medications are likely candidates, whereas recreational drugs are unlikely.

- **Electrocardiogram (ECG)**: an ECG should be done to exclude ischaemia or arrhythmia leading to a low-output state and hypoperfusion.

> Mrs Doolally's investigations were requested and she was found to have a raised WCC and ++ leucocyte esterase and +++ nitrites in her urine. Her other investigations were unremarkable.
>
> **In light of the history, examination, and investigations, what is the diagnosis?**

The urine analysis confirms that Mrs Doolally has a **UTI**, even though clinically she had no suprapubic tenderness. It is not unusual for UTI to present without fever, especially in the elderly who often have difficulty regulating their temperature. Moreover a significant number of patients take antipyretic medications such as steroids, masking infections. It may appear odd that a 'simple' UTI could cause confusion, but you should think of how your own mental ability drops when you have a bad cold with a good going fever. That same drop in mental performance in someone who is already old and frail is why infections that may appear relatively trivial to young adults can cause acute confusion in the elderly. However, it is important to remember that UTIs are common in the elderly and may be coincidental. Therefore you must keep an open mind and be prepared to review the diagnosis if there is no response to treatment.

> **How would you manage Mrs Doolally acutely?**

- **Resuscitation**: as with any acute presentation, you must first assess the need for resuscitation by examining the ABC.
- **Antibiotics**: check your local guidelines for which antibiotics to use for a UTI, as there are different patterns of resistance from common infective organisms (e.g. *Escherichia coli*) depending on where you practice.

- **Confusion**: there are a number of conservative measures you should take in confused patients:
  - Ensure confused patients are not left unattended. Ideally they should be cared for by the same nurse as this helps them orientate themselves in an alien environment.
  - Where possible, put them in a quiet side room.
  - Discontinue non-essential medications as these may be contributing to the confusion.
  - Consider providing fluids and nutrition, as they may be unable or unwilling to maintain a balanced intake. If you suspect thiamine deficiency secondary to alcoholism or malnutrition, you **must** treat (e.g. with thiamine or Pabrinex, a cocktail of vitamins). Thiamine deficiency rapidly causes irreversible cerebral damage and if you wait for the results of your investigations it may already be too late.

- **Sedation**: If the patient becomes aggressive, you may have to resort to sedating them. If so, you can give them:
  - Haloperidol or chlorpromazine. These take about 30–60 minutes to take effect and can have extrapyramidal side-effects; they are therefore to be used with caution in Parkinson's patients.
  - Lorazepam. This acts more quickly, taking 5–10 minutes, and is useful in restoring sleep. However, it may worsen confusion and is also a respiratory depressant.

In the longer term, the management of the confused patient involves treating the underlying cause of their confusion – in this case the UTI. Be wary of non-compliance in confused patients, particularly if they fail to respond to treatment.

Short cases

> Mr Hext is a 65-year-old man who is found to be confused on the ward round the day after resection of his colorectal cancer. His observations and investigations prior to the operation were all normal. There are no signs of infection on inspection of the wound site and he does not look or feel hot or sweaty. His peripheral pulses are present (if a little weak), lung fields are clear, there are no heart murmurs (to suggest endocarditis), and no obvious signs of infection elsewhere. He is not connected to a pulse oximeter, ECG, or blood pressure monitor so you ask for this to be done, and also order some investigations.
>
> **Given his history, what are the possible causes of his confusion that you should be thinking about?**

Post-operative patients are commonly confused; this can be for any number of reasons related to their operation:

- **Hypoxia**: due to any combination of:
  - anaemia from significant blood loss in surgery
  - opiate analgesics leading to a depressed respiratory rate
  - pulmonary embolism reducing gas exchange
  - basal atelectasis
- **Opiates**: direct effect of opiate analgesics on their consciousness
- **Electrolytes**: derangement due to:
  - intra- and post-operative fluid replacement
  - less commonly, renal failure caused by hypoperfusion
- **Infection**: unlikely in this case as there are no signs of infection on examination
- **Sleep loss**: hospitals are noisy and it is even harder to sleep if you are in pain.

2

Mr Burns is a 44-year-old man on the cardiac care unit who becomes confused and aggressive 4 days after suffering a myocardial infarction. Looking at his notes, you find nothing unusual in his observations (pulse, blood pressure, temperature, blood glucose, oxygen saturation), drug history, or blood tests (including inflammatory markers, electrolytes, and liver function). However, you see in his initial clerking that he admitted to drinking 50–60 units a week and has a history of alcoholism.

What should you consider as a first step in this patient? What is the most likely diagnosis? What should you prescribe immediately?

First step: aggressive patients pose a risk to themselves, healthcare workers, and other patients. You should initially consider how to calm him down; if necessary, he may need sedation. However, you should be cautious about prescribing tranquilizers too readily, particularly given the potential cardiac side-effects in a patient with ischaemic heart disease.

Diagnosis: having dealt with the immediate danger, you should proceed with investigating his confusion. The investigations already documented eliminate a number of possibilities. In a man with a history of alcoholism and a 4-day hospital stay, **alcohol withdrawal** is the most likely candidate (severe cases are termed 'delirium tremens' and are associated with a high mortality). Such patients are at high risk of developing Wernicke's encephalopathy due to thiamine deficiency, and this may potentially progress to permanent brain damage.

Immediate prescription: alcohol withdrawal is a medical emergency and can lead to fits and even death. You should prescribe thiamine immediately to prevent irreversible brain damage, and chlordiazepoxide (a sedative) to cope with the withdrawal.

Short case

Mrs Evans is a 47-year-old lady who is brought in by ambulance after her neighbour went around to check on her and found her 'out of sorts'. You try asking Mrs Evans some questions and find her speech is unintelligible. Her neighbour says she lives alone and is self-sufficient, so there is no one to provide any detail as to how long this has been going on for. She does, however, say that she is a regular churchgoer and is teetotal.

Mrs Evans' pulse is 72 bpm, blood pressure 131/83 mmHg, oxygen saturations of 98% on room air, respiratory rate of 13/min, her temperature is 37.3°C. On examination, she is thin but not overly dishevelled, has no signs of a septic focus, and no asterixis. Her pupils are equal and reactive to light. A neurological examination reveals an intention tremor in both hands and significant ataxia such that she can barely stand or walk. Her GCS is 13/15 (Eyes = 4, Verbal = 3, Motor = 6).

You manage to speak to her daughter, who confirms her mother does not drink. She also tells you that she has suffered with bipolar disorder for over 20 years, for which she takes lithium. She is on no other medications.

You request a full set of bloods, including a metabolic and toxic screen, and ask the nurses to conduct a urinalysis when she next passes water. Her blood glucose is 4.2 mM, haemoglobin (Hb) 11.7 g/dL, WCC 4.1×10^9/L, CRP 2 mg/L, Na 132 mM, K 4.2 mM, Cl 101 mM, urea 12.3 mM, creatinine 143 µM, aspartate aminotransferase (AST) 23 U/L, alkaline phosphatase (ALP) 32 U/L, and her TFTs are within the normal ranges, as is her serum alcohol. A CT head scan shows no evidence of haemorrhage or any space-occupying lesion.

What other blood result would you like to know? What is the most likely diagnosis? What other mechanism(s) might be contributing to her confusion?

The differential diagnosis could still include an ischaemic stroke, less easily detected on CT than MRI, but given her relatively young age and the fact that she takes lithium, you should certainly order a **lithium serum level**.

Lithium toxicity could certainly account for both her confusion and renal impairment (as indicated by the raised urea; remember that urea rises out of proportion to creatinine initially because urea is normally reabsorbed in the proximal tubule, whereas creatinine is not). An alternative explanation for her urea and creatinine levels is dehydration. Mrs Evans also has mild hyponatraemia, but this is not sufficient to cause her confusion. Her lithium levels come back and are 3.7 mEq/L (normal range 0.5–1.2).

Her renal compromise and **slight uraemia** could also be contributing to her confusion. Your priority should be to maintain her renal function whilst monitoring her lithium levels until they return to normal. In the longer term, her lithium dose may need changing, although you will also want to investigate her compliance (e.g. was she taking more than her usual dose because she felt down?).

Mrs Bright is a 54-year-old lady who is brought in by ambulance in the early hours of the morning after she was found by her husband wandering the streets. Her husband has come with her, although in her confused state she does not recognize him. She was reportedly behaving aggressively towards the paramedics but is now happy to be in the hospital. You find that she is not oriented in time and scores 5/10 on an AMTS. Her husband tells you that normally she is intellectually very capable (a crossword champion, no less!). He says she was perfectly fine when she went to bed and is distressed at the sudden turn of events. When you ask him, he does recall that she had a headache before going to sleep for which she took paracetamol. She is otherwise fit and well and takes no regular medications. She has never smoked, is not diabetic or hypertensive, has no family history of note (both her parents died in old age), and is not known to have raised cholesterol.

Mrs Bright's pulse is 109 bpm, blood pressure 121/78 mmHg, oxygen saturations of 98% on room air, respiratory rate of 12/min, her temperature is 40.3°C. On examination, she is alert with a GCS of 14/15 (Eyes = 4, Verbal = 4, Motor = 6). There is no dysarthria or impairment of sensation, limb movement, or vision, although she is photophobic and you therefore cannot perform fundoscopy. Her lungs are clear, there is no cellulitis, and no neck stiffness, rash, or herpetic lesions.

A CT is ordered and a lumbar puncture performed. The CT shows no signs of haemorrhage or raised intracranial pressure. The lumbar puncture shows an opening pressure of 28 cm, glucose 1.8 mM, protein 3.2 g/L, WCC 1120/mm^3 (90% neutrophils), red cell count 2/mm^3, and Gram-positive intracellular diplococci.

What is the diagnosis?
Why were you interested in whether she smoked, was diabetic, hypertensive, had any family history, or high cholesterol?

Mrs Bright has **meningococcal meningitis**, based on the results of the lumbar puncture (very high WCC primarily neutrophils, Gram-positive intracellular diplococci, protein >1 g/L, and CSF:blood glucose ratio <0.5, assuming blood glucose is in the normal range of 3.5–5.5 mM). Hers is an atypical presentation (mild headache and photophobia without neck stiffness or rash), but serves as a reminder that meningo-encephalitis can present in a variety of ways and that you should fully investigate a high fever.

Based on the history and examination (i.e. before you got the lumbar puncture results), a stroke was a possibility so you were interested in her risk factors as they inform about the likelihood of this. The lack of focal neurology makes a stroke less likely (and confusion is not a typical feature of stroke), and the CT helps exclude a haemorrhagic stroke.

2

Mr Clifton is a 59-year-old gentleman who is brought in by his son because he is 'not himself'. You try asking him some simple questions but find his speech is unintelligible. His son tells you his father has his own business as an independent property lawyer and is usually 'compos mentis'. They have dinner together once or twice a week, the last time being before the weekend, 3 days ago, when he was perfectly fine. His medical history is notable for lung cancer, for which he is under the care of a multidisciplinary team. His son says it has spread to the adrenals and that the prognosis is not good. He also comments that his father seems to have lost his appetite, which he attributes to a combination of the cancer and his medications, and has been increasingly tired, which he attributes to his low calorie intake. He cannot remember which medications his father takes. He says his father does not drink or smoke, but used to smoke 20 a day for 40 years.

His vitals are: pulse 96 bpm, blood pressure 98/58 mmHg, oxygen saturations of 99% on room air, respiratory rate of 12/min, temperature of 37.5°C. On examination, he is alert with a GCS of 14/15 but confused (Eyes = 4, Verbal = 4, Motor = 6). You note he has a dry tongue and no peripheral or pulmonary oedema. Chest and abdominal examination are otherwise unremarkable. There are no signs of focal neurology.

A bedside blood glucose and urinalysis are unremarkable. His bloods come back shortly after and show: Hb 13.4 g/dL, CRP 3 mg/L, Na 112 mM, K 6.2 mM, Cl 83 mM, urea 9.1 mM, creatinine 78 μM, AST 15 U/L, ALP 32 U/L, with TFTs pending. A toxic screen for alcohol is negative.

How should you investigate a patient with hyponatraemia?

Hyponatraemia is a common cause of acute confusion. **Assuming Mr Clifton's confusion is due to hyponatraemia, what is the likely underlying cause(s)? What should you be wary of when treating Mr Clifton?**

Mr Clifton has **hyponatraemia**, a common cause of confusion (particularly in patients on diuretics and/or with an element of renal failure). The investigation of hyponatraemia is outlined in the flow chart (Fig. 2.1).

You should start by excluding pseudohyponatraemia by measuring the patient's serum osmolality:

- High or normal serum osmolality indicates a 'pseudohyponatraemia', i.e. a low sodium result as an artefact. If the sodium is low, you would expect the overall osmolality to be low (given that sodium is the dominant ion that determines osmolarity). Some machines that measure sodium concentrations in laboratories assume a constant volume of water. If the serum is very concentrated, e.g. with protein or glucose, there will be less water in the vial and therefore less dissolved sodium. This gives rise to an artefactually low sodium reading. Curiously, blood gas analysers, such as those found on many acute wards, are *not* affected by this artefact.

- If the patient has a low serum osmolality, i.e. a true hyponatraemia, you should work out whether they are hypervolaemic, euvolaemic, or hypovolaemic (this distinction is made largely on clinical findings):
  - Hypervolaemic patients have signs of fluid overload, specifically peripheral and pulmonary oedema and a raised jugular venous pressure (JVP). Hypervolaemic hyponatraemia occurs in many conditions, including congestive cardiac failure, hepatic failure, and nephrotic syndrome.
  - Hypovolaemic patients are dehydrated and have the corresponding signs, e.g. low blood pressure, tachycardia, dry mucous membranes, and decreased skin turgor. Hypovolaemia results in hyponatraemia as it stimulates secretion of antidiuretic hormone (ADH) in an attempt to retain fluid, thereby

2

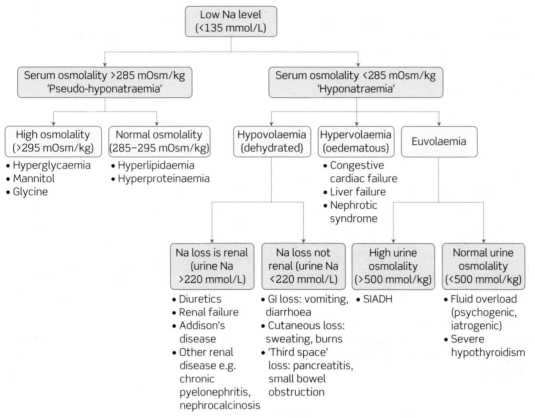

Figure 2.1 Investigating hyponatraemia. Osmolality is the ionic strength of a solution as measured by the lab, osmolarity is the calculated surrogate based on the concentrations of ions.
Based on a diagram by Dr N. Meston, John Radcliffe Hospital, Oxford, with permission.

diluting sodium levels. A urine sodium will identify the site of sodium loss as the kidney or elsewhere:

– urine sodium <220 mM indicates that the kidneys are responding normally to a drop in circulating volume by concentrating the urine. This suggests an extra-renal source of sodium loss, e.g. from the gut (vomiting, diarrhoea), skin (sweating, burns), or into the peritoneal cavity (pancreatitis, small bowel obstruction);

– urine sodium >220 mM implies the kidneys are unable to concentrate urine normally and that salt is being lost in this manner. Causes include diuretics, renal failure, and mineralocorticoid insufficiency (Addison's disease).

• Patients who have neither the clinical signs of hyper- or hypovolaemia should be considered euvolaemic. Measuring their urine osmolality will identify whether this is due to:

– the syndrome of inappropriate ADH secretion (SIADH), where excess ADH allows water to re-enter the serum in the distal tubules impairing the ability of the kidneys to concentrate the urine, leading to a high urine osmolarity (>500 mmol/kg). Note that there are a number of other criteria that must be met before you can make a diagnosis of SIADH; or

– fluid overload (psychogenic polydipsia or iatrogenic), which would be acute, or severe hypothyroidism.

2

In Mr Clifton's case, while lung cancer often causes SIADH (due to ectopic secretion of ADH by small cell lung cancers), the cause is more likely to be **Addison's disease**. First, the hyponatraemia is hypovolaemic (low blood pressure, heart rate at the upper end of normal, no oedema). Although a urinary sodium has not been performed, his high potassium suggests this is due to a failure of the Na/K exchange mechanism in the distal tubule. This happens in adrenal insufficiency (Addison's disease), where a lack of mineralocorticoid (aldosterone) synthesis results in reduced Na/K exchange in the distal tubule with subsequent poor Na and water retention. The adrenals are a common site of metastases from the lungs, although it is unusual for this to result in an Addisonian picture.

You can confirm your hypothesis with a Synacthen test which, if he has Addison's disease, will show no increase in cortisol after stimulation with adrenocorticotropic hormone (ACTH). It is important you perform a brief neurological examination on admission, including fundoscopy to look for signs of brain metastases, which could cause his confusion and may coexist with hyponatraemia.

The management of hypovolaemic severe hyponatraemia is a *slow* infusion of normal saline. You should be wary of correcting his hyponatraemia too rapidly, as this can cause central pontine myelinolysis and death. Thus, you should measure his serum sodium every 2–4 hours and, given this appears to have happened acutely (in the last 3 days), aim to increase his sodium by <2 mM/hour, and by no more than 10 mM/day. You can stop the infusion once he improves symptomatically, usually around 120 mM – there is no need to reach a sodium of 135 mM.

Miss Robertson is a 16-year-old student who is brought in by her parents, having woken up sweating and confused. You talk to her and find she is disoriented in person, place, and time, with an AMTS of 4/10. Her speech is slightly slurred. Her parents tell you that she was recently diagnosed with insulin-dependent diabetes. The family was finding this difficult, particularly the repeated injections and getting the glucose control right. You explain that you must ask about the possibility of recreational drugs and they tell you that as far as they know, she drinks a little but takes no illicit substances. You additionally ask if there were any other symptoms the night before (e.g. complaints of headache or visual problems), but they say she seemed perfectly normal.

You assess her vital observations. Her pulse is 98 bpm, blood pressure 120/71 mmHg, oxygen saturations of 100% on room air, respiratory rate of 13/min, temperature of 37.6°C. You also do a bedside glucose test which reports a level of 2.1 mM.

What is the cause of Miss Robertson's confusion? How should she be treated? What are the risks if she does not receive treatment?

Miss Robertson's confusion (and slurred speech) is caused by **hypoglycaemia** – normal glucose levels are 3.5–5.5 mM. Note that the sweating and rapid pulse rate are due to adrenergic overactivity, which is a consequence of hypoglycaemia. Severe hypoglycaemia, involving seizures or coma, is relatively common in childhood insulin-dependent diabetes, with nearly a third of patients having had at least one severe hypoglycaemic episode. This is particularly common in recently diagnosed diabetics who are still working on their glucose control and who are vulnerable to iatrogenic hypoglycaemia from an insulin overdose. Nonetheless, drug toxicity is the most common cause for teenagers to present to accident and emergency (A&E) as confused or unconscious and you should take care to exclude drugs.

You should take a blood glucose sample to confirm the diagnosis, as BM sticks only provide an estimate. However, hypoglycaemia is a medical emergency so she needs glucose immediately – don't wait for a blood sample to confirm the result before treating, as hypoglycaemia is *much* more likely to kill a patient acutely than hyperglycaemia, so you won't do her any harm by giving glucose. Given that she is able to eat and drink, she should immediately be given a sweet drink or glucose tablets and monitored. As her glucose levels rise her consciousness should also improve. If she were not able to eat or drink (e.g. if she was unconscious), you could give her any of:

- Hypostop gel (dextrose in gel form rubbed into her mouth)
- 50 mL of 20% dextrose IV, repeat up to two times if no recovery after 10–15 minutes, then consider a 10–20% dextrose infusion
- glucagon intramuscularly (IM; children who struggle with hypoglycaemic episodes may have an IM glucagon pen at home).

Note that hypoglycaemia in known diabetics on a long-acting insulin preparation or oral hypoglycaemic agent should be treated with a dextrose infusion (rather than a bolus of dextrose IV).

2

You should check Miss Robertson's blood glucose again after 10–15 minutes. If she has recovered, give her a carbohydrate-based snack (e.g. toast, banana, cereal). If she has not yet recovered, continue treatment and reassess her blood glucose in another 10–15 minutes.

In the longer term, Miss Robertson should be referred for specialist review of her glucose control.

As mentioned above, **seizures** or **coma** may occur in hypoglycaemia.

Viva questions

What functions are tested in the MMSE?

The MMSE tests the following cognitive functions: orientation in space and time, short- and long-term memory, attention, language (comprehension and expression), calculation, and visuospatial ability.

What do you understand by the term 'acute confusional state'?

Acute confusional state is defined in DSM-IV (Diagnostic and Statistical Manual of Mental Disorders, 4th edition) and ICD-10 (WHO International Statistical Classification of Diseases and Related Health Problems, 10th revision) as an observable state of relatively sudden impaired consciousness, cognition (including perception), mood, affect, and behaviour. It is interchangeable with the term 'delirium'.

Which diabetics get ketoacidosis and why? What clinical signs would you expect to see in ketoacidosis?

Ketogenesis is inhibited by even tiny amounts of insulin, so only type 1 diabetics become ketoacidotic. Clinically, signs and symptoms could include:

- polyuria, polydipsia, and a decreased mental state due to hyperglycaemia
- nausea, vomiting, abdominal pain, fatigue, shortness of breath, or Kussmaul breathing due to acidosis
- hypotension and tachycardia due to dehydration
- ketotic or 'fruity' breath.

Confusion and Kussmaul breathing are late signs and should be taken particularly seriously.

How would you distinguish an opiate overdose from a tricyclic antidepressant or cocaine overdose?

Opiates: people take opiates to 'chill out'. An overdose will cause pinpoint pupils and respiratory depression. Needle track marks may be obvious.

Cocaine: people take cocaine for a 'buzz' because it has *sympathetic* like effects. In an overdose, key signs include fixed dilated pupils, sinus tachycardia, hypotension, and pyrexia. Patients may also have respiratory depression and urinary retention.

Tricyclics: tricyclics, on the other hand, have both *sympathetic* stimulatory *and parasympathetic* inhibitory effects, the former particularly on the heart and central nervous system. Patients present with signs of sympathetic stimulation (dilated pupils, sinus tachycardia, brisk reflexes, urinary retention) and parasympathetic inhibition (dry mouth, drowsiness). They may also have upgoing plantar reflexes.

2

What treatment would you give someone presenting with confusion and a history or suspicion of alcohol abuse, and why?

All such patients should be given thiamine (e.g. Pabrinex, which also contains other B vitamins). They should be started on this immediately as prophylaxis for Wernicke's encephalopathy – a complication of alcohol abuse. Wernicke's classically presents as a triad of confusion, ataxia, and ophthalmoplegia, and is potentially reversible in the early stages which is why treatment should be started immediately. Failure to do so results in irreversible damage, known as Korsakoff's syndrome, characterized by amnesia and confabulation. Confabulation is when patients fill in gaps in their memory with fabricated stories.

Traditionally it is said that glucose should *not* be given as it can allegedly exacerbate Wernicke's, although there is little evidence to support this.

In an adult with a head injury, what are the indications for a CT scan? Why do we not scan every patient?

Head injuries can result in life-threatening pathology which can be difficult to detect by other means. For example, patients with an extradural haematoma often have a lucid interval after the incident that precedes progressive neurological deterioration. However, it would be inappropriate to give every patient with a head injury a CT scan, mainly because of the large dose of radiation exposure (there are also resource constraints to consider).

Recent National Institute for Health and Clinical Excellence (NICE) guidelines (Fig. 2.2) outline the indications for CT scanning.

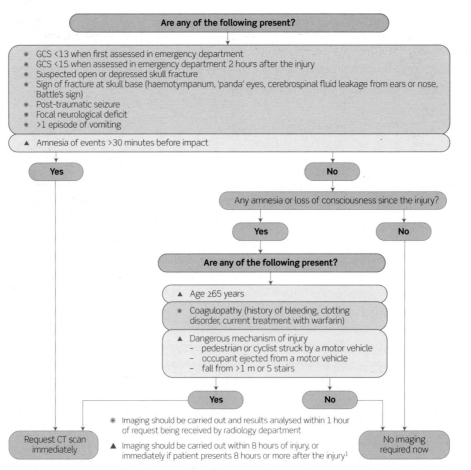

Figure 2.2 National Institute for Health and Clinical Excellence (NICE)(2007) CG56. Head injury. Triage, assessment, investigation and early management of head injury in infants, children and adults. London: NICE. Available from www.nice.org.uk/CG56. Reproduced with permission.

A woman is brought into A&E by two friends because she is confused after having taken an overdose. She says she took 'everything that was in the cabinet' and, having ensured she is stable and does not need resuscitation, you record what she believes this to include. You call the poisons unit at Guy's Hospital in London to check how best to proceed. They recommend supportive measures as necessary (e.g. fluids) and observation for 6 hours. You put a cannula in place and take bloods and then want to give her saline. But as you explain this is what you are going to do, she tells you she is a Jehovah's Witness and doesn't want you to proceed. You explain carefully that giving saline is not against her religion (as it is not a blood product) but she continues to refuse. What should you do?

There are two conflicting ethical principles in this scenario: the obligation on the doctor to do what is best for the patient (beneficence) and the patient's right to choose their own treatment (patient autonomy). Except in the case of life-threatening conditions or where the patient has been assessed as lacking the competence to make their own decisions, adult patients can refuse any treatment. Thus this lady is entitled to refuse treatment, provided you are happy she is competent. It may be worthwhile getting a psychiatric assessment, both to assess her competence and her mental state as she must have suffered some distress to lead her to take an overdose. This was indeed done and, having decided she was competent, she was allowed to leave as per her wishes, before the 6 hour observation period had elapsed and without having any saline.

 For a range of Single Best Answer questions related to the topic of this chapter go to
www.oxfordtextbooks.co.uk/orc/ocms/

Blackout

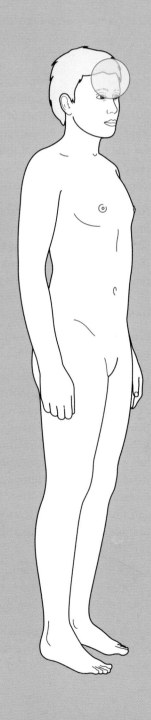

Core case

3

! *Read through the sections in red, covering up the sections in white that follow*
so that you don't see the answer. At the end of each red section, try to answer the
question before reading on.

Core case

> Mr Williams is a 19-year-old student who is brought in by ambulance after collapsing whilst at a university ball. A friend who witnessed the collapse has accompanied him to hospital and confirms that he lost consciousness.
>
> **What are the commonest causes of a transient loss of consciousness?**

Note that the terms 'syncope' and 'loss of consciousness' are not interchangeable as loss of consciousness can be due to either syncopal or non-syncopal causes. Syncope is a form of loss of consciousness in which hypoperfusion of the brain is the cause (from the Greek *syn* (together) and *kopein* (to cut), referring to the fact that the blood flow that joins the brain together with the rest of the body has been cut).

Syncopal causes can be subdivided by mechanism as follows:

- **'Reflex'**: this is believed to involve activation of a primitive reflex that leads mammals to 'play dead' when faced with danger. Their heart rate slows and their blood pressure drops temporarily, reducing cerebral perfusion and leading to syncope. Some people appear to have a low threshold for activating this reflex in specific situations – for example after standing still for a long time, after seeing something frightening (e.g. blood, needles), or when straining (micturition, defaecation).

- **'Cardiac'**: pathologies causing a reduction in cardiac output (such as arrhythmias or outlet obstruction) can also lead to syncope.

- **'Orthostatic'**: orthostatic hypotension basically means low blood pressure on sitting or standing (as opposed to lying flat). When we stand up there is a sudden drop in blood pressure that we compensate for by vasoconstriction, particularly of the 'capacitance' veins in the legs. This reduces the intravascular space, enabling us to maintain the pressure. However, this vasoconstriction takes a few seconds, so to prevent a transient fall in blood pressure every time we stand, there is a temporary increase in heart rate. Patients with reduced intravascular volume (e.g. from dehydration) and/or in whom the normal autonomic response (transient tachycardia and peripheral vasoconstriction) to standing is blunted (e.g. due to drugs or autonomic neuropathy) are vulnerable to blackouts.

- **'Cerebrovascular'**: these are non-cardiac structural causes of reduced cerebral perfusion, i.e. obstructions to the blood flow between the heart and the brain. They are relatively uncommon.

The main causes of a transient loss of consciousness are summarized in Table 3.1, with the most common in large font.

3

Table 3.1 Main causes of a transient loss of consciousness[†]

Syncopal	Non-syncopal
REFLEX **Vasovagal syncope** Carotid sinus hypersensitivity Situational syncope (e.g. micturition)	**Intoxication** (e.g. alcohol, sedatives) Head trauma Metabolic (mainly hypoglycaemia) Non-epileptic 'seizure' (psychologically driven) Epileptic seizure Narcolepsy
CARDIAC **Arrhythmias** Structural cardiac pathology causing outflow obstruction (e.g. aortic stenosis, hypertrophic obstructive cardiomyopathy (HOCM)) Massive pulmonary embolism	
ORTHOSTATIC **Dehydration** **Drugs** (anti-hypertensives, anti-sympathetics) Autonomic instability Baroreceptor dysfunction (in hypertensive patients)	
CEREBROVASCULAR Vertebrobasilar insufficiency Subclavian steal Aortic dissection	

[†] You should also remember that patients may believe they have lost consciousness when in fact they haven't. Such patients may have a psychogenic (non-epileptic) 'seizure' or transient global amnesia (rare!).

The age of any given patient makes particular causes of loss of consciousness much more likely than others.

What is the main cause of loss of consciousness in a patient:
(1) aged 25 years?
(2) aged 55 years?
(3) aged 85 years?

---

1) In young patients, the commonest cause of loss of consciousness is **vasovagal syncope**. Patients describe a warning or pre-syncopal sensation – an odd sensation in the stomach, going pale and clammy, and knowing they are going to lose consciousness.

2) In middle-aged patients, the most common causes of loss of consciousness are **vasovagal syncope** (see above) and **cardiac arrhythmias**. This is because cardiac arrhythmias are usually secondary to ischaemic heart disease, itself more common as patients age and accumulate an increasing burden of atherosclerotic lesions. By this line of reasoning, one would expect cardiac arrhythmias to account for most episodes of lost consciousness in elderly patients as well, but in reality many of the patients who have sufficient ischae-mic heart disease to cause arrhythmias in middle age will succumb to an atherosclerosis-related death (usually cardiac or stroke) before reaching 'old age'. Patients typically describe losing consciousness without any warning or without any obvious trigger (e.g. suddenly passing out whilst sitting in front of the television). Arrhythmias are important as there is a high risk of fatal arrhythmia.

3) In elderly patients, the most common cause of loss of consciousness is **ortho-static hypotension caused by medications**. These include diuretics and angiotensin-converting enzyme (ACE) inhibitors (reduced blood volume and vasodilatation), β-blockers (inability to increase heart rate on standing), α-blockers (inability to vasoconstrict the major capacitance veins), and cal-cium-channel blockers (inability to vasoconstrict and some are negatively inotropic/chronotropic). Many elderly patients are on a number of these drugs simultaneously and find it hard to maintain adequate blood pressure. Patients typically describe losing consciousness after standing up, because their body is unable to compensate for the sudden drop in blood pressure. The condition carries a significant morbidity (from broken bones, loss of confidence and independence) and mortality (from venous thromboem-bolic disease and infections acquired as a consequence of prolonged bed rest after a fall).

> Now that you have your differential diagnosis and some idea of what is most common in a person of Mr Williams' age, you can move on to the history.
>
> **What questions should you ask about the episode of loss of consciousness itself?**

In the history, from both the patient and a witness (if available), you should get a detailed description of what happened before, during, and after the episode. Specifically:

Before

- **Was there any warning?** If there was no warning, the cause is most likely a cardiac arrhythmia or a massive pulmonary embolus. Note that sometimes arrhythmias are preceded by palpitations. Patients with other causes of black-out tend to have some warning (e.g. aura preceding an epileptic seizure, dizzi-ness preceding a vasovagal episode).
- **Were there any precipitating factors** (e.g. exercise, straining, standing up, fear, pain)? Postural triggers suggest orthostatic hypotension. Other precipi-tating factors are consistent with a vasovagal episode. Loss of consciousness caused by head turning suggests carotid sinus hypersensitivity. Blackout

whilst sitting or lying down is suggestive of a cardiac arrhythmia. Passing out when exercising suggests structural cardiac pathology such as aortic stenosis or a cardiomyopathy.

• **Was there any recent head trauma?** This may seem obvious, but patients will not always associate head trauma with an episode of loss of consciousness, especially if there is some delay between the two. Be wary of subdural haemorrhages (particularly in the elderly and alcoholics) which may be precipitated by head trauma days or weeks earlier and may be associated with subsequent seizures.

During

• **How long was the patient unconscious – seconds or minutes?** Blackouts due to a vasovagal episode or an arrhythmia are short-lived, lasting seconds.

• **Did they bite their tongue, move their limbs, or were they incontinent of urine or faeces?** Note that tongue-biting is virtually pathognomonic of an epileptic seizure, whereas twitching and incontinence can be features with other causes, e.g. vasovagal.

After

• **Did they recover spontaneously? If not, how long did it take them to recover? Were they confused after recovery?** A spontaneous recovery argues against a metabolic or neurological cause (other than epilepsy). A slow recovery with confusion suggests an epileptic seizure.

These points are summarized in Table 3.2.

Table 3.2 Summary features of episodes of loss of consciousness

	Epilepsy	Vasovagal (i.e. a faint)	Arrhythmia
Before	May have stereotyped aura (partial seizure); or no warning (general seizure)	Vagal symptoms (sweating, pallor, nausea) May be a precipitant (e.g. fear)	No warning
During	Lasts minutes Stereotyped episodes, same every time Tongue-biting pathognomonic Twitching and incontinence may also occur but not specific	Lasts seconds May twitch or be incontinent	Lasts seconds May twitch or be incontinent
After	Slow recovery, confused for 5–30 minutes	Rapid recovery on sitting or lying	Rapid spontaneous recovery

3

Mr Williams remembers feeling unwell and dizzy before passing out, but seems alright now, half an hour later. His friend tells you that he appeared well earlier in the evening, although he was inebriated. However, immediately before he collapsed his friend says 'the colour drained from his face'. He tells you Mr Williams was unconscious for only a few seconds and was a little surprised but not particularly confused when he came around.

Other aspects of the history can also help in the diagnosis of blackouts.

What would you particularly ask about in the history?

Past medical history

- **Has it happened before?** If it has happened before, you should ask the same questions about previous episodes and if they are increasing in frequency.
- **Diabetes?** This predisposes to vascular disease, hypoglycaemia, polyuria and dehydration, and autonomic dysfunction that can cause orthostatic hypotension.
- **Cardiac illness?** Ask about palpitations and chest pain as well as previous diagnoses. The presence of heart disease is a strong predictor of a cardiac cause of syncope. Arrhythmias may arise following infarction. Left ventricular outflow obstruction may occur secondary to aortic stenosis, HOCM, etc.
- **Peripheral vascular disease?** Ask about claudication in case the patient is not aware of having peripheral vascular disease. Peripheral vascular disease is associated with coronary artery disease, as both are manifestations of the same underlying pathological process – atherosclerosis. It is also associated with cerebrovascular events (transient ischaemic attacks (TIAs), strokes), but these are very rarely a cause of transient loss of consciousness.
- **Epilepsy?** If they have epilepsy, did this episode resemble one of their typical seizures?
- **Anaemia?** This can contribute to hypoxia.
- **Psychiatric illness?** Panic attacks are associated with hyperventilation and loss of consciousness. Non-epileptic 'seizures' are also more common amongst patients with psychiatric comorbidities.

Drug history

- **Insulin? Oral hypoglycaemics?** These will obviously make patients susceptible to hypoglycaemia.
- **Antihypertensives?** (e.g. diuretics, ACE inhibitors, β-blockers, calcium-channel blockers). All can cause hypotension.
- **Vasodilators?** (e.g. glyceryl trinitrate (GTN), isosorbide mononitrate). These can also cause hypotension, particularly in elderly patients.
- **Anti-arrhythmics?** These can paradoxically predispose to arrhythmias.
- **Antidepressants?** Hypotension can be a side-effect with some antidepressants, e.g. tricyclic antidepressants.

Social history

- **Alcohol**? Many people who are intoxicated are brought in as 'loss of consciousness of unknown cause', although some might not have lost consciousness but simply become unable to stand anymore.
- **Stimulant recreational drugs?** Drugs such as cocaine and amphetamines stimulate the heart, causing tachyarrhythmias and potentially a drop in cardiac output.

Family history

- **Sudden death**? Such a history is significant in all cases of unexplained syncope, but is particularly informative regarding exercise-induced syncope. Some cardiomyopathies and arrhythmias are hereditary.

Mr Williams has no past medical history of note, only childhood asthma. He is not taking any medications. He sheepishly admits to consuming more than 8 units of alcohol earlier that evening, but no other recreational drugs.

The history argues in favour of some causes and against others, but you still need to exclude some of the less likely causes as they are potentially very serious.

What signs would you look for on examination?

The examination may be unremarkable, but you should look for the following:

- **Tongue:** a bitten tongue. Make sure you look at the side of the tongue.
- **Dehydration**: signs of dehydration (e.g. dry mucous membranes, tachycardia, hypotension), as this can contribute to hypovolaemia and predispose to cerebral hypoperfusion.
- **Head trauma**: any signs of head trauma (you might expect this to have been mentioned in the history, although perhaps not from this patient if he was overly inebriated!). If there has been head trauma, try to establish whether it came before or after the loss of consciousness, i.e. did they hit their head as they fell?
- **Heart**:
  - A slow or irregular pulse, suggesting heart block or atrial fibrillation.
  - Look at the jugular venous pressure (JVP) for cannon waves. These are exaggerated 'a waves' in the jugular pulse caused by right atrial contraction occurring after ventricular contraction has closed the tricuspid valve. Cannon waves occur in complete heart block, a cause of syncope.
  - A heart murmur. Aortic stenosis can cause outflow obstructions and cerebral hypoperfusion.
- **Carotid bruits**: suggest carotid artery stenosis (although loudness of the bruit has no bearing upon severity of the stenosis).
- **Blood pressure**: check for orthostatic hypotension. Take the blood pressure lying down and within 2 minutes of standing. Orthostatic hypotension is defined as a drop of ≥20 mmHg in systolic blood pressure or ≥10 mmHg diastolic on standing.

3

- **Focal neurological signs**: look for signs of peripheral neuropathy (e.g. due to diabetes mellitus, chronic alcohol abuse) or parkinsonism that may be associated with autonomic dysfunction (e.g. in multisystem atrophy). In the case of suspected seizures, check that there has been a full neurological recovery.

Mr Williams' examination is unremarkable.

What first-line investigations would you request and why?

You should perform the following investigations on anyone with loss of consciousness:

- **Oxygen saturations:** may reveal hypoxia, e.g. secondary to a pulmonary embolism (PE).
- **Bloods:**
  - **Capillary blood glucose:** you should exclude hypoglycaemia. You will also be looking for undiagnosed diabetes which can lead to polyuria and dehydration, and which in established diabetics is associated with autonomic dysfunction that can lead to hypotension and blackouts. Although diabetes mellitus is also a risk factor for cerebrovascular disease, strokes and TIAs rarely cause blackouts.
  - **Full blood count (FBC):** to look for an anaemia that may be a contributing factor.
  - **Urea and electrolytes (U&Es):** exclude an electrolyte abnormality.
- **Electrocardiogram (ECG):** the European Society of Cardiology 2004 Guidelines state that this is only warranted when there is a high pre-test probability of an arrhythmia being a cause (e.g. a young patient with sudden blackout with no warning and for no obvious reason), in which case you might look for evidence of arrhythmia or conduction defect including bundle branch block, a short PR or long QT interval. An ECG can be helpful if it shows an abnormality, but if it is normal it does not exclude a cardiac cause as arrhythmias can be intermittent, particularly if the patient is asymptomatic at the time of the recording. 24-hour ambulatory ECG (Holter) monitoring is rarely helpful as few patients have arrhythmias every day and a positive result is just as likely in elderly patients who have experienced a blackout as in those who haven't. As a consequence, the guidelines suggest such recordings are useful only in patients whose symptoms occur daily.

There are a number of investigations you wouldn't carry out initially on everyone with an episode of loss of consciousness, but only if your history and examination suggest certain diagnoses:

- A cardiac abnormality such as a valve lesion, consider an **echocardiogram**.
- Carotid sinus sensitivity, consider a **carotid sinus massage** (see the viva question on this topic).
- Epilepsy, consider an **electroencephalogram (EEG)** and **brain scan** (computed tomography (CT) or magnetic resonance imaging (MRI)) .

Mr Williams' blood glucose, ECG, FBC, U&Es, and oxygen saturations are normal.

In light of his age, history, and investigations, what diagnosis is most likely?

Bear in mind that in approximately 50% of cases of loss of consciousness no diagnosis is made. Given that the patient is young and has an unremarkable history and normal first-line investigations, the most likely diagnosis is **vasovagal syncope**. A cardiac arrhythmia is unlikely given the patient's age and the lack of family history of congenital heart problems. The normal ECG suggests that there is no congenital heart pathology such as Brugada syndrome. Indeed, cardiac arrhythmias in general are unlikely if there is no history of palpitations, no clinical evidence of heart disease, and an entirely normal ECG.

Your consultant agrees that this is most likely a vasovagal attack and decides to discharge Mr Williams.

What advice would you give him on discharge? Does he need to be followed up, and if so, by who?

Mr Williams has had what is probably a vasovagal attack. You should explain this and give him lifestyle advice, that is to sit or lie down if he feels like he is going to faint. Now is also a good opportunity to encourage Mr Williams to avoid excessive alcohol consumption. You should advise him to see his general practitioner (GP) if he has recurrent episodes, but no follow-up is necessary unless these occur.

Short cases

Short case

Mrs Maxwell is a 37-year-old housewife who has been referred to neurology outpatients by her GP after several episodes of loss of consciousness. The GP wonders if she has epilepsy. The GP's letter adds that Mrs Maxwell is an anxious lady with a history of depression. She has come to outpatients with her husband.

You ask her about the attacks. She describes a series of different events. On one occasion, she says she was having an argument with her 8-year-old son and then woke up on the floor. On another occasion, she was out shopping with her husband and son and collapsed. She also says she has ended up on the floor at home without knowing how she got there. Her husband corroborates a number of these episodes. There never appears to be any warning or precipitant.

Her husband tells you the episodes typically last a few minutes. He says that sometimes she twitches, but not always. Afterwards she appears fine apart from sometimes a headache. She tells you that she frequently suffers with headaches.

Given the history, what is the most likely diagnosis? What investigations should you conduct and why?

Recurrent, unprovoked losses of consciousness in a woman of this age should raise your suspicion of epilepsy. However, this is a life-changing diagnosis and you should be sure before making it. Her history is suggestive of **non-epileptic seizures**: the episodes are not stereotyped, her recovery is relatively rapid, and there is no post-ictal confusion. She also has a background of depression and possibly anxiety, which are commonly seen in patients with non-epileptic seizures.

You should nonetheless exclude epilepsy as it is still a possibility. Accordingly, you should request an EEG (looking for features of epilepsy) and MRI or CT of her brain, to look for any obvious abnormalities that may be triggering the epilepsy.

Mr Woodward is a 69-year-old gentleman who is brought to his GP by a friend after fainting in the street. Mr Woodward has been visiting family for the past couple of days and has been complaining of 'dizzy spells', although this is the first time he has lost consciousness. When asked what he means by 'dizzy spells', he confirms that he means light-headedness rather than vertigo (i.e. there is no rotational component to the sensation). He says this occurs on standing and only started about a month ago. On the occasion on which he lost consciousness, his friend says he came round a few seconds later. He says he wasn't particularly confused afterwards, other than wondering why it happened. His medical history includes hypertension, angina, and benign prostatic hyperplasia for which he takes aspirin, bendroflumethiazide, atenolol, and doxazosin. He has been taking these for several years, except the doxazosin which he started a month ago.

What is the most likely diagnosis? What is the physiological basis for this?

Short case

Mr Woodward has a history of light-headedness associated with standing that suggests **orthostatic hypotension**. The timing of these symptoms coincides with his new prescription of doxazosin for his prostate problems. This is not uncommon; surprisingly few patients associate the onset of new symptoms (side-effects) with the start of a new medication. Mr Woodward has good reason to feel lightheaded when he stands up: the diuretic will reduce his circulating blood volume, and the β-blocker and α-blocker will impair the increase in heart rate and vasoconstriction of the large capacitance veins, respectively, when he stands. Therefore Mr Woodward is probably suffering from iatrogenic orthostatic hypotension. This could be confirmed by comparing the lying versus standing blood pressure, looking for a postural drop in blood pressure.

The key to management is to modify his medications by reducing doses to the minimal effective dose, trying different medications altogether (e.g. a different type of α-blocker or a 5α-reductase inhibitor for his benign prostatic hyperplasia), or trying non-medical management of some of his problems (e.g. a transurethral resection of the prostate (TURP) for his benign prostatic hyperplasia).

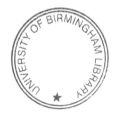

Short case

Mr O'Brien is a 42-year-old estate agent who presents to his GP after several episodes of loss of consciousness over the last 2 months. The episodes occurred whilst he was running or rushing, e.g. for the bus. Each was immediately preceded by sweating. He does not recall any palpitations, nausea, chest pain, or shortness of breath. He tells you that some of these episodes were witnessed and he was told that he was only unconscious for a few seconds. He has not bitten his tongue or been incontinent at any time. He says he recovers rapidly and is able to carry on as normal, although he has been taking it a bit easier.

He has no known history of cardiovascular disease, epilepsy, or diabetes, and takes no medications. His pulse rate is 72 bpm and regular. There is a slow-rising carotid pulse. His apex beat is undisplaced and there are no heaves or thrills. Heart sounds I and II are both audible and there is a loud ejection systolic murmur which radiates to the carotids. His examination is otherwise unremarkable. His blood glucose, ECG, and U&Es are normal. In light of his heart murmur, you order an echocardiogram.

What do you think the echocardiogram would show? How might this account for his episodes of loss of consciousness?

Mr O'Brien's echocardiogram showed severe **aortic stenosis**, consistent with his systolic ejection murmur. His cardiac output was significantly reduced as a result of the outflow obstruction caused by his aortic stenosis. It was this that was predisposing him to blackouts.

There are three main causes of aortic stenosis. In a young patient a congenital bicuspid valve is most common. In the elderly, calcification of the valve commonly leads to stenosis. Rheumatic fever is a third cause of aortic stenosis but thankfully is relatively rare in the UK today. Mr O'Brien's echocardiogram showed a bicuspid aortic valve.

An important differential diagnosis in a young patient presenting like this is HOCM, but this would not account for the slow-rising pulse.

Miss Gokhale is a 15-year-old school student who has come to neurology outpatients with her mother following three suspected seizures in the past 4 months. The first occurred during break time at school, after which she was brought to hospital by ambulance. Two subsequent attacks have taken place, one at home and another at school. Miss Gokhale has no recollection of the episodes, although she knows that she is confused for some time after they occur. Her mother, who spoke to witnesses at school, says that during each attack she 'goes tense and shakes vigorously'. She has not bitten her tongue or been incontinent. The attacks last 5–10 minutes, after which her daughter is confused for around 30 minutes.

What is the most likely diagnosis and why?

Given the stereotyped nature, the lack of vagal symptoms prior to the attacks, and the slow spontaneous recovery with persistent confusion, Miss Gokhale has most likely had **epileptic seizures**. As with the case of Mrs Maxwell above, an EEG and brain CT/MRI was ordered to try to confirm the diagnosis. Neither showed any abnormality. However, epilepsy is a clinical diagnosis and the neurologist felt there was enough in her history to warrant this diagnosis, so she was commenced on anticonvulsants.

A couple of months later, Miss Gokhale comes back to hospital via ambulance whilst fitting. The seizure started at a dinner with her friends over half an hour ago and she has not regained consciousness at any time.

What complication has happened to Miss Gokhale and how should she be managed acutely? What possible causes are there?

Miss Gokhale is in **status epilepticus**. This is a medical emergency and requires urgent attention. As always, you should start by assessing her airway, breathing, and circulation (ABC). As part of this she should be given high-flow oxygen, have monitoring set up (continuous ECG, pulse oximeter, blood pressure cuff), a blood capillary glucose measurement, and two intravenous (IV) lines put in with bloods taken for an FBC, U&Es, Ca^{2+}, and Mg^{2+}. A selective toxin screen and levels of anti-convulsant medications may be appropriate if the history suggests intoxication or non-concordance. Two IV lines are necessary, partly because they can be easily disrupted in patients who are convulsing and also because benzodiazepines (used to try to terminate the seizure) should have a dedicated line. If she is hypoglycaemic you should treat her with 50 mL of 20% dextrose immediately.

Having checked her ABC, you should rapidly assess D and E: disability (Glasgow Coma Scale (GCS) and pupils) and exposure (a quick check for any obvious external signs of injury). Then you should try to end her seizure. Start by giving her 2–4 mg of lorazepam IV as a slow bolus over 2 minutes. If she is still fitting 10 minutes later, you can repeat this. If 10 minutes after that she is still fitting, you should contact an intensive care consultant and start giving her a phenytoin infusion with a loading dose of 18 mg/kg at a rate of 50 mg/min. Be sure to monitor her ECG and blood pressure when starting the infusion for arrhythmias and hypotension (both side-effects of phenytoin given acutely). By this time the intensive care specialists will have taken over and, if she is still fitting 10 minutes later, may decide to give her a general anaesthetic such as thiopentone to terminate the seizure.

Once the acute situation has been dealt with, you should investigate the cause of her seizure. In particular consider:

- Poor compliance with anticonvulsant medications
- Metabolic causes (hypoglycaemia, electrolyte imbalance – renal or liver failure are unlikely in this patient given her age)
- Alcohol or other toxins
- Hypoxia
- Infection (intercurrent infection lowering the seizure threshold in a known epileptic, encephalitis/meningitis)
- Hypertensive encephalopathy
- Cerebral (tumour, head injury, or abscess are all possibilities – stroke, arterio-venous malformation, and vasculitis would be unlikely given her age)

In Miss Gokhale's case, the seizure was terminated with the initial dose of lorazepam. She later revealed that she had stopped taking her medications after a month as she had started to gain weight and felt self-conscious. In addition, she had consumed alcohol at dinner, which may have triggered the seizure.

Viva questions

What are Stokes–Adams attacks? How are they treated?

A Stokes–Adams attack is a sudden transient loss of consciousness induced by a slow or absent pulse and subsequent loss of cardiac output. The underlying problem is either complete (third degree) heart block or sinoatrial disease. Attacks are not associated with a change in posture or any other trigger. They usually last seconds but if they go on for more than 15–20 seconds twitching may occur due to cerebral anoxia. After an attack the patient becomes flushed as the well-oxygenated blood sat in the pulmonary capillaries during circulatory arrest is pumped around. The term Stokes–Adams attack comes from two physicians who described the condition but is not used much nowadays, as the terms 'cardiogenic syncope' or 'syncope due to cardiac arrhythmia' are preferred. Stokes–Adams attacks are treated with a pacemaker.

How would you define epilepsy? How are seizures classified?

Epilepsy is defined as a **tendency to have recurrent, unprovoked seizures**. A single seizure is not enough to diagnose epilepsy. A seizure is defined as transient excessive electrical activity with motor, sensory, or cognitive manifestations discernible to the patient or an observer.

Seizures are broadly grouped as generalized or partial, depending on whether the abnormal electrical activity affects the whole brain from the start (generalized) or is focal, at least initially (partial):

1) **Generalized seizures** can be further subdivided depending on symptoms during the seizure:
   a) **Tonic-clonic ('grand mal')**: patients are initially rigid (tonic phase) and then convulse, making rhythmical muscular contractions (clonic phase)
   b) **Absence ('petit mal')**: usually in children, the patient loses consciousness and appears vacant and unresponsive to observers for up to 30 seconds
   c) **Atonic**: a brief loss of muscle tone, causing the patient to fall to the ground
   d) **Tonic**: like the tonic phase of tonic–clonic seizures
   e) **Clonic**: like the clonic phase of tonic–clonic seizures
   f) **Myoclonic**: an extremely brief muscle contraction (<0.1 second) seen as a jerky movement

2) **Partial seizures** can be divided into those where consciousness is unimpaired (simple) and those where it is impaired (complex). Alternatively they may be classified by the brain area affected, e.g. temporal lobe (*déjà vu/jamais vu*, olfactory/auditory aura, epigastric discomfort), frontal lobe (motor), parietal (sensory), occipital (visual).

Elderly patients presenting to hospital with a loss of consciousness are often seen as an unexciting or unglamorous case, but they are in fact patients who require rapid, effective multidisciplinary team management. Why is loss of consciousness in the elderly so important?

Loss of consciousness in the elderly carries a very high risk of:

- **Morbidity**: elderly patients who lose consciousness and fall are likely to:
  - Injure themselves seriously. Falling can result in head trauma and subdural haematomas; radial fractures that make washing, cooking, and eating difficult; neck of femur fractures that confine them to bed; etc.

    − Lose their confidence. Ask yourself if you would walk confidently down a flight of stairs if the last time you did so you fell down 15 stairs and broke a hip and both ankles. This often leads to significant anxiety or depression, which needs managing.

    − Lose their independence. For example, an elderly patient who has fractured a clavicle and radius may go from living alone to being dependent on carers to wash, get dressed, cook, and feed themselves.

- **Mortality**: loss of consciousness in an elderly patient may not sound life-threatening, but if the patient suffers, say, a neck of femur fracture, they may need a prolonged hospital stay. Whilst an inpatient, their immobility may lead to a deep vein thrombosis and pulmonary embolus. Or they may get pressure sores, which in turn may get infected. They may get urinary tract infections from indwelling catheters, or pneumonia from the lack of movement and small areas of collapsed lung (atelectasis), leading to poor clearance of mucus. A fractured neck of femur continues to be a major (albeit indirect) cause of death in elderly people in the developed world.

- **Cost**: loss of consciousness in the elderly, if accompanied by a fracture, can result in a lengthy hospital stay, prolonged physiotherapy, investment to adapt their house for their new immobility, regular (often daily) visits by carers to help with activities of daily living (ADLs), days off work for caring relatives eager to help, and sometimes moving into a nursing home. All of this entails significant cost to the patient, their family, and the state.

Heart block is a common cardiac cause of loss of consciousness. What is the classification of heart block affecting the atrioventricular (AV) node (i.e. not the bundles or fascicles)? How are the different types distinguished on ECG?

- **First-degree (incomplete) heart block**: every atrial contraction is transmitted to the ventricles, but conduction is slower than normal. It is caused by damage to the AV node (e.g. from ischaemic heart disease, fibrosis, inflammation). On ECG the gap between atrial contraction (P-wave) and ventricular contraction (QRS complex), the PR interval, is >200 ms (one large square on a normally calibrated ECG). This isn't really a 'block', more a 'slowing down'.

- **Second-degree heart block**: some but not every atrial contraction is transmitted to the ventricles. This can be because of excessive vagal stimulation to the AV node or damage to the AV node or bundle of His. Various subtypes are recognized:
  - **Mobitz type I block**: each heart beat shows a progressively increased PR interval until eventually a QRS complex is missed entirely, as if the AV node block is getting progressively worse and then resetting itself. This pattern on an ECG is called Wenckebach. 'Wenckebaching' can be normal in ultrafit athletes.
  - **Mobitz type II block**: this involves random block of the bundle of His such that on an ECG, QRS complexes are found to be missing randomly. It has a high risk of progressing to complete heart block.
  - **Advanced heart block**: this involves a QRS complex missing every second (2:1) or third (3:1) heart beat. AV node conduction is essentially being blocked in an intermittent but regular and predictable manner.

- **Third-degree (complete) heart block**: this results in no conduction at all between the atria and ventricles. On ECG the P-waves are unrelated to the QRS complexes, which are broad. Whilst the atria continue to contract at the pace set by the sinoatrial pacemaker, the ventricles rely on spontaneous conduction originating in the bundle of His to contract at a slow rate of about 40 bpm.

3

What is a tilt table test and what is it used for?

A tilt table test is sometimes used to help determine whether there is a vasovagal cause for blackouts. The patient is placed on a 'tilt table' that swings them from a supine position through 90° to upright. The patient is connected to continuous ECG and blood pressure monitoring and asked to report their symptoms every 3–5 minutes. A baseline is established by monitoring the patient supine for 5 minutes. The patient is then tilted (head up) to between 60° and 90° for between 10 and 60 minutes (a variety of different protocols are used). The test is considered positive if:

- the patient experiences loss of consciousness with a significant fall in blood pressure or heart rate, in which case they are returned to a supine position; or

- symptoms develop.

If an initial test is negative, it can be repeated whilst infusing drugs that increase the susceptibility to the test by vasodilation (e.g. GTN) or bradycardia (e.g. adenosine). This increases the sensitivity but decreases the specificity of the test – under such conditions as many as 45% of control subjects with no history of syncope may have a positive test!

The test is of limited value in patients with situational syncope, e.g. on micturition. It is contraindicated in patients who have orthostatic hypotension.

A false negative rate as high as 30% has been reported, although it is difficult to determine, as there is no gold standard for comparison. Thus a negative test cannot be used to exclude a vasovagal cause.

The low specificity and sensitivity means that this test is seldom used.

What are the main side-effects and interactions of anticonvulsant drugs in general, and specifically: sodium valproate, lamotrigine, carbamazepine, phenytoin?

All anticonvulsants are teratogenic: 2–3% of babies born to patients on one anticonvulsant are affected (around 4–6% if on two or 10% if on three anticonvulsants). Specific drugs are associated with specific defects: sodium valproate with neural tube defects, phenytoin with cleft palate and congenital heart disease. Although the risk of spina bifida from valproate use can theoretically be reduced by high-dose folate supplementation during the first trimester, current National Institute for Health and Clinical Excellence (NICE) advice is to avoid the use of any anticonvulsants during pregnancy where possible.

Carbamazepine and phenytoin interfere with the hepatic metabolism of the contraceptive pill by inducing cytochrome P450, therefore patients on the pill should be advised to double their dose and/or use barrier contraceptives. By the same mechanism they can interfere with warfarin dosing (requiring a greater dose of warfarin for the same target international normalized ratio (INR)).

The specific side-effects include:

- Sodium valproate: weight gain, hair loss and curling, nausea, rash, drowsiness, tremor, drug-induced hepatitis

- Lamotrigine: rash (Stevens–Johnson syndrome), headaches, dizziness, insomnia, vivid dreams

- Carbamazepine: rash, nausea, ataxia, diplopia, agranulocytosis, hyponatraemia

- Phenytoin: acne, rash, ataxia, ophthalmoparesis, sedation, gingival hyperplasia

3

What should you, by law, advise patients with an episode of loss of consciousness about driving?

The Driver and Vehicle Licensing Agency (DVLA) have very clear guidelines on this matter (http://www.dvla. gov.uk/). Your actions depend on the cause of the loss of consciousness. For cars and motorcycles:

- If it was a simple faint with prodromal symptoms and a provoking factor can be identified that is unlikely to recur whilst sitting, there are no driving restrictions and there is no need to advise the DVLA.
- If the loss of consciousness was likely due to a transient loss of blood supply to the brain (syncope) with a *low risk of recurrence*, the patient can drive 4 weeks after the event.
- If the loss of consciousness was likely syncope with a *high risk of recurrence*, the patient can drive 4 weeks after the event if the cause has been identified and treated, or 6 months after if not identified or treated.
- If the loss of consciousness is unexplained and there are no suggestions it was a seizure, the patient cannot drive for 6 months.
- If the loss of consciousness was associated with seizure markers, the patient cannot drive for one (seizure-free) year.

If someone with epilepsy has been on anti-epileptic medication for many years and wants to stop (e.g. due to a desire to be pregnant), they cannot drive for 6 (seizure-free) months after they have stopped.

An elderly patient complains of regular episodes of loss of consciousness at the weekend when he wears his tie to church. Your consultant suspects carotid sinus hypersensitivity. What simple bedside procedure can you do to test this? How is it performed?

You may want to consider performing a **carotid sinus massage**, whereby an ECG and blood pressure are monitored for bradycardia and/or hypotension induced by the carotid sinus massage.

Carotid sinus massage must not be done in anybody with possible atherosclerotic plaques in the carotids, as these may dislodge, causing a stroke. For this reason, Doppler ultrasound examination of both carotids is recommended before doing a carotid sinus massage in any patient with a history of stroke, TIA, or with a carotid bruit on auscultation. Patients should be advised that carotid sinus massage always carries a small but real risk of stroke.

Carotid sinus massage should always be done with a patient connected to a 12-lead ECG, with a large IV cannula *in situ* and a resuscitation trolley (with atropine) at hand, in case the massage triggers a cardiac arrest rather than just a transient blackout. Ideally, one needs beat-to-beat blood pressure monitoring, which was traditionally done invasively but can nowadays be done non-invasively.

During the test, pressure is applied in a firm circular motion to one carotid sinus at a time (where the carotid artery meets the angle of the jaw) for about 5 seconds. You should perform the test both with the patient lying down and standing up.

The procedure is considered positive if symptoms are reproduced during or immediately after the massage, in the presence of asystole longer than 3 seconds and/or a fall in systolic blood pressure of 50 mmHg. There are two possible components to the response: bradycardia and/or reduced blood pressure. Only patients with a significant or predominant bradycardic component may benefit from cardiac pacing.

3

[For budding cardiologists] **What are the following (rare) cardiac causes of loss of consciousness, and why are they important: HOCM; long QT syndrome; Brugada syndrome; arrhythmogenic right ventricular dysplasia?**

These rare causes of loss of consciousness are important as they are associated with sudden cardiac death in young people and athletes.

- **HOCM** is a genetic mutation, either inherited (autosomal dominant) or sporadic, resulting in non-physiological left ventricular hypertrophy. Left ventricular outflow obstruction is due to asymmetrical septal hypertrophy which occludes the outflow tract during systole. This is exacerbated by systolic anterior movement of the mitral valve anterior leaflet. The outflow tract gradient is exacerbated by exercise.

- **Long QT syndrome** is in fact a collection of disorders with different genetic mutations of cardiac ion channels (sodium and potassium). All of them result in prolonged repolarization and a long QT interval on the ECG, particularly on exertion, and are associated with ventricular tachycardia.

- **Brugada syndrome** is caused by a mutation of the cardiac sodium channel gene, at least in some patients. It is often inherited in an autosomal dominant manner. The ECG findings are a right bundle branch block and saddle-shaped ST elevation in V_1–V_3 (the QT intervals are normal). The condition is associated with ventricular dysrhythmias.

- **Arrhythmogenic right ventricular dysplasia** occurs when the myocardium is partially replaced by fatty or fibrofatty tissue. It occurs primarily in the right ventricle, and results in an arrhythmia, hence the name. The ECG is characterized by T-wave inversion in V_1–V_3 (a non-specific finding), right bundle branch block, and an epsilon wave in 50% of cases (a terminal notch at the end of the QRS complex). In addition there may be ventricular ectopics, which can progress to ventricular tachycardia (VT) or ventricular fibrillation (VF).

An implantable cardioverter defibrillator (ICD) device is the only intervention that can prevent sudden death in all of these patients, although β-blockers have some protective value.

For a range of Single Best Answer questions related to the topic of this chapter go to
www.oxfordtextbooks.co.uk/orc/OCMS/

Neck lump

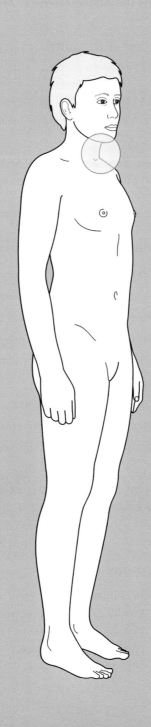

Core cases

! *Read through the sections in red, covering up the sections in white that follow so that you don't see the answer. At the end of each red section, try to answer the question before reading on.*

*Note: we deviate slightly from the trodden path of previous chapters in that we present two core cases. The diagnostic pathway differs for lateral and midline neck lumps and thus we use two core cases to clarify and streamline the approach. As such, the first stage when assessing a patient with a neck lump is to determine whether the lump is **lateral** or **midline**.*

Lateral neck lump

Core case

Mr Haversham is a 76-year-old gentleman who presents to his general practitioner (GP) with a suspected flare-up of gout in his big toe. While taking a history, the GP notices a lump on the side of Mr Haversham's neck.

What is your differential diagnosis for a lateral neck lump?
Try to think of the anatomical structures in the neck, and any pathology that may arise from those structures.

Considering the anatomy and associated pathology, the lump may represent:

Artery: carotid artery aneurysm, subclavian artery aneurysm, chemodectoma

Nerves: neurofibroma, schwannoma

Lymphatics: lymphangioma (simple, cavernous, cystic hygroma)

Lymph nodes: infective, neoplastic (primary or metastatic), granulomatous

Salivary glands: infective, autoimmune, neoplastic

Larynx: laryngocele

Pharynx: pharyngeal pouch

Branchial arch remnant: branchial cyst/sinus/fistula

Skin/superficial fascia: lipoma, epidermal cyst, abscess, dermoid cyst

> **How does the age of the patient influence your differential diagnosis? What are the most common causes of lateral neck lumps in (1) children, and (2) adults?**

The age of the patient has an enormous bearing upon the pathology you should expect to encounter:

1) **In children**, about 75% of neck lumps are benign. Congenital and inflammatory lumps are most common. Thus the differential diagnosis will be weighted in favour of thyroglossal cysts, branchial cleft cysts, cystic hygromas, and lymphadenitis. If malignancy is diagnosed in paediatric neck lumps, it is usually a lymphoma or sarcoma, or sometimes a papillary thyroid carcinoma.

2) **In adults over 40**, as many as 75% of lateral neck lumps are malignant. Of the malignant neck lumps, about 80% are metastases and the rest are mostly lymphomas. In fact, **in the absence of signs of infection, a lateral neck mass in an adult is lymphadenopathy due to metastatic carcinoma (usually squamous) until proven otherwise.**

Which questions should the GP ask about the lump itself?

4

- **How long has the lump been there?** If the lump has been present for less than a few weeks, the likelihood is that it represents infective or inflammatory lymphadenopathy, although some patients will present with malignant neck lumps that have only been noticed within the last few days. If, however, the lump has been present for longer than a few weeks then malignancy must be excluded. Note that congenital neck lumps have often been present for some time, but do not have to have been present since birth. For example, branchial cysts may 'appear' in adults following an episode of infection.

- **Has the lump got bigger, smaller, or stayed the same size?** A lump that is gradually increasing in size must be regarded as a malignancy until proven otherwise. Remember that a progressive increase in size of a malignant neck lump may be reported as a sudden appearance by the patient.

- **Is the lump painful?** Most neck lumps are not painful. The only lumps that are classically painful are acute infective lymphadenitis or an infected branchial cyst.

- **Are there any other lumps?** If the patient has noticed other similar lumps elsewhere on their body (for example, groin or axilla) then it is likely that the lump represents either a systemic disease (e.g. HIV, tuberculosis) or disseminated malignancy (e.g. lymphoma).

Which associated symptoms should the GP ask about?

Given that most neck lumps in adults are enlarged lymph glands, and the most common underlying causes are infection and malignancy, you should ask:

- **Are there symptoms suggestive of infection?** Ask about malaise, fever, rigors, etc. But note that fever, night sweats, and weight loss are also 'B symptoms' of lymphoma. Therefore the time course of symptoms can be useful – an acute history favours infection whereas a more prolonged history favours malignancy. There may also be more 'local' symptoms of infection, such as pain from a dental abscess.

- **Are there any symptoms suggestive of head and neck cancer?** Head and neck cancers are not usually associated with weight loss or malaise, but there are a number of other suggestive features. Those to enquire about include: dysphonia, stridor, stertor, breathing difficulty, dysphagia (see Chapter 6), odynophagia, globus, cough, haemoptysis (see Chapter 8), otalgia, unilateral hearing loss, nasal discharge, epistaxis, and lumps or ulcers on the head or face that have increased in size or started to bleed. There is unfortunately no symptom or group of symptoms that is strongly correlated with early head and neck cancer – this list is merely a guide. Perhaps the only exception is carcinoma of the glottis, for which a change in voice or hoarseness is a highly sensitive (but non-specific) symptom.

> **Other than symptoms, are there any aspects of the history that may make an infective or malignant process more likely? Think about risk factors.**

4

- **Infection**: Has the patient had a recent infection (in particular an upper respiratory tract infection)? Is there a history of contact with someone known to have infectious disease? Recent trauma or an insect bite to the neck? Cat scratches or bites (resulting in cat-scratch fever, due to *Bartonella*)? Or a recent history of foreign travel?
- **Malignancy:** Is there a known current or previous cancer, or a family history of head and neck cancer? Has the patient previously had radiotherapy to the neck? Have they ever been a smoker and/or do they have a high alcohol intake?

> **Why is it important to ask about social history in the context of a neck lump?**

Smoking and high alcohol consumption are strong independent risk factors for the development of head and neck cancer, thus you must *always* ask about them.

> The GP asks Mr Haversham about the lump in his neck. He explains that it has been there for several months and that he didn't think it was worth going to see his doctor about something so small that was causing him no pain. When specifically asked whether the lump has increased in size, Mr Haversham explains that it has probably doubled, but reiterates that it causes him no bother. He is not aware of any other unusual lumps on his body.
>
> With the exception of his painful big toe, Mr Haversham has felt well recently. He has not been feverish and has not been aware of any insect bites or trauma to his neck. He has not been abroad for over a year and has not been in contact with anyone unwell. The GP runs through a quick checklist of oral, nasal, otological, pharyngeal, and laryngeal symptoms, but finds no abnormalities.
>
> Mr Haversham takes no regular medications and has no known allergies. He enjoys a glass of wine each day, and is a smoker with a 30-pack-year history (i.e. 20 cigarettes a day for 30 years).
>
> The GP explains to Mr Haversham that it would be wise for him to examine the lump on his neck. When approaching the examination of a neck lump, the first stage is to localize the lump.
>
> **What specific information should the GP glean about the location of the lump?**

There are three key questions to address that will enable the GP to narrow thier differential diagnosis considerably:

1) **Is it superficial or deep?** Superficial lumps include lipomas, abscesses, epidermal cysts, and dermoid cysts.

2) **Is it in the anterior or the posterior triangle of the neck** (i.e. in front of or behind the sternocleidomastoid)? If we only consider deep structures, we can usually allocate lesions to the anterior or posterior triangle as follows:
   - **Anterior triangle[†]:** branchial cyst/sinus/fistula, carotid body tumour (chemodectoma), carotid artery aneurysm, salivary gland, laryngocele
   - **Posterior triangle:** cystic hygroma, cervical rib, pharyngeal pouch, sub-clavian aneurysm.

3) **What is its relationship to muscle?** Asking the patient to nod their head against resistance will tense the sternocleidomastoid muscle on both sides of the neck (this also demonstrates which triangle the lump is in). Shrugging the shoulder against resistance will contract trapezius. Any lump that is underneath the muscle will be concealed when the muscle contracts.

[†] While we acknowledge that thyroid masses are strictly in the anterior triangle, and that a single nodule in the lateral aspect of a thyroid lobe may present as a lateral lump, we have omitted discussing them in this first case for the sake of simplicity.

What other features of the lump should be characterized during palpation?

- **Is it tender and/or warm?** The only neck lumps that are classically tender and/or warm are infected or inflammatory masses. An important exception in at-risk patient groups is a tuberculous adenitis. In the acute phase this may present with painless lymphadenopathy and overlying erythema, whereas progressive disease can present with a discharging sinus or a 'cold' abscess.

- **Is it solid or fluctuant?** There are various textbook descriptions of degrees of lump firmness that correspond to different causes of cervical lymphadenopathy, but in practice it can hard to distinguish a supposedly 'hard' from a 'rubbery' lump. Classically, lumps can be divided into:
  - **Hard lumps:** malignant lymph nodes
  - **Rubbery lumps:** chronic inflammatory lymph nodes (e.g. tuberculosis) or lymphomatous nodes
  - **Soft lumps:** acute inflammatory lymph nodes
  - **Fluctuant lumps:** branchial cysts, cystic hygromas, pharyngeal pouches, laryngoceles, cold abscesses, epidermal cysts, dermoid cysts, lipomas.

- **Is it pulsatile?** Subclavian or carotid aneurysms are pulsatile. Chemodectomas are often pulsatile but not necessarily so.

- **Is it mobile?** This question relates principally to lymphadenopathy. The majority of lymph nodes are relatively mobile. Malignant lymph nodes may be tethered to adjacent structures, while tuberculous nodes may appear matted together.

Is there anything other than the lump that the GP should examine?

It is always important to examine the entire neck systematically. For many of the isolated causes of a neck lump (such as a chemodectoma or pharyngeal pouch), examining the neck and characterizing the lump is likely to be sufficient. However, lymphadenopathy and parotid masses require further assessment. The remainder of the clinical examination will be dictated by the history and examination findings thus far. The following is a possible guide:

- If **infectious lymphadenopathy** is suspected:
  - Examine the throat, paying particular attention to the tonsils.
  - Systematically examine all lymph nodes of the head and neck.

- If **malignant lymphadenopathy** is suspected:
  - Examine the scalp, face, ears, mouth, and nose for a potential squamous cell carcinoma or melanoma. Otalgia in the absence of any pathology detected by otoscopy is suggestive of malignancy (with referred pain to the ear).
  - Systematically examine all lymph nodes of the head and neck.
  - Examine the breasts (in women) and the lungs.
  - Consider palpating for hepatosplenomegaly if lymphoma or chronic lymphocytic leukaemia is suspected.
  - Perform a full abdominal examination if Virchow's node (left supraclavicular node) is palpable.
  - To complete the search for malignancy it will be necessary to use a fibreoptic endoscope to examine the nasal cavity, nasopharynx, oropharynx, and hypopharynx – but this is beyond the scope of the GP examination.

- If there is a **parotid swelling:**
  - Examine the integrity of the facial nerve. This nerve sits between the deep and superficial lobes of the parotid, and a palsy may result from an invasive malignant tumour (but not from a benign adenoma, which is non-invasive).
  - Examine the oral cavity for displacement of the soft palate by a tumour involving the deep lobe of the parotid.

> The GP examines Mr Haversham's neck. There is a prominent lump in the left anterior triangle. The lump lies just anterior to the superior third of sternocleidomastoid. The lump is not concealed by muscular contraction. It is approximately 4.5 cm × 3 cm in size, elliptical in shape, and has a smooth surface and borders. It is not tender or warm, has a hard consistency, is non-pulsatile and non-mobile, appearing to be tethered to adjacent structures. There are no other palpable lesions in the neck.
>
> **Based upon the history and examination findings thus far, what is the likely anatomical origin of this lump?**

It is most likely that this swelling represents **lymphadenopathy**. It is not tender or warm, suggesting that it is not an acute inflammation or infection. It is not obscured by muscular contraction, thus it is superficial to the muscles. It is firm, and therefore not a cystic structure or a lipoma. Put together, this all suggests it is a non-inflammatory lymph node. Most worrying of all, however, is the fact that this firm lump appears tethered to surrounding structures – a 'red flag' sign for a malignant lymph node.

> The GP examines Mr Haversham's scalp, face, ears, mouth, and nose, but detects nothing abnormal.
>
> **How should the GP proceed? Are there any initial investigations that may help determine the cause of the lymphadenopathy?**

This lump must be regarded as **squamous cell carcinoma that has metastasized to the lymph nodes** until proven otherwise. Mr Haversham should be referred urgently to a specialist head and neck cancer clinic.

There are two initial investigations that are routinely used:

1) **Ultrasound.** The shape, size, echogenicity, and vascularity of lymph nodes can be used to distinguish pathological nodes from normal superficial nodes. Furthermore, malignant nodes have relatively typical ultrasound appearances.

2) **Fine needle aspiration (FNA).** This is used to provide a cytological diagnosis. FNA may be ultrasound-guided. Core biopsy risks spreading any malignancy and thus it is always preferable to do an FNA. Note that lymphoma may be suggested by FNA, but that core biopsy is usually required to confirm the specific subtype.

FNA of Mr Haversham's neck lump revealed squamous cell carcinoma. A thorough examination of his oral cavity, coupled with fibreoptic nasolaryngoscopy, revealed a primary tumour in 'coffin corner' at the posterior tongue/floor of the mouth. It is notoriously difficult to detect tumours in this region, hence the rather macabre nickname.

Midline neck lump

Mrs Luther is a 53-year-old housewife who presents to her GP because she is becoming increasingly self-conscious about a lump in the front of her neck.

What is your differential diagnosis for a midline neck lump?
Split the differential into thyroid and non-thyroid masses (Table 4.1).

Core case

Table 4.1 Differential diagnosis for midline neck lump

Thyroid	Non-thyroid
Physiological goitre[†]	Lipoma
Multinodular goitre[†]	Dermoid cyst
Graves' disease	Epidermal cyst
Hashimoto's thyroiditis	Abscess
Thyroglossal cyst	Lymphoma
Thyroid cyst	
Solitary adenoma	
Carcinoma	
Subacute thyroiditis (de Quervain's, Riedel's)	

† Goitre simply means an 'enlarged thyroid gland'. Physiological goitre refers to its natural enlargement during puberty and pregnancy. Multinodular goitre refers to areas of focal hyperplasia within the thyroid gland that cause it to enlarge in a nodular manner.

4

The key when assessing a midline neck lump is to determine whether the lump is of thyroid origin and, if so, whether it is malignant.

Which questions should the GP ask about the lump itself?

- **How long has the lump been there?** The 'sudden' appearance of a midline lump is suggestive of acute haemorrhage into a thyroid cyst or, more rarely, a fast-growing thyroid carcinoma (anaplastic) or subacute thyroiditis. Thyroglossal cysts have often been present for some time but may 'appear' in adults following an episode of infection. Duration is of little help when attempting to distinguish between the remaining benign and malignant thyroid masses.

- **Has the lump got bigger, smaller, or stayed the same size?** Haemorrhage or infection of an existing lump may produce rapid increases in size. The majority of thyroid neoplasms are slow-growing, with the exception of anaplastic carcinoma.

- **Is the lump painful?** Most midline neck lumps are not painful. Subacute thyroiditis, infected thyroglossal cysts, or acute haemorrhagic cysts are often painful. Hashimoto's thyroiditis may result in discomfort, particularly when swallowing, but few patients would describe this as pain. Thyroid cancer is usually painless, but anaplastic carcinoma can cause pain due to infiltration of surrounding structures (such as ear pain due to vagus nerve involvement).

- **Are there any other lumps?** A thyroid swelling in association with cervical lymphadenopathy must be regarded as malignant until proven otherwise.

Which associated symptoms should the GP ask about?

- **Are there any symptoms suggestive of hyper- or hypothyroidism?** These are listed in Table 4.2. (Note that the term 'thyrotoxicosis' is interchangeable with hyperthyroidism.)

- **Are there any symptoms suggestive of compression or invasion?** A midline neck lump such as a goitre may become so large that it exerts a pressure

---

Table 4.2 Symptoms suggestive of hyper- or hypothyroidism

Hyperthyroid	Hypothyroid
Irritable/nervous/restless	Apathetic/blunting of thought/fatigue
Increased appetite but weight loss	Weight gain
Diarrhoea	Constipation
Heat intolerance	Cold intolerance
Palpitations	
Oligomenorrhoea	

effect on adjacent structures and causes symptoms such as stridor, dyspnoea, dysphagia, and/or discomfort during swallowing. Changes in the quality of the voice may be due to malignant invasion of the recurrent laryngeal nerve and/or vocal cords, but are also common in hypothyroidism due to oedema of the vocal cords.

* **Are there symptoms suggestive of infection?** Ask about malaise, fever, rigors, etc.

Are there any particular aspects of (1) the past medical history and (2) family history that the GP should enquire about?

4

---

1) Past medical history:
   - **Any autoimmune disorders?** Both Graves' disease and Hashimoto's thyroiditis occur more commonly in patients with other autoimmune disorders such as type 1 diabetes mellitus, pernicious anaemia, vitiligo, and Addison's disease.
   - **Known risk factors for thyroid malignancy?** Previous radiation to the neck is a risk factor for the subsequent development of papillary thyroid carcinoma.

2) Family history:
   - **Autoimmune disease?** There may be a familial predisposition to such disorders.
   - **Hereditary forms of thyroid carcinoma?** Approximately 25% of medullary thyroid carcinoma (MTC) is familial. Familial MTC may either be inherited in isolation, or as part of a multiple endocrine neoplasia (MEN) syndrome.

Mrs Luther comments that the lump has been present for several months. She happened to notice it while putting on her make-up, but explains that it has never been painful. She thinks that it has increased in size since she first noticed it, but feels that she is probably self-conscious to a degree that isn't necessarily warranted by the size of the lump. She is not aware of any other lumps.

The GP asks direct questions about any symptoms of thyroid dysfunction, breathing difficulty, change in voice, and fever. Mrs Luther replies that she has none of these symptoms. There is no significant past medical history or family history. She takes no regular medications and has no allergies. She is a non-smoker and enjoys moderate alcohol intake at weekends.

The GP proceeds to examine the lump.

What should the GP determine about the location and characteristics of the lump?

---

* **Location:**
  - **Superficial lump?** Lipoma, epidermal cyst, dermoid cyst or abscess.
  - **Deep lump?** Thyroid gland.
* **Relationship to other structures:**
  - **Moves on swallowing?** Thyroid gland (attached to pre-tracheal fascia).
  - **Moves on tongue protrusion (i.e. deglutition)?** Thyroglossal cyst (attached to hyoid bone).
  - **Tethered to neighbouring muscle or skin?** Malignancy or Riedel's thyroiditis.

4

- **Character of the lump:**
  - **Diffuse, smooth enlargement?** Physiological goitre, Graves', Hashimoto's, or de Quervain's thyroiditis. In the latter it is also tender.
  - **Solitary, solid nodule?** Malignancy more likely.
  - **Solitary, cystic nodule?** Thyroglossal, epidermal, dermoid, or thyroid cysts.
  - **Multiple nodules?** Multinodular goitre (focal hyperplasia) more likely.

Note that it is difficult to distinguish these possibilities accurately from clinical examination, thus some form of imaging is always needed to confirm or refute your impression.

What else should the GP examine?

- **Is there any cervical lymphadenopathy?** This should raise suspicions of thyroid malignancy, but may also reflect infective causes of neck swelling. The thyroid gland drains to lymph nodes along the carotid sheath.

- **What is the extent of any thyroid swelling?** Bear in mind that the enlargement of the thyroid may extend retrosternally. The GP may wish to examine Mrs Luther with her neck extended, to percuss for retrosternal extension of the lump, or to try and elicit Pemberton's sign (elevating the arms above the head results in facial venous congestion and cyanosis due to thoracic inlet obstruction by a retrosternal mass).

- **Are there any signs of hyper- or hypothyroidism** (Table 4.3)?

Table 4.3 Signs of hyper- or hypothyroidism

Hyperthyroidism	Hypothyroidism
HAND SIGNS:	
Fine tremor	Bradycardia
Tachycardia/atrial fibrillation	Slow, deep voice
Sweating	Dry, coarse skin
Palmar erythema	Loss of outer third of eyebrows
Thyroid acropachy (clubbing)	Oedematous looking face
Onycholysis	Slow reflexes
EYE SIGNS:	
Lid lag	
Lid retraction	
Exophthalmos (in Graves' specifically)	
Chemosis	
Ophthalmoplegia	
OTHER:	
Thyroid bruit	
Wasting/proximal myopathy	
Pre-tibial myxoedema (in Graves' specifically)	

Mrs Luther has a 2 cm × 3 cm nodule to the left of her trachea, in the lower third of her neck. The lump is deep and moves when Mrs Luther is asked to swallow – thus it appears that this is a nodule in the left lobe of the thyroid gland. The nodule is firm and non-tender to palpation. The right lobe of the thyroid is not palpable, and there appear to be no other nodules. There is no cervical lymphadenopathy and Mrs Luther is clinically euthyroid.

Which simple investigations should the GP request?

Clinical examination has poor sensitivity for thyroid status and thus the GP should request biochemical tests of thyroid function. Mrs Luther's thyroid status will have a considerable influence upon her further investigation and management. Firstly, note that the presence of a goitre (which Mrs Luther doesn't have) says nothing of a patient's thyroid status – they could be hyper-, hypo-, or euthyroid, and thus you must confirm their status in order to manage them appropriately. Secondly, thyroid status is critically important when considering thyroid nodules because patients with malignancy are almost always euthyroid – hence a diagnosis of hyperthyroidism in a patient with a thyroid nodule should be seen as a 'good' sign.

As a first step, the GP should request:

- **Thyroid-stimulating hormone (TSH)**: in all patients with a thyroid lump. Elevated levels are usually consistent with hypothyroidism while suppressed levels are usually consistent with hyperthyroidism[†]. The GP may request additional tests of thyroid function according to the initial TSH result:
  - if TSH is low request **free tri-iodothyronine (T_3)** and **free thyroxine (T_4)**
  - if TSH is high request **thyroid peroxidase antibodies** (Hashimoto's).
- **Serum calcitonin**: only if there is a significant family history of thyroid cancer. MTC is a tumour of the calcitonin-secreting parafollicular C-cells, thus calcitonin can be used as a serum marker.

[†] The relationship of TSH to thyroid status will differ if the abnormality originates at the level of the anterior pituitary or hypothalamus, but these patients would not present with a thyroid mass, and in any case this is very rarely the cause of thyroid disturbance.

The GP requests a serum TSH, which is later reported as 3.9 mU/L.

Should Mrs Luther be referred to an endocrine surgeon or endocrinologist?

Broadly speaking, if a patient has evidence of altered thyroid function they should be referred to an endocrinologist as thyroid cancer is very rare in this group. By contrast, euthyroid patients with thyroid nodules (either solitary nodules or dominant nodules in multinodular goitres) should be referred to an endocrine surgeon in the first instance. Thus, Mrs Luther should be referred to an **endocrine surgeon**.

Mrs Luther is referred to an endocrine surgeon. She is euthyroid and clinical examination has revealed a single firm nodule in the left lobe of the thyroid.

What further investigation(s) is the surgeon likely to request?

The first-line test for the investigation of thyroid nodules is FNA. Ultrasound may be used to guide aspirations, and can provide an estimate of nodule size and an assessment of whether the nodule is solid, cystic, or mixed (solid and mixed nodules have a higher likelihood of malignancy).

There is relatively little indication for **radionuclide scanning** nowadays. These scans use isotopes (^{99}Tc or ^{123}I) to indicate whether a nodule is functioning or not. Nodules are thus reported as either being 'hot' (functioning) or 'cold' (non-functioning). Hot nodules are almost always benign, whereas about 5–20% of cold nodules are malignant. However, given that about 90% of scanned nodules are cold, radionuclide scanning has little specificity for detecting malignancy. A serum TSH assay serves much the same purpose.

There is also little indication for **computed tomography (CT)** scanning or **magnetic resonance imaging (MRI)** in the majority of cases. The exceptions include retrosternal extension of a goitre, invasive tumours, and haemoptysis. As an aside, it is important to avoid the use of iodinated contrast media with CT scans as these can reduce subsequent uptake of therapeutic radio-iodine by thyroid tissue if needed for treatment.

Mrs Luther is examined by a surgeon and an ultrasound-guided FNA of the nodule is performed. The aspirate is reported by the pathologist as a 'follicular lesion/suspected follicular neoplasm'.

Does Mrs Luther have thyroid cancer? How should she be managed?

There are a number of potential outcomes for FNA of a thyroid nodule:

* Insufficient aspirate to make a diagnosis = Thy1
* Benign (e.g. thyroiditis) = Thy2
* Follicular lesion/suspected follicular neoplasm = Thy3
* Suspicious of malignancy = Thy4
* Diagnostic of malignancy = Thy5

Unfortunately, FNA cannot distinguish between a benign **follicular adenoma** and a malignant **follicular carcinoma**. Thus it is not possible to say whether Mrs Luther has cancer or not. As a consequence, most patients whose pathology shows follicular cells will be treated as if they have cancer. There are a number of stages to subsequent management:

1) **Surgery.** Low-risk[†] follicular carcinoma may be treated by thyroid lobectomy whereas high-risk patients are usually offered total or near-total thyroidectomy.

2) **T_3 replacement.** The patient must have replacement thyroid hormone as their thyroid gland has now been removed. However, TSH levels need to be high (hence the patient is hypothyroid) at the time of administration of subsequent radio-iodine (see below), because the high TSH stimulates uptake of radio-iodine. We therefore need to stop the administration of exogenous thyroid hormone prior to radio-iodine therapy, so that TSH is released from

---

† There are various features that are used to allocate patients with differentiated thyroid cancer to either high-risk or low-risk groups. The principal factors contributing to high risk are older age, male gender, poorly differentiated histological features, tumour size (>4 cm), extrathyroidal invasion, and metastatic spread (but not lymph node involvement, unlike in many other cancers).

negative feedback and levels have time to rise. T_3 has a half-life of about 2.5 days and thus can be stopped 2 weeks before radio-iodine therapy. By contrast, if T_4 (which has a half-life of 7–10 days) was used to replace the patient's thyroid hormone, it would need to be stopped about 6 weeks prior to radio-iodine therapy, and the patient would spend longer in an unpleasant hypothyroid state.

3) ^{131}**I ablation**. The radioactive iodine is selectively taken up by thyroid cells, which are then destroyed by the radiation. This is done for all patients who have undergone total or near-total thyroidectomy as a way of eliminating any malignant cells left behind after surgery. T_3 suppression is stopped 2 weeks before treatment so that any remaining thyroid cells take up the ^{131}I. Some countries are investigating an alternative strategy whereby thyroid hormone replacement does not need to be stopped prior to ^{131}I ablation, and patients are given recombinant TSH to stimulate radio-iodine uptake.

4) T_4 **suppression**. Give a dose sufficient to suppress TSH secretion completely (as TSH will stimulate any remaining, potentially malignant, thyroid tissue to regrow). If thyroglobulin (TG) levels then rise above zero in the presence of T_4 suppression, it suggests a return of the malignant thyroid cells.

5) **Follow-up**. This is usually annual clinical examination with measurement of serum TSH and TG.

Fortunately the prognosis for most differentiated thyroid cancer (follicular or papillary) is very good, and the overall 10-year survival rate is approximately 80–90%.

Short cases

Mr Fry is a 23-year-old bartender who presents to his GP concerned about a lump in his neck. On further questioning he reveals that he has noticed a very slight swelling in his neck 'above his Adam's apple' for the past few years. However, the lump has approximately doubled in size over the course of the last week. It is not painful and he is aware of no other lumps. He has recently suffered from an upper respiratory tract infection, and had to take one day off work last week, but is otherwise fit and well. He takes no regular medications and has no known allergies. He smokes 10 cigarettes each day, and consumes about 35 units of alcohol (as spirits) each week.

On examination, there is an upper midline neck lesion measuring 2 cm × 2 cm. When Mr Fry is asked to stick his tongue out or swallow the lump rises up his neck. It does not appear to be attached to the large neck muscles. The lump has well-defined boundaries and a smooth surface. It feels cystic and is non-pulsatile. It is mildly tender to palpation. The overlying skin appears normal. No other lumps are detected on clinical examination.

What is the diagnosis? How do you account for the recent change in the size of the lump?

An upper midline cystic lesion that is attached to the hyoid bone (hence rises when the tongue is protruded) is consistent with a **thyroglossal cyst**.

These are the commonest upper midline neck lesions, and can appear at any age between approximately 4 months and 70 years, but most appear before the age of 30. The vast majority of thyroglossal cysts are midline (about 10% are lateral), and about 75% of these are at the level of the hyoid. The cysts represent abnormalities in the descent of the thyroid gland from the junction of the anterior two-thirds and posterior third of the tongue to its normal position inferior to the thyroid cartilage. The thyroid gland travels down the thyroglossal tract, any part of which may remain and form a sinus or cyst.

The sudden increase in size of the cyst represents infection secondary to the patient's recent upper respiratory tract infection (hence the lump is tender to palpation). It is not uncommon for thyroglossal cysts to present in this way.

Treatment is by surgical resection of the cyst ± the mid-portion of the hyoid bone (Sistrunk's procedure). There are three reasons for excision:

1) eliminating the chance of further infection

2) eliminating the (small) chance of carcinoma in the cyst

3) cosmesis

4

Mrs Slocock is a 47-year-old housewife who presents to her GP with a lump in her neck. She reports that she has recently noticed a slight swelling in the right side of her neck. She first noticed the lump about 6 weeks ago when she happened to feel her neck (for no particular reason) and noted slight asymmetry. She has continued to feel the lump every few days but is unsure whether it has changed in size. The lump is not painful and she is not aware of any other lumps. She reports feeling well, has no significant past medical history, and takes no regular medicines. She has never smoked, but drinks approximately two bottles of wine per week.

On examination there is a 2 cm × 2 cm lump in the deep tissues of the upper right anterior triangle. The lump does not appear to be attached to sternocleidomastoid. It is firm, non-tender, and has a transmitted pulse. It is possible to move the lump from side to side but not up and down.

What is the most likely diagnosis? How should Mrs Slocock be investigated?

The examination findings suggest that Mrs Slocock has a **carotid body tumour** (also known as a chemodectoma). The lump is located in the region of the carotid bifurcation, is mobile from side to side but not up and down (due to its relation with the carotid artery) and has a transmitted pulse. Large vascular carotid body tumours may be truly pulsatile. Carotid body tumours are a type of glomus tumour or paraganglioma (glomus cells are specialized chemoreceptor cells). They are typically slow growing, but large tumours may exert pressure effects resulting in complications such as cranial nerve palsies or Horner's syndrome.

Carotid body tumours require imaging to determine their precise location. Suitable modalities include duplex ultrasound, angiography, and CT/MRI.

Treatment in the majority of patients is surgical excision. However, as these are such slow-growing tumours it is not unusual for conservative management to be adopted in elderly patients.

4

Miss Banfi is an 18-year-old student who presents to her GP with a sore throat, headache, fever, and fatigue. She has felt unwell for 5 days and is concerned that her symptoms have not improved. On further questioning, she has not had a cough and has had no coryzal symptoms. A couple of her peers at college are suffering from the same symptoms. She has otherwise been fit and well. She has recently started using the combined oral contraceptive pill, and has no known allergies. She does not smoke, but drinks approximately 20 units of wine each week. She has never been outside the UK.

On examination, Miss Banfi is febrile. She has enlarged tonsils and multiple palpable lumps in her neck. Miss Banfi was unaware of these lumps until the GP palpated them. There are five firm and tender lumps, all of which are subcutaneous and in the posterior triangle. Three of the lumps are on the left and two are on the right. The lumps are relatively mobile and are not warm or pulsatile. The GP performs an abdominal examination and detects splenomegaly.

What is the likely cause of the neck lumps? Which blood tests could the GP order to clinch a diagnosis? Should the GP prescribe Miss Banfi a course of amoxycillin for her sore throat?

Multiple, firm, subcutaneous lumps in the posterior triangle can be little other than lymph nodes. The fact that they are tender and coexisting with an acute febrile illness makes it highly likely that this is **cervical lymphadenitis**. The combination of sore throat, lymphadenopathy, fever, tonsillar enlargement, and (most importantly) splenomegaly are characteristic of glandular fever, caused by **Epstein–Barr virus** (EBV). Toxoplasmosis and acute cytomegalovirus (CMV) can also cause lymphadenopathy and splenomegaly, but would not account for the sore throat and swollen tonsils.

The GP could order the following blood tests:

* **Full blood count**: looking for leucocytosis and lymphocytosis.

* **Heterophil antibody tests**: the Paul–Bunnell (monospot) test is based on the fact that an EBV antigen is similar to antigens on the red blood cells of many animals but not humans, so that mixing blood from an EBV-positive human patient with animal blood causes the animal's red blood cells to aggregate and precipitate out of solution – something that can be readily appreciated under the microscope. More modern tests use enzyme linked immunosorbent assay (ELISA) to detect the same antibodies. However, both tests rely on anti-EBV antibodies being present and so can be falsely negative during the early stages of infection (the first 2 weeks), before antibodies are produced.

* **Blood film**: looking for lymphocytosis and atypical T-lymphocytes (large with irregular nuclei).

EBV yields a positive result in all three of the above blood tests (as will acute CMV and toxoplasmosis). A more specific test is to detect IgM towards the EBV viral capsid antigen.

The GP should not prescribe amoxycillin or ampicillin for Miss Banfi's sore throat as both of these antibiotics can precipitate a severe rash in patients with acute EBV infection. There is no specific management for glandular fever, although Miss Banfi should avoid any contact sports for a few months as there is a risk of damage to the enlarged and delicate spleen. Miss Banfi may, however, derive symptomatic benefit from analgesics and throat lozenges.

Mr Farquhar is a 22-year-old trainee accountant who presents to his GP with a lump in the left side of his neck. The lump has been present for a couple of weeks and has gradually been increasing in size. Mr Farquhar remarks that he has had a slight swelling in the same place on two previous occasions, but the lump was less prominent and gradually disappeared over the course of a week. On specific questioning, both of these previous episodes corresponded with an upper respiratory tract infection. The last episode was approximately one month ago. His current lump is not painful. His is aware of no other lumps. He is currently well, takes no regular medications, and has no allergies. He is teetotal, does not smoke, and has never smoked.

On examination, there is a single palpable lesion in the left anterior triangle, anterior to the junction of the superior third and inferior two-thirds of sternocleidomastoid. The lump does not move when Mr Farquhar is asked to swallow or stick out his tongue. The lump is smooth, non-tender, fluctuant, and non-pulsatile. It measures approximately 2.5 cm × 2 cm and is not mobile.

Which diagnosis is most likely?

4

It is most likely that Mr Farquhar has a **branchial cyst** – a fluctuant, non-tender lump in the upper third of the neck anterior to sternocleidomastoid. Branchial cysts are congenital epithelial cysts that result from failure of obliteration of the second branchial cleft. Despite being congenital, the cyst may not present clinically until early adulthood. They are usually unilateral, about 60% are in the location described in the case above, and about 80% present as a persistent swelling. The remaining 20% that present as intermittent swellings often coincide with upper respiratory tract infections. It is likely that the two previous neck lumps that Mr Farquhar describes represent such phenomena, but it is also possible that the lumps were reactive lymph nodes.

4

Miss Pelegrini is a 23-year-old waitress who presents to her GP with a 2-month history of a lump in her neck. She does not think that the lump has changed in size, and reports that it is not painful. She is not aware of any other lumps. She has otherwise been fit and well, and reports no systemic symptoms. There is no history of trauma to the neck. She has no significant past medical history, and her only regular medication is the combined oral contraceptive pill. She smokes 20 cigarettes a day, and consumes approximately 15 units of wine each week.

Examination reveals a non-midline 1.5 cm × 1.5 cm lump in the left anterior triangle of her neck. The lump has smooth regular borders and is fluctuant. It is non-tender. The lump cannot be moved separately from the overlying skin, but is mobile over deeper tissues. It does not change position when Miss Pelegrini is asked to swallow or when she is asked to stick her tongue out. There is a punctum overlying the lump, but no other skin changes. There is no cervical lymphadenopathy.

What is the most likely diagnosis? What treatment should Miss Pelegrini be offered?

The examination findings are of a cystic (fluctuant) lump within the skin, hence this is likely to be a **dermoid cyst** or **epidermal cyst**. Dermoid cysts are either formed at embryological lines of fusion (hence a neck dermoid would be midline) or following a puncture injury (as an 'implantation' dermoid). Miss Pelegrini's lump is neither in the midline, nor follows any known trauma to the neck. Coupled with the fact epidermal cysts are more common than dermoids, it is most likely that this is an **epidermal cyst**.

Epidermal cysts are formed when sebaceous glands are blocked – hence they are often associated with a punctum. They can occur on any part of the skin other than the palms or soles, since these areas have no sebaceous glands.

Epidermal cysts may be **excised** – partly for cosmetic reasons, and partly to avoid the possibility of infection. The cyst is excised under local anaesthetic. An incision is made adjacent to the punctum, and the cyst is removed with the capsule intact. If the entire cyst is not successfully removed it is liable to recur.

Miss Phelps is a 32-year-old lifeguard who presents to her GP with a midline neck lump. The lump has been present for a couple of months, but Miss Phelps is not sure whether it has changed in size. The lump is not painful, and Miss Phelps is not aware of any other lumps. On direct questioning, she reports that she has become rather irritable towards her boyfriend recently. Her appetite has increased, although she has gained no weight. In addition, she reports that her eyes have started to feel rather 'gritty' and wonders whether she may be developing hayfever. Miss Phelps is otherwise well. She has no significant medical history and takes no medications. She smokes about 10 cigarettes daily, but does not drink alcohol. There is no significant family history.

On examination, Miss Phelps has a diffuse midline swelling in the lower third of her neck. The lump measures approximately 6 cm across. It is non-tender, and moves upwards when Miss Phelps is asked to swallow. The lump is smooth and there are no palpable nodules within it. There is no cervical lymphadenopathy.

Miss Phelps' pulse is 105 bpm, regular. Her palms are rather sweaty. The GP notes that she has exophthalmos and is also able to demonstrate lid lag.

What is the likely diagnosis? Would you like to request any investigations? How should Miss Phelps be managed?

Miss Phelps probably has **Graves' disease**. She has a smooth goitre, is clinically hyperthyroid, and also has signs of thyroid eye disease. In the context of hyperthyroidism, eye signs only occur with Graves' disease. Interestingly, smoking increases the risk of Graves' eye disease and thus Miss Phelps should be advised to stop smoking.

The next step should be to confirm Miss Phelps' thyroid status by requesting serum **TSH** and, possibly **free T$_3$** and **free T$_4$**. A suppressed serum TSH level with elevated free T$_3$ and free T$_4$ would support the diagnosis.

Miss Phelps should be referred to a specialist endocrine clinic. There are four broad treatment options available to her:

1) **Antithyroid medication**: drugs such as carbimazole and propylthiouracil are used for control of symptoms for up to about 18 months in the hope of remission. Those who recur need definitive treatment with either radio-iodine or surgery. Patients taking carbimazole need to be warned of the rare but serious risk of agranulocytosis, and must be advised to seek urgent medical attention if they develop signs of infection.

2) **β-Blockers**: remember that thyroxine essentially makes tissues more sensitive to adrenaline and noradrenaline, hence β-blockers counteract the symptoms of hyperthyroidism.

3) **Radio-iodine (^{131}I)**: but about 10% of patients will be hypothyroid within 5 years. In addition, Graves' eye disease is a relative contraindication to radio-iodine, and women of child-bearing age must be warned not to become pregnant within 6 months of receiving treatment.

4) **Total thyroidectomy** and subsequent lifelong replacement therapy with levothyroxine.

Viva questions

What are the anatomical boundaries of the anterior and posterior triangles of the neck?

The boundaries of the anterior triangle are the inferior ramus of the mandible, the anterior border of sterno-cleidomastoid, and the midline of the anterior neck. Clinically speaking, lumps superficial, within, or deep to sternocleidomastoid are also considered to be within the anterior triangle.

The boundaries of the posterior triangle are the posterior border of sternocleidomastoid, the superior border of the clavicle, and the anterior border of trapezius (see Fig. 4.1).

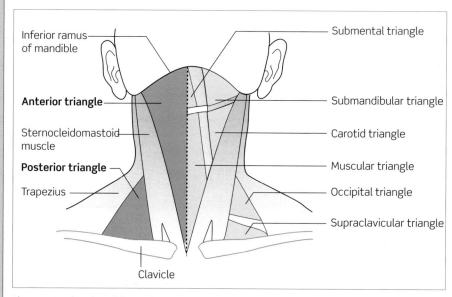

Figure 4.1 Triangles of the neck.

A patient presents with intermittent painful swelling of the parotid gland on one side of his face. Which single question will you ask him about precipitants of the swelling?

The key question is to ask the patient whether the painful swelling is related to eating. This history is typical of sialolithiasis – salivary gland calculi. Calculi may get stuck in the salivary duct(s), causing outflow obstruction. Increased salivary production during eating produces increased back-pressure into the gland which results in painful distension.

What are the characteristic features of the MEN syndromes?

The MEN syndromes represent a predisposition to specific endocrine tumours and are inherited in an autosomal dominant fashion. There are three main syndromes:

1) MEN-1
   - Parathyroid (hyperplasia or adenoma)
   - Pituitary (prolactinoma or growth hormone-secreting tumour)
   - Pancreas (insulinoma, gastrinoma, non-functional)

2) MEN-2A
   - Thyroid (MTC)
   - Adrenal (phaeochromocytoma)
   - Parathyroid (hyperplasia or adenoma)

3) MEN-2B
   - Thyroid (MTC)
   - Adrenal (phaeochromocytoma)
   - Mucocutaneous neuromas

4

What is the Ann Arbor classification for staging lymphoma?

There are four principal stages to the Ann Arbor classification:

i)   Lymphoma in a single region, usually one lymph node.

ii) Lymphoma in two separate lymph node regions on the same side of the diaphragm.

iii) Lymphoma on both sides of the diaphragm ± the spleen.

iv) Disseminated extra-nodal disease.

Turner's syndrome (45 XO) is associated with which neck lump?

Cystic hygromas are strongly associated with Turner's syndrome.

Sjögren's syndrome is a risk factor for which neck lump?

Patients are at increased risk of non-Hodgkin's lymphoma.

4

What is the surface anatomy of the thyroid gland?

The isthmus of the thyroid gland lies inferior to the cricoid cartilage, over the second and third tracheal rings – lower than most people think. The lateral lobes extend superiorly as far as the middle of the thyroid cartilage, and inferiorly as far as the sixth tracheal ring. See Fig. 4.2.

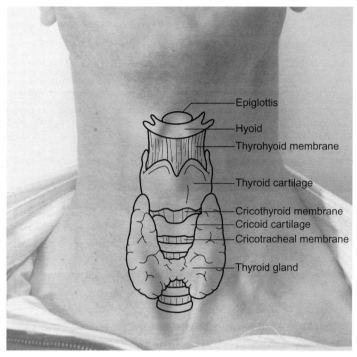

Figure 4.2 Surface anatomy of the thyroid gland.

What is the pathophysiology of (1) Graves' disease and (2) Hashimoto's disease?

1) Graves' disease is an autoimmune non-destructive, stimulatory thyroid disease. The underlying mechanism is antibody-mediated stimulation of the TSH receptor (sometimes referred to as type V hypersensitivity). It presents as **hyperthyroidism and exophthalmos** (due to infiltration of the extra-ocular muscles by immune cells).

2) Hashimoto's disease is an autoimmune destructive thyroid disease. Antithyroid antibodies are present, including antibodies to the TSH receptor but they are non-pathogenic. The underlying mechanism is T-cell-mediated destruction of the thyroid gland (type IV hypersensitivity). It usually presents as **hypothyroidism.**

Which histological types of thyroid neoplasia are there? Which are most common?

The following are all types of thyroid neoplasia:

- Papillary (~60%)
- Follicular (including Hürthle cell tumours) (~25%)
- Medullary (~5%)
- Lymphoma (~5%)
- Anaplastic (rare)
- Metastases (rare)

What are the indications for prophylactic thyroidectomy?

There is a significant risk of MTC in children with a family history of MEN-2A, MEN-2B, or familial MTC (FMTC). The underlying mutations in the *RET* proto-oncogene are inherited in an autosomal dominant manner (chromosome 10q). In contrast to sporadic MTC, the familial form is more likely to be bilateral and metastasize early. As such, it is recommended that these children undergo prophylactic thyroidectomy and lifelong replacement with levothyroxine therapy. The timing of surgery depends upon the underlying condition. Current British Thyroid Association/Royal College of Physicians guidelines recommend surgery at the following ages:

- MEN-2A: before 5 years
- MEN-2B: before 1 year
- FMTC: after 10 years

More precise indications for age-related prophylactic thyroidectomy are being considered based upon the actual codons inherited.

What are the potential complications of thyroidectomy?

As with any surgical procedure, we can divide complications into those specific to the particular operation, and complications of surgery in general:

1) Potential complications specific to thyroidectomy:
   - **Injury to the recurrent laryngeal nerve(s)**. Risk 1 in 100. Unilateral damage produces a weak, hoarse voice. Bilateral damage may require tracheostomy.
   - **Injury to the superior laryngeal nerve(s)**. Risk 1 in 20. Damage leads to difficulties adjusting the pitch of phonation – for example difficulty shouting or singing.
   - **Transient voice changes**. Risk 1 in 10. Occurring in the absence of nerve injury, and lasting 3–6 months.
   - **Transient hypocalcaemia**. Risk 1 in 6. Due to bruising of the parathyroid gland.
   - **Hypoparathyroidism**. Risk 1–2 in 100. Due to parathyroid gland damage.
   - **Hyperthyroid storm**. Very rare. If hyperthyroid patients are not adequately medicated prior to surgery, large concentrations of thyroid hormones may be released during surgery. Mortality may be as high as 20–30%.
   - **Post-operative haemorrhage and airway compromise**. Very rare, but very serious.

2) Potential complications of surgery in general:
   - Infection.
   - Hypertrophic or keloid scarring.
   - Thromboembolism (deep vein thrombosis (DVT) or pulmonary embolism (PE)).
   - Anaesthetic complications (e.g. inadequate analgesia, respiratory depression, urinary retention, cardiac depression).

How does the tachycardia seen with hyperthyroidism differ from the tachycardia seen in generalized anxiety states?

The tachycardia associated with hyperthyroidism can be distinguished from anxiety-driven tachycardia in two ways:

1) **Rhythm**: hyperthyroidism is often associated with atrial fibrillation, particularly in older patients.
2) **Timing**: tachycardia due to hyperthyroidism will persist while the patient is sleeping, while tachycardia due to anxiety should disappear.

In euthyroid patients with a solitary nodule on clinical examination, what features of the history and examination will raise your suspicions of thyroid malignancy?

There are a number of features that increase the likelihood that a thyroid nodule is malignant:

1) Demographic factors
   – Male sex
   – Age <20 years or >70 years

2) History
   – Rapid growth
   – Compression symptoms (e.g. dysphagia, dysphonia, hoarseness)
   – Previous neck irradiation
   – Family history of MEN or familial MTC

3) Examination
   – Firm, hard nodule
   – Fixity to adjacent structures
   – Cervical lymphadenopathy

For a range of Single Best Answer questions related to the topic of this chapter go to
www.oxfordtextbooks.co.uk/orc/ocms/

Haematemesis

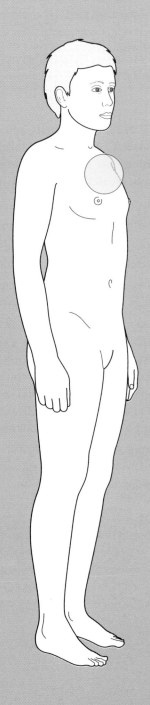

Core case

!   *Read through the sections in red, covering up the sections in white that follow
so that you don't see the answer. At the end of each red section, try to answer the
question before reading on.*

It is 3 a.m. and an ambulance arrives at accident and emergency (A&E) carrying Mr Chris Tucker, a 42-year-old man of no fixed abode. He has blood down his chin and over his shirt, but is alert and orientated. The emergency services were called out by the staff of a local night shelter. Mr Tucker was trying to gain access to it but this was denied due to his intoxication. As he argued with the staff, he began to vomit. The staff saw he was vomiting blood and called for an ambulance. The paramedics state that *en route* to the hospital he retched and brought up a few spoonfuls of blood plus clots. Mr Tucker is immediately placed in the resuscitation room.

How will you manage this patient?

First of all, **call for help.** You cannot manage an emergency alone – it involves teamwork. Call for help and involve your seniors.

Second, this patient has potentially lost a lot of blood. Start with ABCDE – Airways, Breathing, Circulation, Disability, Exposure.

Airways: ensure these are patent. Beware of blood in the oropharynx in a patient with haematemesis. If necessary, use a Yankauer sucker to remove the blood.

Breathing: is the patient able to talk? Are there any signs of respiratory distress (tachypnoea, use of accessory muscles, stridor, gurgling)?

Circulation: does he have a pulse? Is he in shock (tachycardia, narrow pulse pressure, postural hypotension)?

Disability: what is the patient's Glasgow Coma Score (GCS)? Always calculate this in an emergency as a GCS $\leq$ 8 (or rapidly dropping towards that point) means the patient will soon be unable to maintain their own airway and needs intubating urgently. If you can't remember the components of a GCS in an emergency, use the AVPU score (patient is Alert, responds to Voice, responds to Pain or is Unresponsive), where an av<u>P</u>u score (i.e. a patient who is responding to painful stimuli but not voice) is roughly equivalent to a GCS = 8.

Exposure: The patient may have suffered multiple trauma and have various sites of blood loss. Always expose the patient or you'll be caught out by unsuspected wounds.

Mr Tucker looks dishevelled and is obviously inebriated. He starts to tell you about his days in the army as the team take his vital observations, suggesting his airway is clear and he is breathing. He has a heart rate (HR) of 130 bpm, respiratory rate of 30/min and blood pressure (BP) of 86/52 mmHg (supine). His oxygen saturations are 97% on air. His GCS is 15/15 and full exposure of his body reveals yellow (old) bruising over his forearms but no other obvious signs of trauma.

What is your next step?

Mr Tucker is in **shock**, i.e. he has an inadequate circulating volume, often defined as a BP <90/60 mmHg. He needs fluid resuscitation:

- **Get intravenous (IV) access:** insert a large bore (14G–16G) cannula into each antecubital fossa.

- Take bloods for:
  - Full blood count (?how anaemic is this patient – although note that it takes time for haemodilution to cause a drop in haemoglobin concentration or haematocrit as both red blood cells and plasma volume are lost equally when bleeding).
  - Clotting (?bleeding tendency that needs correcting).
  - Urea and creatinine (?hypovolaemia/acute renal failure – also an elevated urea would indicate a significant gastrointestinal (GI) bleed (effectively a large protein meal) that had gone on long enough to be digested and broken down into urea).
  - Electrolytes (?electrolyte disturbance from vomiting). K^+ may be elevated due to destruction of ingested red blood cells.
  - Liver enzymes (?liver disease, a major cause of oesophageal varices and therefore of haematemesis).
  - Cross-match four to six units of blood (check local guidelines on haematemesis).

- Volume resuscitation:
  - **Give up to 2 L of warmed normal saline** (as 250 ml aliquots) stat (i.e. allowed to go in as rapidly as possible under gravity monitoring HR and BP for response).
  - **Consider giving 1 or 2 units of blood**[†] if there is fresh blood on digital rectal examination (suggesting ongoing bleeding) or signs of shock despite giving the normal saline, such as a postural drop in BP of >15 mmHg, or a systolic BP <100 mmHg. Use O, Rh-negative blood if type-specific blood has not yet arrived.

- **Monitoring**: insert a urinary catheter (to monitor renal function) and central venous pressure (CVP) line if[†]:
  - **Elderly and shocked patient**: >60 years old and systolic BP <100 mmHg or Rockall score ≥3.
  - **Severe cardiac, respiratory, or renal disease**.
  - **Patient requires more than four units of blood**.
  - **Initial Rockall score ≥4**.

[†] Local protocols regarding the need to transfuse blood or insert a CVP line can vary between hospitals.

> Two large-bore cannulae are inserted, bloods are taken, and 2 L of warmed normal saline started. Mr Tucker is observed carefully for 5 minutes. His HR is now 110 bpm and his BP has risen to 100/61 mmHg.
>
> **What is you next step now that the patient is stable?**

You need to establish where the blood came from, as it can be easy to confuse *haematemesis* (vomiting blood) with *haemoptysis* (coughing up blood), particularly when only small amounts of blood are being brought up.

Mr Tucker is adamant that he has not been coughing up the blood, but rather vomiting it. This, plus the paramedics' description of retching and bringing up blood with clots (due to the action of stomach acid on blood), is highly suggestive of haematemesis: upper GI haemorrhage manifesting as vomiting of blood.

What are the causes of haematemesis?

Haematemesis is due to bleeding in the upper GI tract (proximal to the ligament of Treitz that demarcates the boundary between the duodenum and jejenum). Potential causes are:

> Oesophagitis/gastritis/duodenitis
> Bleeding peptic ulcer (gastric or duodenal)
> Oesophageal varices
> Mallory–Weiss tear
> Oesophageal cancer
> Gastric cancer
> Arteriovenous malformations
> Bleeding diathesis
> Trauma to oesophagus or stomach
> Vascular angiodysplasia in oesophagus or stomach (e.g. Dieulafoy lesion, scleroderma ('watermelon stomach'), hereditary haemorrhagic telangiectasia)
> Boerhaave's oesophageal perforation
> Haemobilia
> Aorto-enteric fistula

The consultant asks you to calculate Mr Tucker's Rockall score.

What is the Rockall score and what is it used for?

The Rockall score[1] was developed to predict the risk of rebleeding and mortality in patients with upper GI haemorrhage, but is often used as an indicator for severity that helps guide urgency of endoscopy. The scoring system is given in Table 5.1.

[1] Rockall TA, Logan RF, Devlin HB, Northfield TC (1996). Risk assessment after acute upper gastrointestinal haemorrhage. *Gut*, **38**: 316–321.

Table 5.1 The initial Rockall scoring system (pre-endoscopy)

	0 points	1 point	2 points	3 points
Age	<60 years	60–79 years	≥80 years	
Shock		HR >100 bpm	Systolic BP <100 mmHg	
Comorbidities			Heart failure, ischaemic heart disease, any major comorbidity	Renal failure, liver failure, disseminated malignancy

The criteria in Table 5.1 are used to calculate the initial Rockall score, which is based on clinical findings alone. In addition, there are criteria based on findings at endoscopy that serve to calculate the final Rockall score (a combination of pre- and post-endoscopy findings) (Table 5.2).

Table 5.2 The final Rockall score (post-endoscopy)

	0 points	1 point	2 points	3 points
Stigmata of recent haemorrhage			Blood in the upper GI tract, adherent clot, visible, or spurting blood vessel	
Diagnosis	Mallory–Weiss tear, no lesions identified	All other diagnoses	Malignancy of upper GI tract	

Haematemesis carries an overall mortality of 10% and is therefore a very serious condition. You need to establish whether Mr Tucker is a candidate for emergency endoscopy.

What are the indications for an emergency endoscopy in a patient with haematemesis? What other investigations would you request?

Guidelines on how urgently this should be performed vary between hospitals but the general view is that an emergency endoscopy (i.e. as soon as possible) is required if there is:

* suspicion of continuing upper GI bleeding
* suspicion of oesophageal varices as the cause of bleeding
* an initial Rockall score ≥3. If the score is >6, the patient probably needs surgery rather than endoscopy, although the decision to take someone to theatre is not made on the Rockall score alone, or
* if the patient has an aortic graft – in this case you should suspect aorto-enteric fistula until proven otherwise.

In addition to an oesophagogastroduodenoscopy (OGD), you should consider the following investigations for haematemesis patients:

* **Erect chest radiograph.** A perforated peptic ulcer may cause both haematemesis and a pneumoperitoneum (although peptic ulcers tend to either bleed or perforate, but rarely do both). You may also see a left-sided pleural effusion if there has been a Boerhaave's perforation.
* **Computed tomography (CT) scan of the chest–abdomen.** All patients with a known aortic graft (e.g. to repair an aortic aneurysm) require a CT of the chest–abdomen to rule out an aorto-enteric fistula.

5

To determine if Mr Tucker qualifies for an emergency endoscopy, you take a history. You are interested in trying to establish the aetiology of his haematemesis and, in particular, whether he has oesophageal varices.

What questions will you specifically ask on the history?

Presenting complaint and systemic enquiry

* **How much blood has the patient vomited?**
* **What exactly was the character of the vomit?** Fresh blood suggests an upper GI bleed. 'Coffee grounds' suggests blood that has been partially digested by stomach acids but might be confused with faeculent vomiting, as may occur with small bowel obstruction.
* **Melaena (tarry black stools) or frank blood in stool?** Suspect ongoing upper GI haemorrhage. Melaena is due to an upper GI haemorrhage and digestion of the blood during GI transit. Haematochezia is fresh blood in the stools. It is usually due to lower GI haemorrhage but can be due to an upper GI haemorrhage if the bleeding is profuse or the GI transit time fast (note that blood can act as a cathartic, reducing transit time).
* **Did forceful vomiting trigger the haematemesis?** Suspect a Mallory–Weiss tear or Boerhaave's perforation.
* **Recent weight loss?** Suspect upper GI malignancy.
* **Problems swallowing?** Suspect oesophageal malignancy.
* **Easy bruising, distended abdomen, puffy ankles, lethargy?** Suspect liver failure. This could explain a bleeding tendency and/or, if the liver is cirrhotic, explain oesophageal varices.
* **Epigastric pain?** Gnawing epigastric pain suggests gastric carcinoma. Epigastric pain worse on touching his toes suggests gastro-oesophageal reflux disease (GORD).

Past medical history

* **Previous upper GI haemorrhage?** How was it managed?
* **Heartburn or epigastric pain?** Suspect a bleeding peptic ulcer or bleeding oesophagitis/gastritis/duodenitis.
* **History of GORD?** If no diagnosis of GORD, history of reflux or waterbrash? Chronic GORD causes oesophagitis and, ultimately, Barrett's oesophagus and adenocarcinoma.
* **Aortic repair with grafts?** Suspect an aorto-enteric fistula until proven otherwise.
* **Bleeding tendency?** Suspect a clotting problem that needs correcting.
* **Chronic liver disease?** Suspect both a bleeding tendency and oesophageal varices.

Drug history

* **Anticoagulants** (e.g. warfarin)? Suspect a clotting problem.
* **Regular non-steroidal anti-inflammatory drugs (NSAIDs), aspirin, steroids, or bisphosphonates?** Suspect peptic ulcer disease.

- Remember that many drugs can cause liver toxicity long term (**e.g. methotrexate, α-methyldopa, amiodarone**).
- **β-Blockers** may mask the signs of shock by preventing a tachycardia in a patient who is hypovolaemic.

Social history

- **Excessive alcohol consumption?** Increases the risk of cirrhosis leading to oesophageal varices, gastritis, and peptic ulcer disease.
- **Smoking?** Increases the risk of peptic ulcer disease and upper GI malignancy.
- **IV drug use? Tattoos?** Suspect chronic viral hepatitis leading to liver cirrhosis.

Mr Tucker is unsure whether the vomiting triggered the haematemesis or whether it was haematemesis from the very beginning. He tells you that he had drunk four 2-L bottles of cider that day and admits that he drinks about two 2-L bottles of cider every day. He frequently has heartburn but denies any reflux. He smokes 'as much as [he] can' and admits to having taken illicit drugs in the past, saying 'you name it, I've done it'. He has never had any surgery and there's been no change in his stools or weight. He does not take any regular medications.

What will you look for on examination?

Look for the following in particular:

On inspection

- **Tattoos? Needle track marks? Piercings?** All are risk factors for chronic viral hepatitis which can cause cirrhosis (in turn causing a bleeding tendency and/or oesophageal varices).
- **Signs of liver disease**: jaundice, scratch marks (jaundice is itchy), bruising, spider naevi (more than four), palmar erythema, Dupuytren's contracture of the palm, gynaecomastia, ascites, ankle oedema, caput medusae? Suspect liver cirrhosis.
- **Purpura?** Suspect thrombocytopaenia (e.g. immune thrombocytopenic purpura (ITP), chronic liver disease).
- **Thoraco-abdominal scar?** Has the patient had an abdominal aortic aneurysm (AAA) repair with a graft?
- **Cachexia?** Suspect malignancy.

Abdominal palpation

- **Hepatomegaly?** Suspect liver disease.
- **Splenomegaly?** Suspect portal hypertension (usually, but not always, due to liver cirrhosis).
- **Epigastric tenderness?** Suspect peptic ulcer disease or gastritis/duodenitis.
- **Epigastric mass? Supraclavicular lymphadenopathy (Virchow's node)?** Suspect malignancy.

Digital rectal examination

- **Haemorrhoids?** Suspect portal hypertension. Remember that internal haemorrhoids are not palpable.

5

* **Melaena or haematochezia?** Confirms a GI bleed. Melaena is due to upper GI bleed. Haematochezia is usually a lower GI bleed but can rarely be due to upper GI bleeds and a rapid GI transit time. Faecal occult blood testing may be performed but rarely affects management.

Mr Tucker is jaundiced, has signs of recent IV drug use, and several tattoos. He is thin, but not cachectic. He has palmar erythema and at least 10 spider naevi over his chest and shoulders (see Fig. 5.1). A digital rectal examination is unremarkable.

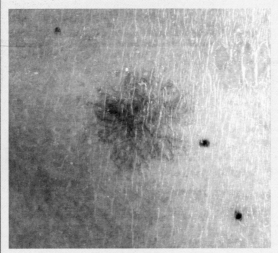

Figure 5.1 Photograph of spider naevi on the chest.

What will you tell the gastroenterology registrar about Mr Tucker's need for an urgent endoscopy?

Mr Tucker is a 42-year-old male of no fixed abode and significant alcohol abuse who presented with haematemesis. He is stable and shows no signs of ongoing upper GI bleed. He has an initial Rockall score of 5 due to a systolic BP <100 mmHg at presentation and signs of liver failure (spider naevi, palmar erythema). There is also a suspicion of oesophageal varices due to the liver disease (high alcohol intake, jaundice, caput medusae, IV drug use, tattoos). Because of this, he needs an **emergency endoscopy**.

The gastroenterology registrar agrees that an emergency endoscopy is required. Meanwhile, the erect chest radiograph and blood results become available. The erect chest radiograph is normal. The blood results show:

Hb	12.7 g/dL
RBC	3.2×10^{12} cells/L
WCC	5×10^9 cells/L
Platelets	105×10^9 cells/L
MCV	112 fL
Albumin	20 g/L
Bilirubin	62 µM
ALT	105 U/L
AST	94 U/L
ALP	52 U/L

GGT	230 U/L
Serum amylase	56 U/L
Urea	9.1 mM
Creatinine	102 μM
Na	136 mM
K	4.1 mM
PT	21.5 seconds
APTT	52 seconds

(Hb, haemoglobin; RBC, red blood cell [count]; WCC, white cell count; MCV, mean corpuscular volume; ALT, alanine aminotransferase; AST, aspartate aminotransferase; ALP, alkaline phosphatase; GGT, gamma-glutamyl transferase; PT, prothrombin time; APTT, activated partial thromboplastin time)

What do these blood results suggest? Are there any further investigations you will request in light of his history, examination, and initial blood results?

Mr Tucker's blood results show:

- **Macrocytic anaemia**: the high MCV is consistent both with alcohol consumption (although the mechanism by which this causes macrocytosis remains unclear) and vitamin B_{12} or folate deficiency anaemia. Note that the haemoglobin is borderline low. Haemorrhage causes a proportional loss of blood volume and blood contents, so the concentration of red cells and haemoglobin won't change until at least 24 hours after a haemorrhage, by which stage the kidneys will have retained fluid but red blood cells will not yet have been replaced. The very slight anaemia is more likely due to malnutrition – this patient is homeless and therefore at high risk of malnutrition and deficiency of folate and/or vitamin B_{12}.

- **Low albumin**: this is most likely due to chronic liver disease but could be due to malnutrition (insufficient protein in diet), malabsorption, or renal nephrotic syndrome (losing albumin via kidneys).

- **Raised liver enzymes** (ALT, AST) suggesting damage to hepatocytes, which would be consistent with alcohol abuse and liver cirrhosis.

- **Raised bilirubin**. This explains the jaundice.

- **Raised GGT**, particularly in the absence of any changes to ALP, is consistent with alcohol abuse.

- **Prolonged clotting times**: clotting factors II, VII, IX, and X (which mainly affect the PT but also the APTT) are made by the liver, hence prolonged clotting times are consistent with liver disease. More importantly, it suggests a bleeding tendency which may cause, and will certainly exacerbate, any upper GI bleeding.

- **Raised urea**: in the presence of normal renal function (e.g. normal creatinine), this is known as 'pre-renal uraemia'. In this case, it is probably a reflection of increased protein ingestion due to blood in his GI tract.

You should arrange for the following investigations:

- **Viral hepatitis and HIV serology**. Given Mr Tucker's tattoos and evidence of IV drug use, he should be screened for viral hepatitis and HIV. Remember that HIV testing requires explicit consent.

- **Urinalysis**. Mr Tucker has low albumin so you should rule out proteinuria, which would suggest a nephrotic syndrome (losing protein via the kidneys).

It is difficult to accurately identify the aetiology of haematemesis until endoscopy is performed.

How would you manage any haematemesis patient whilst they await endoscopy? Is there anything you would do differently or in addition in the case of Mr Tucker, and why?

All patients awaiting endoscopy for haematemesis should be managed as follows:

- **Regular observation**. Hourly to begin with. Every 30 minutes if ↓BP or ↑HR.
- **Nil by mouth**. The patient must remain nil by mouth until the endoscopy is performed. Stomach contents will obstruct the view at endoscopy and carry a significant risk of aspiration into the lungs during the procedure.
- **Fluids**. All patients will need ongoing IV fluids as they are nil by mouth and potentially still bleeding.
- **Correct coagulopathy**. If your clotting screen has identified a clotting abnormality, you should attempt to address this.

Mr Tucker should additionally be managed for his suspected chronic liver disease and oesophageal varices using the SIGN Guidelines 2008:

- **Reduce portal hypertension**. Glypressin is an ADH agonist that reduces mesenteric blood flow and thus reduces portal pressure. An IV infusion is effective in about 80% of patients.
- **Antibiotic cover**. If the patient has suspected liver disease (as in this case), they should also receive fairly broad-spectrum antibiotics (e.g. ciprofloxacin) prior to endoscopy, as up to 50% of patients with liver disease and upper GI bleeding develop sepsis.

Finally, given Mr Tucker's history of alcohol abuse and potential malnourishment, you should consider:

- **Thiamine**. To prevent Wernicke's encephalopathy in someone who is potentially malnourished.
- **Monitoring for alcohol withdrawal symptoms**. If present, give chlordiazepoxide.

What forms of imaging could be used if endoscopy failed to reveal the source of bleeding?

- **Angiography**. A femoral catheter is sited and used to inject a contrast agent into the coeliac axis and superior mesenteric artery. In this way, actively bleeding vessels can be visualized.
- **Laparotomy**. In some cases (especially with posterior peptic ulcers), it is necessary to proceed to laparotomy to visualize and stop the bleeding.

The endoscopy is performed and reveals a bleeding, distended oesophageal vein in the distal oesophagus.

How will the gastroenterologist manage the bleeding oeosphageal varix?

The gastroenterologist needs to **stop the bleeding** (Fig. 5.2). This can be done by:

- **Endoscopic band ligation**. This is the preferred method for stopping a bleeding oesophageal varix. Rubber bands are placed on the end of the endoscope and used to ligate the bleeding vessel and any other obviously distended vessels.

- **Endoscopic sclerotherapy**. This is usually not performed first line in oesophageal varices as it can induce necrosis of the oesophageal mucosa and is less effective than banding.

- **Balloon tamponade**. A tube is passed down into the stomach. A terminal balloon is inflated in the stomach to keep the tube in place and the stomach is aspirated of its contents. A second balloon along the length of the tube is inflated to apply pressure to the bleeding vein and induce haemostasis. This technique is associated with a rebleed rate of 50% and serious complications (oesophageal ulceration and aspiration pneumonia) in 15–20%. Thus it is reserved for when endoscopic band ligation has failed or is not possible because of blood obstructing the view.

- **Transjugular intrahepatic portosystemic shunt (TIPS or TIPSS)**. This complex procedure involves passing a catheter down the jugular vein and creating a shunt from a hepatic vein to the portal vein to relieve the portal hypertension. If this is not possible, a portosystemic (aka portocaval) shunt can be placed surgically (see below).

- **Portocaval (portosystemic) shunt**. This surgical technique involves placing a shunt between the portal and systemic circulation, thus bypassing the liver and reducing the portal hypertension that is causing the oesophageal varices.

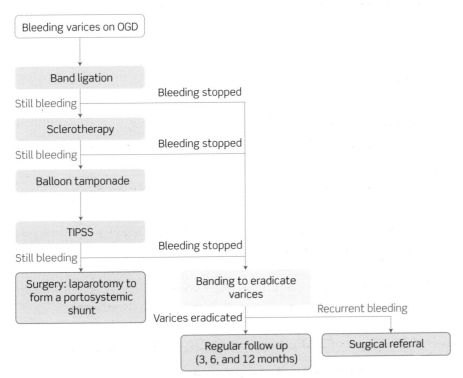

Figure 5.2 The management of bleeding oesophageal varices.

Remember that a major role of the liver is to metabolize many substances absorbed by the gut into the portal circulation ('first-pass metabolism') so that the blood is 'detoxified' before entering the systemic circulation. By placing a shunt that bypasses the liver, many toxins absorbed by the gut will enter the systemic circulation and can trigger an encephalopathy. Because of this, portocaval shunts are now rarely performed.

> **What long-term management might be offered to Mr Tucker for his portal hypertension?**

- **Lifestyle advice.** It is essential you tell him to stop drinking alcohol and smoking. Although the likelihood of success in changing such deeply embedded habits is small, the recent dramatic events may help reinforce the need for such changes in Mr Tucker, particularly if the advice is given by a doctor.
- **Keep his BP low.** This minimizes the chances of oesophageal varices rebleeding. Typical agents used include propanolol or isosorbide mononitrate (especially if β-blockers are contraindicated, e.g. in asthma).
- **Antibiotics.** A 1-week course of antibiotics (e.g. ciprofloxacin) should be considered in patients with liver cirrhosis and upper GI bleeding, as 50% of them will develop sepsis.
- **TIPS/TIPSS.** See above.
- **Treat encephalopathy.** The liver usually removes lots of dietary toxins from the blood before they reach the systemic circulation. If this filtering does not occur due to liver failure or portosystemic shunts, the patient is at risk of encephalopathy. If patients develop encephalopathy, they can be placed on a very low protein diet and given lactulose or enemas to decrease GI transit time and minimize GI absorption. Lactulose also reduces the pH in faeces, making the environment more hostile to ammonia-producing bacteria.

Short cases

The following is a clerking from A&E for a patient:

16/05/2008   12:15pm   Emergency Department

Tanya Dimitriopolous   48   Female

B.I.B.A.

PC/   Haematemesis ++

HPC/   Feeling fine till this AM (11:00). Sudden urge to vomit.
           Vomit (×2) contained "dark clots" but no frank blood.
           Has not opened bowels today. ° melaena ° PR blood recently.

PMHx/   Chronic back pain.
           Appendicitis (appendicectomy aged 16)
           TAH BSO for fibroids (2yrs ago)

Rx/   Ibuprofen 800mg tds

SHx/   ° smoke (never)
           EtOH "occasional glass of wine"

FHx/   Nil of note. 2 children aged 11 and 16, both well. Parents alive and well.

O/E   Alert but pale and anxious.
           Airway: patent
           Breathing: tachypnoeic (30/min)
           Circulation: BP 91/62 = >500 mL Hartmann's given stat.

CVS	Resp	Abdo	Neuro
° murmurs	° LN, trachea central	° organomegaly ° hermias ° masses BS present DRE = melaena	CN I→XII normal GCS 15/15 Upper + lower limb neuro normal

Imp/   xxxxxxxxxxxxx
           xxxxxxxxxxxx

Plan/   Bloods: FBC, clotting, U&Es, creatinine, liver enzymes, albumin, amylase.
           Cross match 4 units
           Fluids: 500 mL Hartmann's, check BP in 30 min ⟶ 115/85
           CXR erect ⟶ NORMAL
           Hand over to medics

                                              JDNash F2 1519

Sidebar note:

B.I.B.A. = brought in by ambulance
TAH BSO = total abdominal hysterectomy and bilateral salpingo-oophorectomy
BS = bowel sounds
GCS = Glasgow Coma Score
CN = cranial nerves
DRE = digital rectal examination
LN = lymph nodes

5

> **What is the *most likely* diagnosis?**

5

The presence of 'dark clots' in vomit is strongly suggestive of blood that has been modified by stomach acid, and thus of an upper GI bleed. This would also explain the melaena (dark faeces due to blood modified during intestinal transit). The most likely diagnosis for any upper GI bleed in someone who takes regular ibuprofen and has heartburn is a **bleeding peptic ulcer**. However, as was stated in the core case, note that it is difficult to diagnose the aetiology of upper GI bleeds accurately until endoscopy is performed.

An OGD was performed and revealed an actively bleeding peptic ulcer in the fundus of the stomach. The bleeding was stopped using an endoscopic adrenaline injection around the ulcer, and an infusion of omeprazole (a proton pump inhibitor) was started after the endoscopy to reduce the risk of rebleeding. Biopsies were taken and revealed that the ulcer was positive for *Helicobacter pylori*. Mrs Dimitriopolous was discharged on a course of triple therapy (a proton pump inhibitor and a combination of two antibiotics) for eradication of *H. pylori*. She was asked to stop taking ibuprofen and was instead started on regular paracetamol, with a view to adding codeine if her back pain was not controlled.

Mr Doherty is a 28-year-old gentleman who presents to his local A&E with haematemesis and chest pain. He was celebrating his 'stag do' the previous night with his friends. After a particularly spicy vinda- loo, they went clubbing and consumed copious alcohol. They were kicked out when Mr Doherty started to throw up. His friends find this hilarious but Mr Doherty looks pained. He tells you that his chest hurts a lot and that he has vomited 'at least six times' since they left the nightclub. The last two times he has vomited blood and that is why he has come to hospital, much to the disappointment of his friends who seem keen to continue the party in the hospital until security turns up and asks them to leave.

Mr Doherty's past medical history is unremarkable and he takes no regular medications. He smokes 'socially' but is adamant that he only drinks at weekends, although he admits this is frequently 'more than is healthy'. He denies taking any illicit drugs. He has not had any epigastric pain, heartburn, or noticed any changes in his bowel habit.

On arrival at A&E, his ABCs are checked and found to be stable. A chest radiograph was normal. Indeed, the only findings of note are his obvious inebriation, a purple appearance to his face due to burst superficial capillaries from vomiting, and persistent chest pain.

What diagnosis should you consider in Mr Doherty's case?

Mr Doherty has presented with chest pain and haematemesis after many episodes of forceful vomiting. A **Mallory–Weiss tear** of the oesophageal mucosa, or the rare but more serious diagnosis of Boerhaave's perforation of the oesophagus, should be considered. Given that his observations and chest radiograph were normal in A&E, a Boerhaave's perforation is less likely. Ultimately, an OGD will be needed to confirm or exclude the diagnosis.

Mrs Jones-Harcourt is a 42-year-old housewife who presents to A&E because she is vomiting copious amounts of blood. She was at a cocktail party with some friends when one of them noticed a trickle of blood coming out of her left nostril. She then began to vomit blood and is now very distressed, as her clothes are covered in blood. She continues to bring up blood as the emergency staff attend to her. A large-bore IV cannula is inserted into each antecubital fossa, bloods are taken for investigations, and 500 mL aliquots of normal saline are given stat until her BP normalizes. Once her observations are stable, she is given water to wash out her mouth and her face is wiped clean. The attending doctor asks her to lean forward and notices that blood is still coming out of her left nostril.

What is the cause of this lady's haematemesis? How should it be managed?

The presence of blood coming out of this lady's nose should make you strongly suspect a **nose bleed (epistaxis)**, with most of the blood falling back into the pharynx where it is causing vomiting. (Figure 5.3 shows a diagram of the blood supply to the nose.)

Anterior nosebleeds from Little's area account for 90% of epistaxis but rarely cause haematemesis. These can often be resolved by asking the patient to sit up with her head leaning forward (this prevents blood flowing back into the pharynx) and pinch the front of the nose firmly for 10 minutes ('Trotter's method'). If this fails it may be necessary to apply an adrenaline-soaked pack to the bleeding area or to cauterize the source of blood using a silver nitrate coated stick.

Posterior nosebleeds from branches of the sphenopalatine artery are less common but more serious and more likely to result in haematemesis, as the blood is more likely to drip back into the pharynx. They should be dealt with by an ear, nose, and throat (ENT) specialist who can pack the bleeding area using either a vasoconstrictor-soaked gauze or a catheter with a balloon.

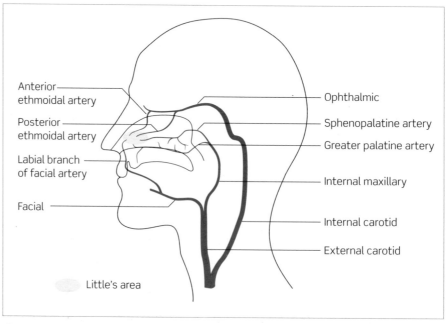

Figure 5.3 Diagram of the blood supply to the nose.

Viva questions

What are the main risk factors for peptic ulcer disease?

- *Helicobacter pylori*
- Smoking
- Alcohol
- NSAIDs and aspirin
- Blood group O
- Hypercalcaemia
- Physiological stress (not psychological stress)
- Burns (Curling's ulcers) or brain trauma (Cushing's ulcers[†]).

[†] Remember that Harvey Cushing was a neurosurgeon.

Why are alcoholics particularly vulnerable to haematemesis?

Alcoholics have a tendency to suffer haematemesis for several reasons:

1) **Anatomy**. As their liver becomes damaged and fibrosed, blood flows through less freely. Consequently, the circulation must find ways that bypass the liver. These are called portosystemic anastamoses (links between the hepatic/portal and systemic circulations). They occur at:
   - the oesophagus, giving rise to oesophageal varices;
   - the umbilicus, giving rise to caput medusae;
   - the rectum, giving rise to rectal varices;
   - the diaphragm; and
   - the retroperitoneum.
2) **Physiology**. Alcoholics are at risk of cirrhosis. This impairs the liver's ability to function, including its ability to synthesize clotting factors. Consequently, alcoholics tend to have an impaired clotting function and a tendency to bleed. Alcohol is also an irritant to the oesophageal and gastric mucosa, thus predisposing alcoholics to oesophagitis, gastritis, and peptic ulcers.
3) **Behaviour**. Alcoholics are more prone to vomiting and therefore to Mallory–Weiss tears, Boerhaave's perforation, and tearing an oesophageal varix.

What is the Child–Pugh score used for?

The Child–Pugh score is used to assess the severity of liver cirrhosis. The higher the score, the more likely it is that the patient has portal hypertension, oesophageal varices, and ultimately, haematemesis.

5

Can you draw a simplified clotting cascade?

A good way of drawing the clotting cascade is to start from the bottom – this is the most important part, the easiest to remember, and this way you are less likely to get tied up in detailing which factors activate which other factors. The clotting cascade can be activated by the extrinsic pathway (measured as the PT and affected by warfarin and liver disease) or the intrinsic pathway (measured as the APTT and affected by heparin, haemophilias, and von Willebrand disease). Figure 5.4 shows a simplified diagram of the blood clotting cascade.

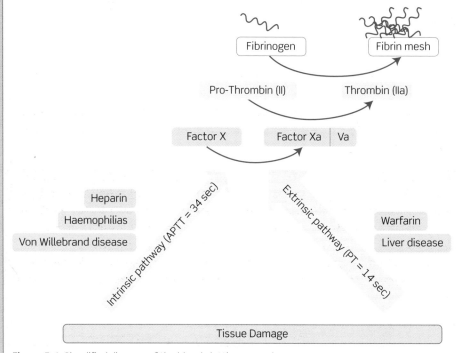

Figure 5.4 Simplified diagram of the blood clotting cascade.

What are the risks and complications associated with blood transfusions?

Immune-mediated complications

* **Febrile reaction:** due to the immune system attacking foreign platelets or white cells. The patient becomes febrile but the problem is self-limiting and the management is supportive.

* **Urticarial reaction:** due to the immune system attacking foreign serum proteins. The patient develops skin erythema, hives, and itching but no fever. Treatment is with antihistamines.

* **Acute haemolytic reaction:** due to mismatch of ABO blood group alleles. The patient rapidly becomes cold, feverish, nauseated, and has chest and/or flank pain. Stop the blood transfusion and use fluids and mannitol (diuretic) to flush out the products of haemolysis.

* **Delayed haemolytic reaction:** due to mismatch of alleles of non-ABO blood groups (e.g. Duffy, Kell, Kidd, etc.). Patient slowly develops malaise, jaundice, and fever. Treatment is supportive and the symptoms are self-limiting.

- **Anaphylaxis:** typically due to immunoglobulin A (IgA)-deficient patients who have anti-IgA antibodies attacking the IgA in the transfused blood. The patient becomes breathless and hypotensive. Potentially fatal, treatment is with adrenaline (0.5 mg intramuscularly (IM)) and corticosteroids.

- **Pulmonary oedema:** thought to be due to antibodies in the transfused blood causing the patient's white blood cells to aggregate and clog up the pulmonary capillaries. The patient becomes severely breathless. Treatment is with respiratory support.

- **Purpura:** due to the patient developing antiplatelet antibodies. The lack of platelets leads to non-blanching haemorrhages in the skin (purpura). Treatment is by plasmapheresis to remove the offending antibodies. More likely in women who have given birth and thus potentially been exposed to platelets with different antigens (from the baby).

Non-immune complications

- **Coagulopathy:** massive transfusion of red blood cells can dilute clotting factors and platelets to the point where the blood is unable to clot. Treated by transfusing platelets and/or fresh frozen plasma.

- **Infection:** infection with viral hepatitis, HIV, Creutzfeld–Jakob disease (CJD) prion, etc. are all possible but thankfully rare with modern transfusion services. HIV and viral hepatitis are screened for but CJD prion is currently not screened for.

Christine is a 57-year-old lady who presented to her local A&E with haematemesis. She was found to have oesophageal varices secondary to advanced alcoholic cirrhosis. After a long consultation with the hepatologists, she enrolled in a programme to stop drinking alcohol and is on a waiting list for a liver transplant. She visits her GP for a follow-up appointment and says that she has been abstinent of alcohol for the last 2 months. The GP notices that her latest blood results show a slight rise in her GGT level and asks if Christine has been drinking anything at all. She bursts into tears and confesses that she had a bottle of wine over the weekend to celebrate her husband's birthday.

Is Christine still eligible for a liver transplant?

The demand for healthy livers for transplantation far exceeds supply, despite advances in hepatology that have allowed a single liver to be divided and donated to multiple recipients. The general perception is that liver transplants should be prioritized so that patients with liver pathology that is 'out of their control' (e.g. primary biliary cirrhosis) get priority over patients whose 'chosen lifestyle' has damaged their liver (e.g. alcoholism, viral hepatitis C from IV drug use). This is not a moral judgement but relates to the likelihood of the transplanted liver being damaged.

For this reason, many liver transplant services require that patients with cirrhosis from alcohol abuse enrol in a programme of alcohol cessation and must be abstinent for a certain period of time (typically 3–6 months). Patients unable to meet these criteria are likely to 'spoil' their precious new liver through further alcohol abuse, when the liver could have gone to someone else. However, there is little evidence that patients with alcohol dependence who complete a 3–6 month abstinence programme have significantly lower rates of post-transplant alcoholism than patients who don't complete these programmes. Nonetheless, the consensus is that a patient who is unable to abstain from alcohol for 3–6 months prior to a liver transplant should not be eligible for the new liver.

It is important to distinguish between a 'slip' and a 'relapse'. It is possible that Christine has had a one-off slip that has not occurred before and will not occur again, in which case one could argue that she is still eligible for a liver transplant. It is also possible that Christine has in fact relapsed into alcohol abuse, in which case she would no longer be suitable for a liver transplant. It would perhaps be suitable to reassess Christine in a few weeks' time with repeated blood tests for alcohol levels and GGT. If she is still drinking, she will have to be removed from the transplant list. If not, the GP will have to use his or her professional judgement about whether to report the one-off 'slip' in her alcohol abstinence.

For a range of Single Best Answer questions related to the topic of this chapter go to
www.oxfordtextbooks.co.uk/orc/ocms/

Dysphagia

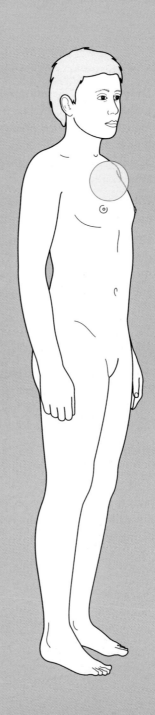

Core case

! *Read through the sections in red, covering up the sections in white that follow so that you don't see the answer. At the end of each red section, try to answer the question before reading on.*

> Mrs Sweeney is a 76-year-old retired greengrocer who presents to her general practitioner (GP) because she is having difficulty swallowing.
>
> Different patients mean different things when they say 'swallowing difficulty'. What could Mrs Sweeney mean?

When a patient says 'swallowing difficulty', they could mean:

* **Dysphagia:** difficulty swallowing. If they really mean dysphagia, try to understand when exactly it feels as though the food 'gets stuck'. Those with high dysphagia (oro-pharyngeal and upper oesophageal) describe difficulty initiating a swallow or immediately upon swallowing. Those with low dysphagia (lower oesophageal) feel the food getting stuck a few seconds after swallowing.

* **Odynophagia:** painful swallowing. Odynophagia may be due to malignancy, but is more commonly a feature of infection such as candidiasis.

* **Globus:** the common sensation of having a lump in the throat without true dysphagia. Globus is very common and its aetiology is poorly understood – however, only a small proportion of affected patients will seek medical help and it is an entirely benign condition.

> **What is your differential diagnosis for dysphagia?**
>
> Dysphagia is an impairment of swallowing and thus can involve any structure between the mouth and the lower oesophageal sphincter. Try to organize your differential *anatomically* into 'high dysphagia' (oropharyngeal and upper oesophageal) and 'low dysphagia' (lower oesophageal), and think about whether the underlying mechanism is *structural* or *functional* (Table 6.1).
>
> **Which diagnoses are the most common?**

Broadly speaking, high dysphagia is more likely to be due to generalized/systemic neuromuscular disease, whereas low dysphagia is more likely to be due to a local obstructing lesion.

Table 6.1 Differential diagnosis of dysphagia

	Functional	Structural		
		Luminal	Mural	Extrinsic
High dysphagia	Stroke Parkinson's disease Myasthenia gravis Multiple sclerosis Myotonic dystrophy Motor neuron disease		Cancer Pharyngeal pouch Cricopharyngeal bar	
Low dysphagia	Achalasia Chagas disease Nutcracker oesophagus Diffuse oesophageal spasm Limited cutaneous scleroderma (CREST)	Foreign body	Cancer Stricture (caustic or inflammatory) Plummer–Vinson syndrome Schatzki ring Congenital atresia[†] Post-fundoplication	Mediastinal mass Retrosternal goitre Bronchial carcinoma Thoracic aortic aneurysm Pericardial effusion Ortner's syndrome Dysphagia lusoria[†]

Common conditions are depicted in a larger font.

[†] These are congenital conditions that would therefore present at an early age.

> In a patient of Mrs Sweeney's age, is there any particular diagnosis that you must rule out?

New-onset dysphagia in middle-aged to elderly patients is carcinoma until proven otherwise.

> What questions would you like to ask specifically about the swallowing?

- **What is the duration of the symptoms?** This is a key question – cancer typically presents with a short history of days to weeks, whereas chronic motility disorders such as achalasia present with symptoms lasting months to years.

- **Is the dysphagia progressive or intermittent?** Progressive dysphagia is highly suggestive of a stricture (benign or malignant), whereas intermittent symptoms are more characteristic of motility disorders.

[†] Note that patients may be able to describe foods becoming stuck at a particular level of their oesophagus, but that this reported level often correlates poorly with the true level of the obstruction.

* **Is the dysphagia to solids, fluids, or both?** If the patient is able to swallow fluid as per normal but has difficulty with solid food items (which feel as if they are sticking[†]) this points towards a mechanical obstruction, i.e. a stricture (benign or malignant). Of course, as the stricture becomes more severe then the dysphagia may start to involve fluids as well. Equally it is possible for oesophageal cancer to present as a sudden 'absolute' dysphagia if a morsel of food lodges above a critically narrowed lumen – in which case the patient cannot even swallow saliva. If the dysphagia is initially more pronounced for fluids over solids then this suggests a motility disorder (e.g. achalasia or a neuromuscular condition).

What associated symptoms should you also ask about in the history?

* **Is there any coughing?** Coughing that occurs immediately after swallowing suggests that there is a problem with the coordination of swallowing events and thus points towards disorders such as stroke and Parkinson's disease. By contrast, if coughing occurs some time after a meal, this implies regurgitation of food retained within a pharyngeal pouch, or gastro-oesophageal reflux disease.

* **Is there any choking?** This too suggests a functional problem with the oropharyngeal phase of swallowing.

* **Is there any gurgling or dysphonia?** Patients with a pharyngeal pouch can often be heard to make gurgling noises if they attempt to speak soon after eating or drinking. It may also be possible to see a visible bulging of the neck.

* **Is there heartburn or waterbrash?** The presence of these two symptoms is highly suggestive that the dysphagia is related to reflux disease, with or without a stricture.

* **Weight loss:** this is the cardinal 'red flag' for oesophageal cancer, although of course any cause of dysphagia will ultimately result in weight loss if the dysphagia is sufficiently severe.

* **Nocturnal cough/wheeze:** while these symptoms are more commonly due to asthma, gastro-oesophageal reflux, or post-nasal drip, they can also be a feature of achalasia because stasis of food and saliva in the oesophagus can result in aspiration.

* **Neurological symptoms** should be enquired about in any patient who has features suggestive of a functional dysphagia, e.g. difficulty coordinating swallowing, slow eating, extra effort required to eat/chew, tiredness after eating, and early dysphagia for liquids.

* **Rheumatological symptoms** may be relevant in the context of limited cutaneous scleroderma (previously known as CREST syndrome), in which patients may suffer from a combination of Calcinosis, Raynaud's, (o)Esophageal dysmotility (the E in CREST refers to the American spelling of oesophagus), Sclerodactyly, and Telangiectasia.

Why is past medical/surgical history relevant?

The two key medical conditions to enquire about are **gastro-oesophageal reflux disease (GORD)** and **peptic ulcers**. However, the patient may not have a proven diagnosis of either of these conditions and may simply complain of a combination of dyspepsia and/or waterbrash. GORD and peptic ulcers are directly implicated in the aetiology of two of the most common causes of dysphagia:

- **GORD** predisposes to oesophageal adenocarcinoma and non-malignant strictures of the oesophagus. A history of GORD due to a sliding hiatus hernia is also significant if the patient has had a fundoplication operation to tighten the lower oesophageal sphincter. Post-operative dysphagia is a potential complication of such a procedure if the wraps are made too tight.
- **Peptic ulcers** can also lead to scarring and strictures around the gastric cardia and lower oesophagus.

There may also be a history of a progressive neurological disease such as multiple sclerosis or Parkinson's disease.

Why is a detailed drug history of particular importance when investigating dysphagia?

6

Drugs can contribute towards dysphagia in two main ways:

1) Firstly, drugs such as calcium-channel blockers and nitrates, which relax smooth muscle, can cause or exacerbate reflux symptoms by decreasing oesophageal tone.
2) Secondly, drugs such as non-steroidal anti-inflammatory drugs (NSAIDs), steroids, and bisphosphonates predispose to peptic ulceration.

On further questioning, Mrs Sweeney describes how she has had progressive difficulty swallowing solid foods – particularly meat – over the past 3 weeks. She says that the chunks of food feel as if they are getting stuck midway down her throat, but she has no difficulty with the actual chewing movements.

She has not suffered from any coughing or choking after eating. She has not noticed any changes in her voice or any gurgling after eating or drinking.

When asked directly about any weight loss, she says that she has probably lost a few kilos as her clothes feel somewhat loose, but says that she is not surprised at this because she feels that she is able to eat so little.

Her past medical history is significant for GORD, for which she takes regular omeprazole, and polymyalgia rheumatica, for which she takes daily prednisolone. Her GP has also prescribed calcium, vitamin D, and a bisphosphonate to be taken as bone-protecting therapy while she is taking regular steroids.

The GP examines Mrs Sweeney. What are the relevant aspects of the physical examination?

There is relatively little that can be gained from the examination of a patient with dysphagia, but there are five features that are particularly relevant:

1) **Cranial nerve pathology:** this is particularly important if there are features in the history that suggest a functional dysphagia as the patient may have bulbar palsy for example.
2) **Signs of gastrointestinal (GI) malignancy:** patients with oesophageal carcinoma may be markedly cachectic, and may have a palpable Virchow's node. If there is a carcinoma extending into the cardia of the stomach this may be palpable in thin patients.

3) **Neck mass:** It may be possible to palpate a large pharyngeal pouch in thin patients, and this may even gurgle on palpation. A goitre may also be palpable, causing the dysphagia by extrinsic compression.[†]

4) **Features of CREST syndrome** (described above).

5) **Koilonychia:** suggests severe iron-deficiency anaemia which can cause Plummer–Vinson syndrome (oesophageal webs).

> Mrs Sweeney has a cachectic appearance. Abdominal examination reveals a palpable lymph node in the left supraclavicular fossa but is otherwise unremarkable.
>
> **What is the most likely diagnosis to account for Mrs Sweeney's dysphagia?**

The short history of a progressive dysphagia that is more pronounced for solids than fluids, occurring on a background of GORD in an elderly patient, and coupled with examination findings of cachexia and lymphadenopathy, is highly suggestive of **oesophageal carcinoma**. This is statistically more likely to be adenocarcinoma given that this subtype accounts for about 65% of oesophageal carcinoma in the UK.

> The GP refers Mrs Sweeney urgently to an upper GI surgeon.
>
> **What are the different types of investigation used for dysphagia, and what are the indications for each?**

There are four main investigations for dysphagia and you should be aware of the indications for each:

1) **Barium swallow:**
   - This is a cineradiographic study which monitors the passage of a bolus of barium contrast medium from the upper to the lower oesophageal sphincter of a supine patient. Various lesions have characteristic appearances on barium swallow (see Figs 6.1–6.4). Patients may also be asked to swallow an effervescent agent to produce a double-contrast study that is better at visualizing mucosal lesions. Note that a barium swallow is not the same thing as a barium meal – the latter follows the passage of barium through the stomach and into the duodenum.
   - Barium swallow is useful in investigating patients who may have a high lesion. During endoscopy this region is intubated blindly, and in the presence of a pharyngeal pouch or high oesophageal cancer there is a risk of injury or perforation. It is also indicated in patients with features suggesting achalasia (e.g. intermittent symptoms, difficulties with fluids and solids).

2) **Endoscopy:**
   - Allows visualization of luminal and mural lesions, as well as the opportunity to biopsy and treat lesions. Various procedures, such as stricture dilatation, stent insertion, laser coagulation, and Botox injections can all be carried out endoscopically.

[†] Note that there are various other conditions that can cause dysphagia by extrinsic compression of the oesophagus, such as Ortner's syndrome or bronchial carcinoma, but it would be unusual to search for signs of such conditions in the first instance. It is more likely that these would be retrospective diagnoses made once a barium swallow shows extrinsic compression.

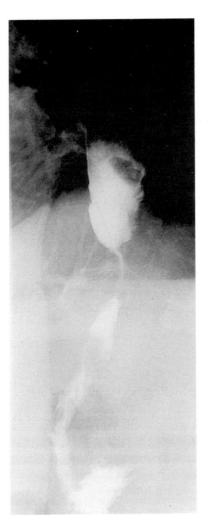

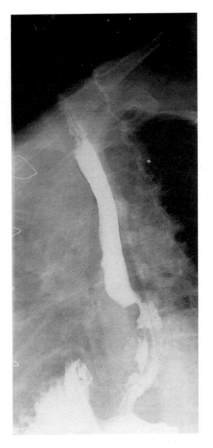

Figure 6.2 Barium swallow showing extrinsic compression of the lower oesophagus by an extraluminal mass. With kind permission from Dr R. Graham.

Figure 6.1 Barium swallow showing a mid-oesophageal stricture consistent with oesophageal cancer.

  – Endoscopy is a more sensitive and specific test than double-contrast barium swallow and is often the first-line investigation for low dysphagia.

3) **Videofluoroscopy:**
  – Essentially a modified form of barium swallow in which upright patients are given barium in liquid, solid, or semi-solid form. A speech therapist modifies the swallowing technique throughout the study.
  – Most suited to patients with a functional high dysphagia.

4) **Manometry:**
  – Assesses the pressures in the lower oesophageal sphincter and the peristaltic wave in the rest of the oesophagus.
  – Manometry is the key investigation for diagnosing a motility disorder and distinguishing between the different types of motility disorders (e.g. achalasia and nutcracker oesophagus). It is indicated when barium swallow and/or endoscopy are unremarkable, suggesting a cause other than mechanical obstruction.

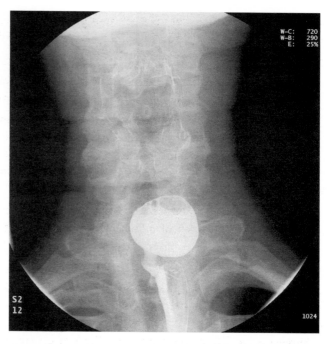

Figure 6.4 Barium swallow (anterior–posterior projection) showing a pharyngeal pouch.
With kind permission from Dr R. Graham

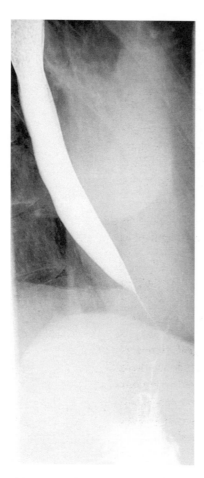

Figure 6.3 Barium swallow showing the classic 'bird's beak' appearance of oesophageal achalasia.

Mrs Sweeney was seen by an upper GI surgeon within a fortnight. An outpatient oesophagogastroscopy was performed and an irregular ulcerative lesion on a background of 'velvety' epithelium was seen in the distal 5 cm of oesophagus. Multiple biopsy samples were taken. Histology revealed high-grade dysplastic columnar epithelium, with penetration of the basement membrane.

What is the diagnosis and how should Mrs Sweeney be managed?

Mrs Sweeney has oesophageal **adenocarcinoma** on a background of **Barrett's oesophagus** (hence the velvety epithelium in the distal oesophagus). She should be referred to a specialist multidisciplinary cancer team comprising surgeons, pathologists, anaesthetists, radiologists, oncologists, and specialist nursing support.

The first thing to do with a cancer patient is to grade and stage the malignancy. Remember that you grade the tumour histopathologically (the more the cells deviate from normality, the higher the grade) and stage the patient by determining how far the cancer has spread anatomically.

The team will assess the stage of Mrs Sweeney's cancer to establish whether the tumour is operable and whether she is fit for surgery. Oesophagectomy is associated with the highest mortality of any elective surgical procedure, and only about a third of patients are deemed suitable for surgery due to advanced disease or comorbidity. Various imaging modalities may be required for **staging:**

1) **Endoscopic ultrasound (EUS):** useful for assessing intramural versus transmural disease, and for detecting local lymph node involvement.

2) **Spiral computed tomography (CT) chest/abdomen:** is the principle modality for staging the tumour. If the scan reveals inoperable or metastatic disease then there may be no advantage in further assessment of the primary. Some centres also use **positron emission tomography (PET) scanning** for tumour staging.

3) **Laparoscopy:** may be used to exclude peritoneal deposits if scanning indicates a significant burden of infradiaphragmatic disease but radical treatment is still planned.

If the tumour is judged to be suitable for radical treatment, it is necessary to also perform a **fitness assessment** for surgery with a combination of lung function tests, arterial blood gas (ABG), electrocardiogram (ECG), exercise tolerance test ± echocardiogram.

Surgery is the definite treatment modality for early stage oesophageal adenocarcinoma. Adjuvant chemotherapy (after the surgery) is poorly tolerated, but there is a role for neo-adjuvant chemotherapy (before the surgery) to shrink the tumour pre-operatively. The majority of patients diagnosed with oesophageal cancer are unsuitable for surgery (either because of the advanced tumour stage or patient comorbidities) and multidisciplinary palliative care is therefore required.

What is Mrs Sweeney's prognosis?

The overall prognosis for oesophageal cancer is usually poor. As with other cancers, prognosis is stage-dependent. For the minority of cancers that are caught at stage 1 (no invasion of muscularis propria and no nodal involvement) the 5-year survival is about 80%. Unfortunately 70% of patients present with lymph node involvement, and in these patients 5-year survival is about 15% even with modern treatments.

Short cases

Miss Aggrawal is a 27-year-old lawyer who presents with a 2-year history of mild dysphagia to both solids and liquids. She says that she has no problems with coordinating swallowing in her mouth, but feels that food and drink are sticking on their way down to her stomach. She has not noticed any choking or gurgling related to eating and is not aware of any weight loss.

She has visited her GP twice in the last year, complaining of heartburn and a nocturnal cough. These were attributed to GORD and asthma, respectively, despite no assessment of her peak flow, and she was offered acid-suppressing medication and a bronchodilator inhaler. Neither of these therapies has eased her symptoms, however. She takes no other medications and is otherwise fit and well.

Given Miss Aggrawal's dysphagia to liquids, her GP performs a thorough examination of her peripheral nervous system and cranial nerves, but nothing abnormal is noted. Abdominal and neck examinations are also unremarkable.

The GP refers Miss Aggrawal for a barium swallow. This shows a dilated oesophagus with a beak-like terminal narrowing. Manometry is also performed and shows an elevated lower oesophageal sphincter pressure with incomplete relaxation of the sphincter and aperistalsis in the body of the oesophagus.

What is the most likely diagnosis? What are the treatment options for Miss Aggrawal?

The history, examination, and investigation findings suggest **achalasia**. Compare this presentation of a young patient, with no loss of weight, and a long history of symptoms, with the classical cancer presentation of an older patient with weight loss and rapidly progressive dysphagia. The bird's beak appearance on barium swallow is classical for achalasia, but it is necessary to perform manometry to distinguish achalasia from other motility disorders such as nutcracker (hypertensive) oesophagus.[†]

It is likely that both Miss Aggrawal's 'GORD' and 'asthma' were symptoms of her achalasia, hence the lack of response to medications.

There are a number of treatment options available to Miss Aggrawal, although it is important to appreciate that no treatment can restore peristaltic function to her oesophagus and thus her swallowing will never completely return to normal. Treatments are aimed at loosening the lower oesophageal sphincter:

* **Pneumatic balloon dilatation** achieves good results in the majority of patients, and about 60% are free of dysphagia at 5 years. Most patients will require repeat treatments. The main risk is of oesophageal perforation (5%).

* **Surgical (Heller's) myotomy** (longitudinal incision of the muscle fibres of the distal oesophagus) tends to produce better short- and long-term relief of dysphagia, but risks the development of GORD in about 10% of patients. For this reason, there is debate as to whether to perform simultaneous Nissen fundoplication (wrapping the stomach around the lower oesophagus to prevent reflux).

* **Botox injections** produce good results that last up to 1 year, and may be favoured in patients unsuited to interventional therapy.

[†] Note that there are two other small-print diagnoses which may produce identical investigation findings to achalasia: Chagas disease (endemic to Central and South America and due to *Trypanosoma cruzi* infection) and 'pseudo-achalasia' due to an oesophageal carcinoma which infiltrates the myenteric plexus. Endoscopy is required to identify the latter, and should be suspected if there is a <6-month history in an older patient with weight loss.

- **Drugs** such as calcium-channel blockers and/or nitrates may relax the lower oesophageal sphincter sufficiently to produce relief of symptoms, but are not first-line therapies and are primarily reserved for elderly patients with contraindications to surgery or dilatation.

6

6

Mr Giles is a 60-year-old farmer who is brought to hospital by ambulance. He was at a local cattle market when he developed chest pain and his fellow farmers called an ambulance. He was given glyceryl trinitrate (GTN) *en route* to hospital, which relieved his pain, and an early ECG revealed no signs of ischaemia.

On arrival at A&E he is pain free and repeat ECGs are unremarkable. He describes how he has had intermittent central crushing chest pain for the last year. He has been hospitalized twice with the pain, and had an angiogram during his last admission which revealed patent coronary arteries. On further questioning he describes getting episodes of chest pain at least once a week, but that they are responsive to GTN. The pain does not radiate, and it is not induced by exercise.

A functional enquiry reveals that Mr Giles has been troubled by heartburn for 'some years' and takes antacid tablets whenever he feels the need. When specifically asked whether his chest pain ever coincides with a difficulty swallowing food he says 'yes'.

Mr Giles's past medical history is significant for hypertension, for which he takes bendroflumethiazide and ramipril. He is a cigarette smoker with a 12-pack-year history (20 cigarettes a day for 12 years), and enjoys about 10 pints of ale a week.

The A&E registrar examines Mr Giles but does not find anything remarkable. He requests a blood troponin, which is negative, and discharges Mr Giles with a diagnosis of 'non-cardiac chest pain'.

Can you suggest a more refined diagnosis? How would you like to investigate Mr Giles? How would you treat him if your suggested diagnosis is correct?

It is likely that Mr Giles is suffering from **oesophageal spasm**. This is suggested by the fact that he has chest pain that bears no relation to exertion and does not radiate (hence being atypical of cardiac chest pain) and is relieved by GTN spray (the smooth muscle of the oesophagus responds to nitrates). The fact that his coronary angiogram revealed no lesions adds further weight to this diagnosis. The association of the chest pain with intermittent spells of dysphagia clinches the diagnosis – but do not expect all patients with oesophageal spasm to present with dysphagia. Most patients will have a symptom complex involving some or all of chest pain, heartburn, regurgitation, globus, and dysphagia.

The diagnosis could be confirmed by performing **manometry**. There are two main types of spasm that may be seen, although the treatment for both is the same. Diffuse oesophageal spasm produces high-amplitude, simultaneous, prolonged contractions of the oesophageal body, and is sometimes referred to as 'corkscrew oesophagus'. By contrast, nutcracker (or hypertensive) oesophagus produces an abnormally strong peristaltic pressure wave in the oesophageal body, and may be associated with a hypertensive lower oesophageal sphincter.

If Mr Giles does have oesophageal spasm it is likely that his symptoms would be relieved with a **calcium-channel blocker** such as sublingual nifedipine. Alternatively he could continue to use GTN for symptomatic relief. If he is able to identify any foods (such as very hot or cold food) which precipitate the spasm he should be advised to consider avoiding them.

6

Mr Gan is a 64-year-old retired restaurateur who presents to his GP with a 5-week history of progressive dysphagia to solids. He describes how it feels as if food items are getting stuck halfway down his throat. He denies any choking, gurgling, heartburn, or waterbrash. He has, however, suffered from increasing dyspnoea over the past 2 months, and has been coughing for a couple of weeks. The coughing occurs both day and night, and has recently been associated with episodes of haemoptysis. Mr Gan thinks that he has lost about 4 kilos in the past couple of months and describes feeling increasingly lethargic.

He has no significant past medical history and takes no regular medications. He does not drink, but has a 40-pack-year history of cigarette smoking.

On examination, Mr Gan is cachectic. There is hepatomegaly and palpable lymph nodes in his left supraclavicular fossa. Percussion and auscultation of Mr Gan's chest is unremarkable, as is a neurological exam.

In light of Mr Gan's haemoptysis and prolonged dyspnoea, his GP refers him for an urgent chest radiograph. This shows multiple coin lesions and hilar lymphadenopathy. A subsequent CT of his chest and abdomen indicates prominent subcarinal lymph nodes and multiple liver lesions consistent with metastatic lung cancer.

What is the mechanism of Mr Gan's dysphagia?

Mr Gan's dysphagia is caused by **extrinsic compression** of the oesophagus by the prominent subcarinal deposits of secondary tumour. He would be offered palliative care to try and minimize the degree of dysphagia suffered but his prognosis, sadly, is poor.

Viva questions

What is Barrett's oesophagus? How common and worrying is this condition?

Barrett's is metaplasia of the squamous epithelium of the lower oesophagus into columnar epithelium (also known as CLO or columnar lined oesophagus). It is usually associated with inflammation and ulceration of the distal oesophagus, and may be endoscopically visible as an area of 'velvety' epithelium. Barrett's is caused by persistent irritation of the squamous epithelium by GORD; both stomach acid and bile are implicated in the aetiology.

The significance of Barrett's is that it is a precursor lesion to adenocarcinoma, increasing the relative risk 30–40-fold. About 1% of the UK population has Barrett's (although only about 5% of these patients are diagnosed). The incidence of adenocarcinoma developing in these Barrett's patients is approximately 1 per 100 person years. Regular endoscopic surveillance is recommended for patients with known Barrett's; the role of lifelong acid-suppressing therapy (proton-pump inhibitors), antireflux surgery, and endoscopic mucosal ablation is controversial.

What are the risk factors for oesophageal cancer?

There are two main types of oesophageal cancer – squamous cell carcinoma and adenocarcinoma (carcinoid, small cell carcinoma, and leiomyoma are very rare). In recent years there has been a relative decrease in the incidence of squamous cell carcinoma and a corresponding increase in the incidence of adenocarcinoma. Risk factors for these cancers are:

- Squamous cell carcinoma:
  - Alcohol
  - Smoking
  - Dietary nitrosamines (found in pickled/mouldy foods) and nitrates (found in Chinese, Iranian, and South African diets)
  - Aflatoxins
  - Achalasia
  - Plummer–Vinson syndrome (see below)
  - Hereditary tylosis[†]
  - Coeliac disease

- Adenocarcinoma:
  - Barrett's oesophagus (hence any factor which predisposes to reflux oesophagitis)
  - Smoking and alcohol intake are not as important as they are for squamous cell carcinoma

[†] Hereditary tylosis is a very rare autosomal dominant condition, also known as focal non-epidermolytic palmoplantar keratoderma. It manifests as symmetrical keratosis of the palms and soles of the feet.

What is Plummer–Vinson syndrome?

This is a rare collection of features including atrophic glossitis (smooth tongue), cheilosis (cracks at the corner of the mouth), koilonychia, and dysphagia that is associated with iron-deficiency anaemia. The dysphagia is due to the development of a post-cricoid web of hyperkeratinization. Correction of the iron deficiency may lead to a dramatic improvement in the degree of dysphagia, but persistent dysphagia may require balloon dilatation. The syndrome is most common in middle-aged to elderly women and is pre-malignant for cricopharyngeal carcinoma.

The condition is also known as Patterson–Brown-Kelly syndrome (Plummer and Vinson described the condition in America, while Patterson and Brown-Kelly described it independently in the UK).

What is the pathophysiology of achalasia?

Achalasia is caused by an absence of ganglion cells in the myenteric plexus (Auerbach's plexus) of the oesophagus. The consequence is a failure of relaxation of the lower oesophageal sphincter, and aperistalsis in the oesophageal body. The underlying cause of these changes in achalasia is unknown. Chagas disease results in an identical pathophysiology, and infiltrating carcinoma can also produce a 'pseudo-achalasia' by invasion of the myenteric plexus. A congenital absence of myenteric plexus ganglion cells also underlies Hirschprung's disease (megacolon) of the intestine.

A dysphagic patient presents with a hoarse voice and bovine cough. Can you think of any pathologies that may account for all these symptoms?

A hoarse voice and bovine cough are characteristic of **recurrent laryngeal nerve pathology**.

There are two main ways in which dysphagia may be connected with such a palsy:

1) The nerve may be infiltrated by a primary malignancy of the oesophagus or a mediastinal malignancy that is causing dysphagia by extrinsic compression.

2) Ortner's syndrome describes the situation in which the recurrent laryngeal nerve is compressed by the cardiovascular system – most commonly left atrial dilatation secondary to mitral stenosis. Sufficiently severe left atrial enlargement can also cause dysphagia by extrinsic compression.

A patient with oesophageal adenocarcinoma is judged to be an unsuitable candidate for surgery. What palliative treatments may be available for such a patient?

There are various treatment modalities which may be used to provide symptomatic relief from malignant dysphagia, including:

- Intubation with a rigid silastic endoprosthesis or expandable metal stent
- Ablation with laser or argon beam plasma coagulation
- Chemotherapy
- Radiotherapy
- Psychological and social support.

6

How can oesophageal cancer present? What are the most common symptoms?

Oesophageal cancer, whilst still relatively rare, is now the eighth most common cancer in the UK with around 7000 new cases a year. The most common symptoms are:

- Dysphagia (~75%)
- Weight loss (~60%)
- GI reflux (~20%)
- Odynophagia (~20%)
- Dyspnoea (~10%)

Less common symptoms include GI bleeding, fatigue due to anaemia, hoarseness (due to involvement of the recurrent laryngeal nerve), cough, facial flushing due to superior vena cava (SVC) obstruction, and breathlessness due to malignant pleural effusion.

What are the common complications after an oesophagectomy?

Removal of the oesophagus and refashioning of a gullet using the stomach is a major operation. The major complications for the junior house officer to be aware of are:

- **Breakdown of the anastomosis** due to poor blood supply (e.g. tight sutures, tension on the anastomosis), infection, and patient factors (e.g. smoking, diabetes mellitus, old age).

- **Pneumonia** due to poor ventilation secondary to pain, this can be minimized using specialist analgesia (e.g. high thoracic epidural blocks by specialized anaesthetists) and encouraging ventilation (physiotherapy).

- **Cardiac arrhythmia.** Manipulation of the tissue near to the heart predisposes patients to intraoperative and post-operative cardiac arrhythmias.

For a range of Single Best Answer questions related to the topic of this chapter go to
www.oxfordtextbooks.co.uk/orc/ocms/

6

Cough

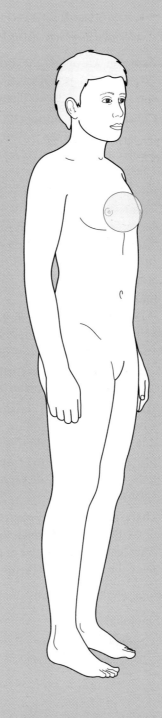

Core case

Mrs Virginia is a 78-year-old lady who presents with a persistent cough.

What specific questions should you ask her in the history?

First, ask open questions about the cough itself:

- **Acute or chronic?** The British Thoracic Society (BTS) defines acute as <3 weeks and chronic as >8 weeks. Between 3 and 8 weeks the cough may be due to recovering acute illness or developing chronic illness.

- **Constant or intermittent?** A cough that is intermittent may suggest an extrinsic trigger (e.g. if the patient only coughs at work there may be an allergy to something in the workplace). A cough that is constant suggests an intrinsic cause.

- **Productive or dry?** The presence of sputum indicates inflammation and/ or infection. Patients with chronic obstructive pulmonary disease (COPD) have chronically inflamed airways and often produce white or clear sputum. Patients with infection have yellow or green sputum. Asthmatics may also produce yellow sputum. Particularly large volumes of green or rusty sputum may be coughed up in bronchiectasis and lung abscesses.

- **Blood?** More specifically:
  - Blood-streaked sputum? Suggests infection or bronchiectasis.
  - Pink and frothy sputum? Suggests pulmonary oedema.
  - Frank blood (haemoptysis)? See Chapter 8. Suggests tuberculosis (TB), lung cancer, pulmonary embolus, bronchiectasis, or other rarer causes (e.g. Wegener's granulomatosis, Goodpasture's syndrome).

- **Timing?** Asthma is classically worse at night. Pulmonary oedema or gastro-oesophageal reflux disease (GORD) can also be worse at night due to the positional effects of lying flat. Patients often report sleeping propped up on pillows to mitigate these effects. Trigger factors such as pets, cold weather, or exercise indicate asthma, as does a worsening in spring/summer.

- **Character?** A wheezy cough suggests airway obstruction due to asthma or COPD. A bovine cough (breathy) is characteristic of vocal cord paralysis. A dry cough is suggestive of pulmonary fibrosis. A gurgling cough is suggestive of bronchiectasis. Pertussis infection causes a 'whooping' cough.

Second, ask directed questions about factors that might be triggering the cough:

- **Smoking?**
- **Asthma?**

- **Allergies?** New pets, new house, new job (exposure to allergens)?
- **Recent rhinitis/sinusitis?**
- **History of GORD?**
- **Drug history?** Certain drugs (e.g. angiotensin-converting enzyme (ACE) inhibitors) can cause a cough.
- **Travel?** The patient may have visited an area of the world where TB is highly prevalent (e.g. Asian subcontinent, Central Asia, sub-Saharan Africa).

Third, ask about factors that might be associated with the cough and give you clues about the underlying cause:

- **Fevers, night sweats, rigors, weight loss?** These suggest malignancy, TB, or another severe infection.
- **Breathlessness?** This would be in keeping with asthma, COPD, pneumonia, or pulmonary oedema but rarer in lung cancer or GORD.
- **Chest pain, particularly pleuritic chest pain?** This may indicate pneumonia, pneumothorax, pulmonary embolism, or viral pleurisy. Equally it may be due to muscle strain secondary to vigorous coughing, or a fractured rib following trauma.
- **Wheeze?** This suggests obstruction of the airways such as that found in asthma, COPD, or tumours compressing an airway.

Mrs Virginia says that she has had a cough for months but that over the last few days she has been 'coughing more, and more muck has been coming up'. She says that the sputum is yellow-green, but there has been no blood. There appear to be no triggers or periodicity.

In her history she reveals that she is a long-term smoker (60 years smoking 10 a day = 30 pack years) and has a diagnosis of COPD. She says she walks a mile a day to the shops and back, and has no history of asthma, allergies, or reflux. She uses inhalers for her COPD ('a dry powder one, a blue spray, and a brown spray') but is not on home oxygen and takes no other medications. Reassuringly, she has had no night sweats, rigors, or weight loss, and is no more breathless than usual. However, she says she has felt a little hot over the last day. She has not been abroad 'since the war', although she went on a Saga holiday in Eastbourne the previous summer.

What is the differential diagnosis of cough? Try thinking about conditions which present acutely or chronically, and whether the cough would be dry or productive (Table 7.1).

Which of these are most likely given this lady's presentation?

Mrs Virginia's complaint is an acute worsening of her productive cough. This therefore narrows the differential down to an infectious cause. Of those, the absence of constitutional features (e.g. weight loss, night sweats) or foreign travel makes TB unlikely.

Table 7.1 Differential diagnosis of cough

	Dry	Productive
Acute	Asthma Rhinitis/sinusitis with post-nasal drip Upper respiratory tract infection (pharyngitis, laryngitis, tracheitis) Drug induced, e.g. ACE inhibitors Smoke/toxin inhalation Inhaled foreign body Lung cancer (causing obstruction of a major bronchus) Pulmonary oedema (secondary to heart failure)	Lower respiratory tract infection (pneumonia, bronchitis) COPD TB
Chronic	Asthma GORD Post-nasal drip Smoking Lung cancer Drug induced COPD Pulmonary oedema (secondary to heart failure) Non-asthmatic eosinophilic bronchitis Psychogenic	Bronchiectasis TB Lung cancer (If congenital: cystic fibrosis or Kartagener's syndrome)

What specific signs should you look for on physical examination that would be consistent with an infectious cause? What other signs might you see, given her COPD?

With regards to her likely infection, you should look for:

* **Systemic features**: Is she febrile? Is she sweating? Is she tachycardic?
* **Respiratory distress**: Is her respiratory rate increased? Is she having difficulty breathing – can she complete sentences, is she using her accessory muscles? Is she peripherally cyanosed? Is she confused (you can assess confusion with an Abbreviated Mental Test Score (AMTS); see Chapter 2)? These give an idea of the severity of her condition.
* **Tender cervical lymphadenopathy**: in a patient with a cough, this suggests infection in the upper respiratory tract.
* **Lungs**: reduced chest expansion, focal dull percussion note, breath sounds (reduced in effusion, bronchial sounding in pneumonia), and vocal resonance.

Vocal resonance distinguishes between consolidation, which increases resonance, and effusion, which diminishes it.

Given her COPD, you should also note any:

- **Chest wall deformities** (e.g. hyperexpansion or 'barrel chest').
- **Intercostal recession**: a sign of severe COPD.
- **Signs of right heart failure** due to her COPD ('cor pulmonale'), such as peripheral oedema, raised jugular venous pressure (JVP), a parasternal heave, a loud or palpable P_2 heart sound, or tricuspid regurgitation.
- **Asterixis**: even though some COPD patients are chronic CO_2 retainers, asterixis can be seen if COPD deteriorates and CO_2 levels rise significantly.

On examination, Mrs Virginia looks sweaty and unwell. She is cachectic and has a 'barrel chest'. Her fingers are tar-stained. She is tachycardic and tachypnoeic with a pulse of 107 bpm and a respiratory rate of 22/min. Her temperature is 38.5°C. She has poor chest expansion, an expiratory wheeze, hyperresonant percussion note throughout but with dullness at the right lung base, and bronchial breath sounds in the same place. Vocal resonance is increased over the area of percussion dullness. You find no lymphadenopathy in the neck. She is not confused, with an AMTS of 9/10.

What investigations would you like to request?

Blood tests:

- **Arterial blood gas (ABG)**: you will want to assess her gas exchange to monitor her progress (she should also be on pulse oximetry) and ensure she doesn't develop respiratory failure. Keep in mind that she has COPD and that her baseline may therefore be different from a 'normal' baseline, e.g. slightly elevated CO_2 levels may be normal for her.
- **Full blood count (FBC)**: the white cell count should be raised in infection, with a neutrophilia if it is a bacterial infection.
- **C-reactive protein (CRP)**: will also be raised if there is an underlying infective process.
- **Urea and electrolytes (U&Es)**: the patient's U&Es may be deranged if she is dehydrated and consequently hypoperfusing her kidneys. Urea is an indicator of severity and influences prognosis.

Imaging:

- **Chest radiograph**: this may reveal areas of consolidation, potentially in a lobar pattern, or a pneumothorax (which are more common in patients with COPD).
- **Electrocardiogram (ECG)**: you must perform this to rule out ischaemia or atrial fibrillation secondary to pneumonia. It may also show right heart strain in some patients with COPD.

Note: **sputum cultures** are rarely useful as the sputum will contain all the commensal flora that is normally found in the upper respiratory tract. However, bronchoalveolar lavage may be performed to get a sputum sample free of this flora and thereby identify the offending organism, but this is only done if a pneumonia does not respond to conventional antibiotic treatment suggesting infection with an atypical organism.

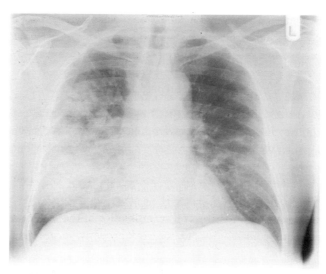

Figure 7.1 Portable antero-posterior (AP) chest radiograph for Mrs Virginia.

Mrs Virginia's chest radiograph is shown in Fig. 7.1. **How would you interpret this radiograph?**

Mrs Virginia's chest radiograph shows an area of dense opacity in the right side of her chest. The dense pattern confined to a discrete area of lung is in keeping with consolidation. Given that the right hemidiaphragm is still visible but the right heart border has been obscured this is therefore likely to represent consolidation in the right middle lobe – which is consistent with the clinical findings on examination.

Mrs Virginia's CRP and white cell count are raised, with a neutrophilia. Her saturations are 95% (on 28% oxygen) and her ABG shows P_aO_2 (arterial partial pressure of oxygen) = 12.4 kPa, P_aCO_2 (arterial partial pressure of carbon dioxide) = 6.2 kPa, pH 7.42, HCO_3^- = 32 mM. Her U&Es show Na 142 mM, K 4.7 mM, Cl 103 mM, urea 9.2, creatinine 122 μM. An ECG showed sinus tachycardia but no other changes.

In light of the history, examination, and investigations, what is the diagnosis? What is the CURB-65 score, what is it used for, and how is it calculated? How should she be managed?

Mrs Virginia has a pneumonia exacerbating her COPD. Her mild hypercapnia should not be a cause of concern as her pH is within the normal range, suggesting the CO_2 retention is chronic and therefore unlikely to be clinically significant.

The CURB-65 score can be used to calculate severity of pneumonia and therefore determine the need for hospitalization. CURB-65 is an acronym for the constituent prognostic factors; the presence of any one scores 1 point, up to a maximum of 5. Patients with a score of 2 or more need to be admitted to hospital.

Confusion (new to the patient), defined as an AMTS of ≤8/10

Urea >7 mM

Respiratory rate >30/minute

Blood pressure <90 systolic and/or <60 diastolic

>65   years old

Mrs Virginia's CURB-65 score is 2. She should therefore be admitted, partly because of the CURB-65 score and partly because elderly patients with pneumonia can deteriorate rapidly. She should be given a broad-spectrum antibiotic in line with local protocol, which should take into account:

- Severity, as assessed by the CURB-65 score
- Comorbidity with COPD
- Hospital-acquired (nosocomial) infection versus community-acquired infection
- Suspicion of unusual organism (e.g. *Pneumocystis jirovecii* in HIV-positive patients, *Pseudomonas* in cystic fibrosis patients)
- Whether she has had any pneumonia treated by antibiotics in the past few weeks (this would suggest the antibiotics did not work properly, so you may need to use different ones)
- Whether or not a particular antibiotic is deemed to predispose to infections such as *Clostridium difficile* colitis.

7

Short cases

> A week after discharge, Mrs Virginia is admitted to A&E again, this time with breathlessness. She is agitated but does not complain of any chest pain. She says the breathlessness came on suddenly while she was sat in her chair at home. An ECG taken in the ambulance showed sinus tachycardia but no other changes. Her oxygen saturations are 92% (on 28% oxygen), her respiratory rate is 28/min, her heart rate 112 bpm, her blood pressure 135/89 mmHg, and her temperature is 37.3°C. On examination, she has unilaterally decreased chest expansion and an area of hyper-resonant percussion, and reduced breath sounds throughout her left lung anteriorly and posteriorly. Her trachea is not deviated.
>
> **What are the complications of pneumonia? What is most likely to have happened in this case?**

The complications of pneumonia include:

* **Spread of infection**: pleural effusion, empyema, abscess, septicaemia
* **Damage to local structures**: bronchiectasis, pneumothorax

Her breathlessness, apyrexia, and examination suggest a **pneumothorax**. Pneumothorax is an uncommon complication of pneumonia but she also has COPD, which could have left her with bullae in her lungs that are prone to rupture (e.g. after a particularly vigorous cough). You MUST exclude a tension pneumothorax by checking for tracheal deviation on examination.

Mrs Virginia had no tracheal deviation and was stable. The signs on physical examination indicated a pneumothorax in her left lung, which was consistent with her chest radiograph. It can be difficult to distinguish a large bulla from a pneumothorax on a single chest radiograph, so in this case a comparison was made with the radiograph from her previous admission. If a previous radiograph is not available for comparison, CT of the chest will distinguish between the two. Mrs Virginia's pneumothorax was decompressed using a chest drain.

Miss Wilson is a 33-year-old nurse who has been referred to the respiratory clinic by her GP with a 3-month history of a dry cough. The GP's letter notes that she has never smoked and has no previous history of respiratory illness, reflux, or any allergies, but has a high body mass index (BMI).

You take a history in which Miss Wilson confirms all of this. She adds that her cough got worse in the spring, but can think of no other exacerbating factors. She says that sometimes she wakes up at night coughing. She has not had a fever, night sweats, or rigors. She has had no chest pain. She does not have a wheeze, is no more breathless than usual on exertion, and is not breathless at rest.

What diagnoses are most likely? If you are the registrar seeing her in outpatients, what investigations would you conduct and what would you be looking for?

The three most common causes of chronic cough in a non-smoker are **asthma**, **post-nasal drip**, and **GORD**. Asthma is a likely cause in this lady, despite the lack of allergies or atopy (e.g. eczema) and her age (asthma is most common in children and the elderly).

As such, in addition to listening to her lungs, you should perform spirometry or peak flow measurement to assess her lung function. The BTS guidelines for diagnosing asthma suggest using measurements of either peak expiratory flow (PEF) or forced expiratory volume in 1 second (FEV_1) – both of these are reduced in obstructive airways disease such as asthma and COPD. However, asthma is characterized by variability in PEF and FEV_1, either in response to treatment (e.g. with an inhaled short-acting bronchodilator) or spontaneously (e.g. diurnal variation). Demonstrating the following variations can be used to diagnose asthma:

- PEF: ≥20% and 60 L/min variation on ≥3 days a week over a fortnight (recorded in a PEF diary).

- FEV_1: ≥15% and 200 mL increase after a short-acting bronchodilator (e.g. salbutamol) or trial of steroid tablets (e.g. prednisolone 30 mg/day for 14 days), or ≥15% decrease after 6 minutes of exercise. These can be compared with predicted normal values for someone of a given gender, height, and age (see Fig. 7.2).

It is important to request a chest radiograph as well, to exclude any unusual but more serious causes such as lung cancer, but we would not expect to see any abnormality indicating asthma.

On examination, Miss Wilson's lungs sound clear, with no added sounds. However, her FEV_1 is 2500 mL and improves to 3600 mL after salbutamol. This 44% (and greater than 200 mL) increase following administration of a β_2-agonist together with the history strongly suggests asthma, and she is started on a trial of salbutamol inhalers. Post-nasal drip is still a possibility but is largely a diagnosis of exclusion. If inhalers do not work after a trial period, you may wish to try antihistamines and/or nasal decongestants. Finally, reflux (GORD) is still also a possibility, particularly given her high BMI, although she does not give any history of heartburn or regurgitation. In your letter to her GP you may want to add that if treatment for asthma and post-nasal drip do not work, Miss Wilson could try antacids, histamine H_2 antagonists, or proton-pump inhibitors.

Peak expiratory flow in normal adults

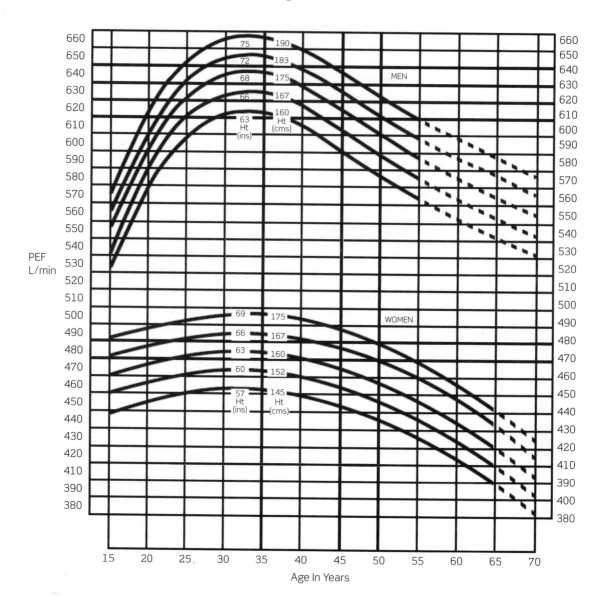

Figure 7.2 Peak expiratory flow in normal adults.

Adapted with permission from Nunn AJ, Gregg I (1989). New regression equations for predicting peak expiratory flow in adults. *BMJ*, **298**: 1068–1070.

7

Mr Hughes is a 48-year-old office worker who comes to his GP complaining of a chronic dry cough. He has had it for the last few months and thought it was a cold, but has come in as it hasn't resolved and is annoying his work colleagues and wife. His coughing spells occur throughout the day and night, with no predictable triggers. On questioning, he comments that he often has heartburn and wakes up with a sore throat.

He is a non-smoker, drinks about 15 pints of lager a week, and has a high body mass index. His past medical history includes an inguinal hernia repair and childhood asthma, although he has not had to use an inhaler since he was a teenager. He also suffers from hayfever in the summer but has no other allergies. He has no new pets or other recent changes to his environment (new job or house). He does not have a history of diagnosed GORD despite his heartburn. His only recent travel was to Spain, and he has had no fevers, night sweats, rigors, or weight loss. His examination is unremarkable and spirometry is normal.

What diagnosis is most likely? How would you test your hypothesis?

Mr Hughes' cough is dry and chronic, and he is a non-smoker. Normal spirometry is not inconsistent with intermittent asthma, but his high BMI and heartburn should make you suspicious that his cough is caused by **gastro-oesophageal reflux** irritating his larynx, despite the lack of a formal diagnosis. You could start a **therapeutic trial** with a proton-pump inhibitor for GORD and arrange a follow-up appointment in clinic. You should also advise weight loss, as this may bring symptomatic relief. Mr Hughes was started on such a trial and after 3 months his cough had resolved.

7

Mrs Aurelie is a 52-year-old lady who complains of a cough during a follow-up visit to her GP. Her GP has recently diagnosed her with hypertension. She has had the cough for a few weeks, but has had no sputum or haemoptysis, fever, breathlessness, chest pain, or wheeze. She has never smoked and does not have a history of asthma or GORD. She has no allergies. She takes enalapril for her hypertension and alendronate, calcium, and vitamin D for osteoporosis prevention because she had a hysterectomy and bilateral salpingo-oopherectomy when she was aged 43. Examination of her respiratory system is entirely normal.

What is the most likely cause of Mrs Aurelie's cough?

Mrs Aurelie has had a non-productive cough for the past few weeks. She has also recently been diagnosed with hypertension and started on enalapril. In the absence of any clues in the history or examination to suggest an alternative diagnosis, it is most likely that her cough is due to the ACE inhibitor (enalapril) that she is taking, as ACE inhibitors can cause a dry cough in 10–20% of patients. This is because ACE is also responsible for breaking down the inflammatory bradykinins in the lungs. Thus, inhibition of ACE leads to a build up of bradykinins and lung inflammation, triggering cough.

Her GP changed her prescription from enalapril to an angiotensin II receptor blocker (e.g. losartan, candesartan, valsartan), which offer the same renal protection but do not cause a dry cough. Mrs Aurelie's cough had disappeared by the time she was next seen by her GP a few weeks later.

7

Mr Morris is a 78-year-old retired man who presented at his GP's surgery with a persistent cough. He says he has had a smoker's cough for 40 years, but that in the last few months it has got worse. He had gone to his GP because his wife was being kept awake by his coughing at night. The cough is non-productive and he has had no fever, chest pain, night sweats, or any significant weight loss that he is aware of – although he admits that he is thin anyway and never weighs himself. He is not known to be asthmatic, has no known allergies, and does not suffer from reflux. He is on no medications and jokes that 'the cigarettes keep me healthy'. He has smoked 20 a day since he joined the army for national service in 1949. He is partial to a beer or two but rarely goes to the pub these days (less than once a week).

Mr Morris' pulse is 80 bpm, blood pressure 130/82 mmHg, respiratory rate 13/min, temperature 37.3°C. On examination, he is thin but does not appear cachectic, and is comfortable at rest. He appears well perfused with a capillary refill time of <2 seconds. There is no cervical lymphadenopathy or any other peripheral stigmata of respiratory disease, although there is heavy tar staining of the fingers of his right hand. Chest expansion, percussion, and auscultation are all unremarkable.

The GP refers Mr Morris to the hospital for a chest radiograph and respiratory opinion. The chest radiograph shows a large mass at the right hilum.

What is the most likely diagnosis?

Mr Morris most likely has **lung cancer**. Although he has had a (smoker's) cough for a long time, the recent change should alert you to possible pathology. Given that the cough is non-productive and that on examination he is afebrile and has no respiratory signs, an infective process appears unlikely. In light of his history of lifelong smoking, lung cancer is a definite possibility. This is made even more likely by the chest radiograph.

Assuming a diagnosis of lung cancer is confirmed by biopsy, it will most likely be a **squamous cell carcinoma** because of the hilar location. This will be investigated in more detail by the specialist team. The GP was right to be suspicious and order a chest radiograph.

Mr Thomas is a 27-year-old retail manager who is referred to the respiratory clinic for investigation of his persistent cough. His referral letter documents an episode of pneumonia 9 weeks ago, which was treated by the GP with antibiotics. He made a good recovery, but the cough became dry and persisted. The cough does not vary with time of day and is not associated with exercise or any other triggers. There is no history of asthma, allergies, or gastro-oesophageal reflux. He has never smoked and takes no regular medications.

Mr Thomas' pulse is 64 bpm, blood pressure 120/72 mmHg, oxygen saturations 98% on room air, respiratory rate 11/min, temperature 36.8°C. There are no peripheral stigmata of respiratory disease and chest expansion, percussion, and auscultation are all unremarkable. Lung function tests performed in the respiratory clinic are normal.

What is the most likely cause of his persistent cough? What are the treatment options?

Patients with pneumonia, particularly viral pneumonia, can have a persistent post-infectious cough some time after the infection has subsided. Judging from the history and the negative findings on examination and lung function testing, this looks to be the most likely cause.

There are a number of treatment options available:

- **Antitussives (cough suppressants)?** If an underlying cause cannot be identified, these may offer symptomatic relief (e.g. if sleep is being disrupted). These operate via two mechanisms: (1) depressing the brainstem 'cough centre', e.g. codeine, pholcodine; (2) reducing peripheral receptor sensitivity, e.g. benzocaine (a local anaesthetic). Unfortunately, there is currently no high-quality evidence to suggest that cough suppressants actually work, despite their widespread use. Furthermore, the opiate cough suppressants are associated with side-effects such as constipation, particularly with codeine but less so with pholcodine, and may be associated with dependence.

- **Inhaled corticosteroids?** The evidence is mixed on the efficacy of corticosteroids. It is thought that in some patients chronic cough is associated with airway inflammation, even in the absence of asthma, and that corticosteroids suppress this inflammation.

- **Inhaled ipratropium bromide?** This is an anticholinergic that blocks the efferent limb of the cough reflex, and may also decrease stimulation of cough receptors. This has been shown to be of benefit in patients with persistent cough after an upper respiratory tract infection.

7

Viva questions

How might your management have been altered if Mrs Virginia had a history of weight loss, night sweats, blood-streaked sputum, and had just returned from Pakistan, where she had lived most of her adult life working as a teacher?

Such a history would make you suspect a diagnosis of **TB**. TB is contagious, airborne, difficult to treat, and potentially fatal. Patients suspected of having active TB are isolated in a side room until the diagnosis is either excluded by three negative sputum samples or confirmed and treatment commenced.

Which patients should not necessarily be given 100% oxygen and why?

Patients with COPD are at risk of becoming hypoxaemic for a number of reasons:

- The airways contain significant amounts of mucus that impairs ventilation.
- The lungs are hyperinflated, making them less efficient at moving air.
- The hypoxic vasoconstriction mechanism is blunted. This usually ensures that areas of lung that are poorly ventilated are supplied with less blood, so that gas exchange only occurs in well-ventilated areas. If this mechanism no longer works well, blood travels through poorly ventilated areas of the lung and is not well oxygenated.

When COPD patients become hypoxic, it is tempting to administer 100% oxygen. However, in a minority of COPD patients, it has been observed that administration of 100% oxygen to combat hypoxaemia can be detrimental, leading to patients developing hypercapnia (high CO_2) which obtunds them and can eventually make them comatose. Traditional teaching states that this is because some COPD patients no longer rely on detecting high CO_2 levels to stimulate breathing (as is normally the case in people without COPD) but rather rely on low O_2 levels ('hypoxic drive'). Giving too much oxygen in these cases can actually remove the stimulus to breathe. However, experiments suggest this is not the case, as hypercapnia develops in COPD patients given O_2 without any significant drop in ventilation rate, so clearly their stimulus to drive is not reduced. The current hypothesis is that too much oxygen further diminishes the hypoxic vasoconstriction effect that usually prevents poorly ventilated areas of lung being perfused with blood. In other words, it is believed that giving too much oxygen results in blood being diverted ('shunted') to areas of the lungs that in COPD patients are incapable of efficient gas exchange, thus diverting blood from the areas of lung that are still able to exchange gas efficiently.

For this reason, COPD patients who become hypoxaemic are administered oxygen using 'Venturi' masks, which allow oxygen to be delivered at safer, smaller, fixed ratios (from 24% to 40%) such that the lungs are better ventilated, but not so much so that the COPD patient can become hypercapnic.

> **You see a patient in clinic with lung cancer who has a bovine cough. Can you explain this symptom?**

It is likely that this patient has a **recurrent laryngeal nerve (RLN) palsy**. Such a palsy is more common on the left than the right. The left branch of the RLN loops around the arch of the aorta and thus has a longer intrathoracic course (and hence is more likely to be affected by chest pathology) than the right branch – which loops around the right subclavian artery. Damage to the recurrent laryngeal nerve is most commonly due to malignancy (e.g. a Pancoast apical lung tumour) or surgery (e.g. neck surgery).

For a range of Single Best Answer questions related to the topic of this chapter go to
www.oxfordtextbooks.co.uk/orc/ocms/

7

Haemoptysis

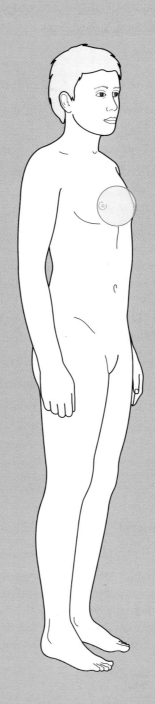

Core case

! *Read through the sections in red, covering up the sections in white that follow so that you don't see the answer. At the end of each red section, try to answer the question before reading on.*

Mr Philip Morris is a 72-year-old retired electrician who presents to his general practitioner (GP) after coughing up blood. He is not coughing up any blood at present, appears well, and is able to talk calmly about what has happened.

The first step should be to establish if this is truly haemoptysis.

What might haemoptysis be confused with by the patient? How will you tell if it really is haemoptysis?

You need to ensure that you are not mistaking haemoptysis with:

* **Haematemesis:** brownish-red blood that is vomited from the gastrointestinal (GI) tract.

* **Epistaxis (nosebleed):** particularly posterior nosebleeds.

* **Bleeding gums:** combined with a cough, this may be confused with true haemoptysis.

To tell if it is really haemoptysis, you can ask the patient where they think the blood is coming from (they may say it initially dripped from their nose), its colour (darker, coffee-ground appearance suggests partially digested blood), any history of nosebleeds, nausea, vomiting, gastric disease, or alcoholism. For the latter, asking if he is an alcoholic is unlikely to yield a valid response. Instead, you can try the CAGE questions to detect alcohol dependence. An answer of 'yes' to two or more of the following questions is a fairly accurate detector of alcohol abuse and dependence:

Have you ever felt you need to Cut down on your drinking?

Have people Annoyed you by criticizing your drinking?

Have you ever felt Guilty about your drinking?

Have you ever needed an Eye-opener to steady your nerves in the morning?

Why should you worry particularly about haemoptysis?

Haemoptysis should always be investigated thoroughly for two reasons:

1) It may be the presenting symptom for life-threatening lung disease.

2) Massive haemoptysis, variably defined as anything from >100 mL to >1000 mL over 24 hours, may be life-threatening itself, usually through asphyxiation but potentially also shock.

Haemoptysis is thus a 'red flag' symptom and any patient with haemoptysis requires a full diagnostic work-up.

What diagnoses should you be concerned about?

These can be grouped together under a surgical sieve – we have used INVITED MD:

Infective: pulmonary tuberculosis (TB), bronchitis, pneumonia, lung abscess, mycetoma

Neoplastic: primary lung cancer, metastatic lung cancer

Vascular: pulmonary infarction, left ventricular failure, bleeding diathesis, arteriovenous malformation, vascular–bronchial fistula

Inflammatory: Wegener's disease, Goodpasture's syndrome, systemic lupus erythematosus, hereditary haemorrhagic telangiectasia (Osler–Weber–Rendu syndrome), polyarteritis nodosa, microscopic polyangiitis

Traumatic: iatrogenic (lung biopsy, post-intubation), wounds (broken rib)

Endocrine: (none)

Degenerative: bronchiectasis

Metabolic: (none)

Drugs: warfarin (bleeding diathesis), crack cocaine use

The most common causes are infection and exacerbations of chronic obstructive pulmonary disease (COPD), but these should never be assumed to be the cause. Lung cancer is a 'must exclude' diagnosis in a presentation of haemoptysis.

Note that up to a third of cases of haemoptysis have no identifiable cause.

What questions should you ask Mr Morris about the haemoptysis?

- What is he coughing up?
  - **Frank blood**: this is suggestive of a vascular problem such as a ruptured blood vessel (invasive cancer, bronchiectasis, TB, mycetoma), a ruptured arteriovenous malformation, or a vascular–bronchial fistula.
  - **Blood-streaked sputum**: any infection of the lungs can cause this; however, in the context of chronic production of large volumes of sputum this would suggest bronchiectasis.
  - **Pink frothy sputum**: this suggests pulmonary oedema (secondary to, for example, left ventricular failure or severe mitral stenosis).
- **How much is he coughing up?** Try to help the patient quantify this by comparing with amounts they might know – a teaspoon, a tablespoon, an eggcup, or more – especially as even a small amount of coughed-up blood will be alarming and seem like a lot to many patients. Massive haemoptysis can be caused by erosion of a pulmonary blood vessel.
- **How suddenly did it start, and has it got worse progressively?** Sudden onset is consistent with pulmonary embolism (PE) or erosion of a cancer into a large pulmonary blood vessel. Gradual onset argues for a progressive condition such as lung cancer or bronchiectasis.

8

Mr Morris tells you he has been coughing up frank blood. He feels it is a lot. When you try to quantify it, he tells you that he has found blood spotting on his handkerchief throughout the day, but he finds it difficult to quantify how much. It seems to have developed fairly rapidly, although he has had a smoker's cough for years. You are also able to confirm that the blood is bright red and almost certainly from the lungs.

What symptoms apart from coughing up blood might you ask Mr Morris about? Think of key clues that would help you narrow your differential diagnosis.

8

+ **Cough productive of sputum?** Indicates lower respiratory tract infection (pneumonia, bronchitis, TB), bronchiectasis, or lung cancer.

+ **Fever?** More commonly associated with a lower respiratory tract infection. Night sweats may indicate TB or carcinoma.

+ **Weight loss?** This is associated with lung cancer and TB. You should consider whether the weight loss was planned or not, but significant weight loss in a relatively short period is rarely the result of dieting and exercise and should therefore be investigated.

+ **Pleuritic chest pain?** Pleuritic chest pain can arise following a PE or pneumonia that has spread to the pleura.

+ **Shortness of breath?** Try to quantify this in terms of exercise tolerance: How far can they walk before they get breathless? Can they climb a flight of stairs without getting breathless? Sudden-onset shortness of breath can be caused by PE, whereas a more gradual time course would be consistent with heart failure.

+ Are there any **extra-pulmonary manifestations** of lung cancer such as:
  − **Bone pain?** (bone metastases)
  − **Dull, aching, swollen wrists/ankles?** (hypertrophic pulmonary osteoarthropathy (HPOA), a rare disorder most commonly seen in patients with lung cancer)
  − **Cushingoid features, muscle weakness, oedema, skin hyperpigmentation?** (if there is a small cell carcinoma secreting ectopic adrenocorticotropic hormone (ACTH))
  − **Polyuria, polydipsia, hypotonia, hyporeflexia, muscle weakness?** (hypercalcaemia secondary to bone metastases or PTH-related peptide (PTHrP)-secreting lung cancer)
  − **Muscle weakness?** (especially proximal muscles i.e. difficulties standing and walking), autonomic dysfunction (e.g. **dry mouth, constipation, urinary retention?**) Eaton–Lambert syndrome is a rare neuromuscular disorder most commonly seen in patients with small cell lung cancer.

+ Has he had **haematuria and/or oliguria?** There are a number of *rare* conditions that can affect both the lungs and kidneys (causing a 'pulmonary–renal syndrome'). The main causes of this are:
  − Goodpasture's syndrome, an autoimmune condition where autoantibodies attack the lungs and the glomeruli in the kidneys. This is important to identify early since the patient progresses rapidly to irreversible renal failure
  − Vasculitides, e.g. Wegener's granulomatosis, microscopic polyangiitis, polyarteritis nodosa
  − Systemic lupus erythematosus.

Mr Morris has had a cough for years, but it is only productive when he is unwell. He has not been unwell recently, although he notes that he has unintentionally lost weight – he estimates a stone (about 6.5 kg) in the last 6 months. He has no pleuritic chest pain, but gets breathless after climbing just one flight of stairs at home. He attributes this to his age, and lack of exercise. He has had no urinary symptoms.

What features about Mr Morris' past history will help you narrow your differential diagnosis even further?

- **Smoking history?** Smoking is the most significant risk factor for lung cancer. Quantify how much he smokes or smoked using the average number of cigarettes smoked a day and the number of years smoked, i.e. when he started and, if relevant, quit. Someone who smoked 10 cigarettes a day for 30 years is said to have smoked for 15 pack years (10 cigarettes = 0.5 packs; and 0.5 × 30 years = 15 pack years).

- **Exposure to asbestos or other inhaled industrial substances?** For example silica (i.e. stone cutter's dust), coal, radon, arsenic, haloethers, polycyclic aromatic hydrocarbons. Such exposure is a risk factor for lung cancer and, in the case of asbestos, mesothelioma.

- **Prior lung disease?** This may indicate a chronic condition, such as TB or bronchiectasis, or a vulnerability to repeated infections (e.g. pneumonias) that you may wish to investigate further.

- **Did he grow up abroad or travel recently?** If yes, which country? Has he been vaccinated for TB? TB is endemic in many countries, particularly the Asian subcontinent and southern African states, and patients can be relatively asymptomatic for extended periods of time.

- **Does he have risk factors for a deep vein thrombosis (DVT)/pulmonary embolus (PE)?** These include prolonged stasis (bed rest or long-haul flight), blood vessel damage from recent trauma or surgery, malignancy causing hypercoagulable blood, other clotting abnormalities, or a history of previous venous thromboembolism. Also ask about a painful swollen limb, particularly leg, which could be a DVT leading to a PE.

- **Is he on anticoagulant medications or does he have a known bleeding diathesis (tendency)?** These can increase the risk and/or magnitude of internal haemorrhage.

Mr Morris is a smoker with a 50-pack-year history, having started when he was conscripted into the navy and given cigarettes each week as part of his compensation (a common story in his generation). As a retired electrician, he has almost certainly had some exposure to asbestos, but denies ever having worked too closely with it as he was primarily concerned with residential housing. He has no history of lung disease. He has not travelled beyond the UK 'for many years' and has not been immunized against TB. He has no risk factors for a DVT/PE other than his smoking history. He is not taking aspirin or warfarin.

The GP conducts a full physical examination, beginning by simply inspecting Mr Morris. The GP then examines his hands, head, neck, and chest. The examination is completed by checking his abdomen and his neurological status. Think of how the diseases mentioned in your differential might manifest during the examination:

What signs should the GP particularly look out for on examination of this gentleman?

- General inspection from the end of the couch:
  - **Hoarse voice**: ?invasion of recurrent laryngeal nerve by cancer
  - **Purpuric rash** or **petechiae**: ?vasculitis affecting lungs
  - **Cushingoid appearance** (moon face, buffalo hump on neck, fat on abdomen, wasted limbs): ?lung cancer secreting ACTH
  - **Cachexia**
- Hands:
  - **Clubbing**: ?lung cancer, lung abscesses, bronchiectasis
  - **Tar stains**: ?smoker
  - **Wasting of the dorsal interossei**: ?invasion of T1 nerve root by apical lung cancer (Pancoast tumour)
- Arms:
  - **Hypotonic, hyporeflexive, weak arms**: ?hypercalcaemia due to bone metastases from lung cancer
- Face:
  - **Swollen face**: ?obstruction of superior vena cava by tumour
  - **Bleeding from oral or nasal mucosa**: ?source of blood, i.e. not true haemoptysis
  - **Saddle nose**: ?Wegener's granulomatosis
  - **Horner's syndrome** (miosis, ptosis, and anhydrosis, i.e. small pupil, droopy eyelid, and lack of sweating): ?invasion of the sympathetic supply to the face by apical lung cancer
  - **Jaundice**: ?liver cancer which has spread to the lungs or vice versa
  - **Focal neurology**: ?brain metastases from lung cancer
- Neck:
  - **Cervical lymphadenopathy, non-tender**: ?TB, bronchial carcinoma
  - **Left supraclavicular lymphadenopathy (Virchow's node)**: ?GI malignancy which may have metastasized to the lungs
  - **Tracheal deviation**: ?lung collapse secondary to a large mass such as a tumour or abscess
- Chest:
  - **Asymmetrical lung expansion**: ?lung pathology in side of reduced expansion
  - **Dullness to percussion**: ?pneumonia, lung abscess, pleural effusion due to cancer
  - **Stridor**: ?tumour or foreign body obstructing bronchus
  - **Crackles**: ?pneumonia, left ventricular failure, bronchiectasis
  - **Pleural rub**: ?mesothelioma, pleuritis from pneumonia, distal PE causing infarction and associated pleurisy
- Abdomen:
  - **Hepatomegaly**: ?liver malignancy which can spread to the lungs, and vice versa
- Legs:
  - **Unilateral signs of DVT?** A DVT may have caused a PE. Look for a unilaterally inflamed leg, unilateral pitting oedema, tenderness over the deep veins or distended, non-varicose superficial veins.

8

> Mr Morris' pulse is 78 bpm, his blood pressure is 132/66 mmHg, his respiratory rate is 14/min and his temperature is 36.5°C.
>
> The positive findings on examination of Mr Morris include tar stains on his hands and a palpable liver edge 2 cm below the ribs. There were no abnormal findings on examination of Mr Morris' respiratory system.
>
> Mr Morris gets referred to the respiratory clinic as an outpatient. He is referred urgently because of his haemoptysis, weight loss, and hepatomegaly. You are the Registrar at this clinic and you confirm the history and examination findings obtained by the GP.
>
> **Which investigations should you request and why?**

- **Oxygen saturations**, which form part of the vital observations and help you to understand the severity of the underlying pulmonary disease causing the haemoptysis.
- **Blood tests:**
  - **Full blood count (FBC)** looking for anaemia, which reflects the magnitude and duration of bleeding or which may be a manifestation of an underlying malignancy. You are also looking for a raised white cell count indicating an infectious or inflammatory process.
  - **C-reactive protein (CRP)** which will be raised in infection, inflammation, and some cases of malignancy.
  - **Clotting screen**, for a bleeding disorder which may be exacerbating if not directly causing the haemoptysis.
  - **Urea and electrolytes (U&Es)** for renal involvement, as in Goodpasture's syndrome or Wegener's granulomatosis, which can affect the kidney and the lung.
  - **Calcium, phosphate, and alkaline phosphatase (ALP)** for bone metastasis from a primary lung cancer.
  - **Liver enzymes** for liver involvement of a cancer.
- **Urine test:** urinalysis looking for haematuria, suggesting pulmonary–renal syndrome.
- **Imaging:** chest radiograph

Note: if TB is suspected, strenuous efforts should be made to obtain specimens or tissue from which to culture the organism (particularly given the growing prevalence of resistant strains). The skin sensitivity tests (Heaf, Mantoux) and newer T-cell based assays (e.g. Quantiferon, ELIspot) are only useful to determine latent TB infection and tell you nothing about disease activity. As many people are infected but not diseased, these tests are of little diagnostic value. They are used in contact tracing to see if somebody who has been exposed to open TB has become infected.

> **What signs would you be looking for on chest radiograph?**

- **Mass lesion/nodule:** carcinoma, TB, granuloma, abscess, vasculitides, e.g. Wegener's granulomatosis
- **Diffuse alveolar infiltrates:** pulmonary oedema
- **Hilar lymphadenopathy:** carcinoma, infection (if accompanying infiltrates), TB

- **Lobar or segmental infiltrates:** pneumonia, PE, obstructing carcinoma, TB
- **Patchy alveolar infiltrates:** bleeding disorders, Goodpasture's syndrome, idiopathic pulmonary haemosiderosis

Mr Morris' oxygen saturations are 95% on room air. His FBC shows a haemoglobin concentration of 14.5 g/dL, a white cell count of 4.6×10^9 cells/L, a CRP of <2 mg/L, a urea of 5.8 mM, a creatinine of 68 µM, and a corrected calcium of 2.54 mM. Urinalysis is unremarkable. In light of his history and examination, computed tomography pulmonary angiogram (CTPA) and a skin test for TB are not requested. His chest radiograph is shown in Fig. 8.1.

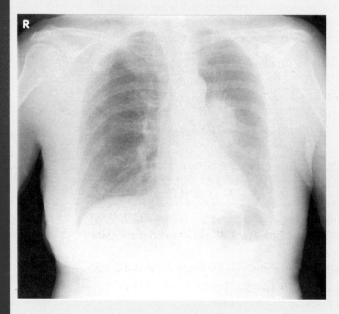

Figure 8.1 Chest radiograph for Mr Morris.

What is the most likely diagnosis? What should your next step be?

The chest radiograph shows a mass lesion sometimes called a 'coin lesion' in the patient's left hilum. This, in combination with his history (smoker, haemoptysis, and weight loss) and examination (hepatomegaly), is strongly suggestive of **lung cancer** (although there is a broader differential diagnosis for a coin lesion; see the Viva questions).

You need to confirm and classify the diagnosis with **cytology of sputum and bronchoscopic washings**. If the lesion is peripheral, one might opt for a **CT-guided percutaneous fine needle biopsy**. The reason is that cancer is ultimately a pathological diagnosis: clinical features can make you strongly suspect malignancy, but only a pathological sample will confirm it.

You also need to **stage** the cancer with a **CT scan**, looking for local spread and lymph node involvement, and a **bone scan**, looking for bone metastases.

> **What features make the other diagnoses listed at the start less likely?**

- TB
  - No history of chronic productive cough, fevers, or night sweats. However, he has unintentionally lost weight. He has not travelled abroad for years (although he may have latent TB).
  - On examination, he is apyrexic. There is no evidence of consolidation or a pleural effusion.
  - White cell count and CRP within the normal range.
  - No features on chest radiography suggesting TB (e.g. calcification).

- PE
  - Remember that this is a diagnosis of exclusion, as its presentation can be very varied and it is therefore not possible to diagnose clinically.
  - No history of sudden-onset pleuritic chest pain or breathlessness, although his exercise tolerance is poor. The only risk factor is smoking; he has not had a swollen limb recently, been immobile for a prolonged period, had trauma or surgery recently, has no previous history of venous thromboembolism or any clotting disorder, was not known to have a malignancy, and, although we didn't ask, is almost certainly not on the contraceptive pill or hormone replacement therapy!
  - Examination findings of good oxygen saturations on room air (95%) and no tachycardia, confirmed by a normal electrocardiogram (ECG).

- Pneumonia
  - No history of fever or cough productive of sputum. No pleuritic chest pain. Does not account for weight loss.
  - On examination, resonant percussion note and clear lung fields (no crackles), no tachycardia or tachypnoea, plus good saturations on room air.
  - White cell count and CRP within the normal range.

- Bronchiectasis
  - No history of chronic cough productive of sputum, as in classic bronchiectasis, although this does not exclude bronchiectasis. No wheeze and no dyspnoea at rest although, as mentioned, his exercise tolerance is poor. No history of recurrent respiratory illness. Not typically associated with weight loss.
  - On examination, no clubbing, no crackles or wheeze.

> **If the chest radiograph had not shown anything, what further investigations might you have considered?**

If risk factors for cancer are present, e.g. male, over 40 years of age, significant smoking history, you may wish to consider a **CT scan**. If this is still inconclusive, you may also consider further tests including PET and fibreoptic bronchoscopy.

How should Mr Morris be managed, both acutely and in the longer term?

As always, you should check his need for resuscitation (**Airway, Breathing, Circulation, ABC**). From the examination we know that he is in a stable condition. Were his haemoptysis more serious, you would want to stop the bleeding and prevent aspiration of blood as well.

In the longer term, having had his diagnosis confirmed and his tumour staged, on an outpatient basis, Mr Morris should be referred to the multidisciplinary team (MDT) for management. Management will depend on the results from histology (grade) and the stage (spread) of the tumour as discussed in the Viva questions.

8

Short cases

Mr Johnson is a 55-year-old engineer who presents to A&E with haemoptysis. He has coughed up a tea-spoonful of blood, which was a dark red colour, on each of the last 3 days. He has not had fever, weight loss, or breathlessness. However, he has had some chest pain on deep inspiration over the last day, which is not reproduced by pressing on his ribs. He does not recall any trauma to his ribs. He is a non-smoker, has had no exposure to industrial antigens, or previous lung disease. He grew up in Scotland and has never been outside Europe. He recalls having a sore, swollen calf a few days ago but it resolved on its own so he did not go to the GP. His only risk factor for venous thromboembolism is stasis on the long bus journeys he is making every week back home to Scotland.

On examination, his pulse is 94 bpm and regular, his blood pressure 122/64 mmHg, his respiratory rate 12/min and his temperature 35.9°C. His oxygen saturations, however, are 91% on room air. There are no other signs of cyanosis or stigmata of respiratory disease. His bloods show a haemoglobin concentration of 15.2 g/dL, a white cell count of 5.2×10^9 cells/L, a CRP of <2 mg/L, a urea of 6.1 mM, a creatinine of 58 µM, and a calcium of 2.45 mM. Urinalysis and an ECG are unremarkable.

In light of the above, what diagnoses would you like to exclude? Is there a clinical algorithm or scoring system that would help?

Mr Johnson's history and examination do not clearly point to any diagnosis, but the long bus journeys may have predisposed to a DVT (which would explain the swollen calf) and the chest pain and low oxygen saturations suggest lung pathology, such as a PE. You therefore should exclude a **PE**.

When you suspect PE based on the history (the clinical examination will rarely show anything more than a tachycardia and/or mild fever), you should refer to the **Wells' criteria** to determine, based on your clinical findings, the best investigation. The criteria are listed in Table 8.1 with their scores.

Table 8.1 The Wells' criteria for pulmonary embolism (PE)

Criteria	Points
Clinical signs and symptoms of DVT	3 points
PE is the most likely diagnosis	3 points
Heart rate >100 bpm	1.5 points
Immobilization >3 days or surgery in the last 4 weeks	1.5 points
Previously diagnosed DVT or PE	1.5 points
Haemoptysis	1 point
Malignancy diagnosed in the last 6 months	1 point

A score of ≥4 merits a CTPA (or perfusion scan) to investigate further; a score of <4 only justifies a D-Dimer test to *exclude* a PE.

It is worth noting that the Wells' criteria have been criticized because one of the weightier elements is subjective: whether PE is the most likely diagnosis. This can be the difference between low and moderate risk. An alternative clinical prediction tool has been recently developed, the revised Geneva score (2006), which does not rely on the clinician's judgement. It may come to replace the Wells' criteria if it is validated.

Mr Johnson has a Wells' score of 4 (symptoms of a DVT and haemoptysis). His D-dimer was >500ng/mL so he had a CTPA, which confirmed a PE. He was prescribed a prolonged course of anticoagulants and discharged.

8

Miss Gautam is a 19-year-old woman who presents with haemoptysis. She tells you she suffered from a lot of chest infections when she was growing up in Bangladesh. However, she has come to you because in the last week her sputum has become stained with bright red blood. There has been no more than an eggcup of blood at most. She has not had coryzal symptoms or felt feverish, but has felt 'not 100%' and had night sweats. She has also lost around a stone [about 6.5 kilos] in weight in the last 6 months, although she says she has been dieting and exercising. She denies any chest pain or shortness of breath.

She is a non-smoker, has no history of exposure to industrial agents, or diagnosed lung disease. She grew up in Bangladesh until the age of 16, when she moved to the UK with her family. She has not been vaccinated against TB. She is on the combined oral contraceptive pill but is taking no other medications, and has no other risk factors for venous thromboembolism.

On examination, she has a temperature of 39.2°C, a pulse of 89 bpm, blood pressure of 109/66 mmHg, respiratory rate of 12/min, and oxygen saturations of 96% on room air. There are no peripheral stigmata of respiratory disease. Her chest expansion is slightly reduced on the right hemithorax, and percussion over the right lower hemithorax is dull. Auscultation of the right lower lung field reveals reduced breath sounds, some crackles, and increased vocal resonance.

Her bloods come back with a haemoglobin concentration of 10.3 g/dL, a white cell count of 7.2×10^9 cells/L, a CRP of 11 mg/L, a urea of 5.6 mM, a creatinine of 47 µM, and a Ca of 2.38 mM. Urinalysis and an ECG are unremarkable.

You send off blood cultures and request a chest radiograph. While you are waiting for radiology to do this, your Consultant asks you to present the case with your working differential diagnosis and management plan.

What is the diagnosis you are most concerned about? Given this, what specific actions should your management plan consider?

Short case

8

With her history of growing up in the Indian subcontinent and chronic cough (in the absence of smoking), haemoptysis, night sweats, and weight loss, you should be most concerned about **pulmonary TB**, although pneumonia is also a possibility. The suspicion of TB is reinforced by examination and investigation findings consistent with an infection (temperature, raised white cell count, and CRP) and consolidation (reduced expansion, dullness to percussion, reduced breath sounds, crackles, increased vocal resonance). The mild anaemia suggests a chronic disease process. This is likely a reactivation of the TB or post-primary infection. Reactivation of TB typically (although not always) affects the upper lobes because *Mycobacterium tuberculosis* is a highly aerobic bacterium and the apices are the most oxygenated part of the lungs.

In addition to reviewing her need for resuscitation (ABC), you need to:

1) Ensure that microbiology know to look for acid-fast bacilli (i.e. using a Ziehl–Nielson or silver stain). Bear in mind that *M. tuberculosis* is a very slow-growing bacterium and it can therefore take many weeks before a positive result is obtained on culture.

2) TB is a notifiable disease so you must notify the authorities for contact tracing. They may vaccinate contacts with Bacille Calmette–Guérin (BCG) and, rarely, provide prophylactic therapy.

3) Place the patient in isolation to prevent further spread.

4) Test her for HIV, as although she most likely acquired TB during her childhood she may have acquired it more recently secondary to HIV infection which has implications for prognosis and management.

5) Look for signs of spread to other organs. Check particularly for meningeal irritation, bone or joint pain particularly in weight-bearing joints (e.g. Pott's fracture in the spinal column), dysuria or pelvic pain (genitourinary infection), or abdominal pain.

6) If the diagnosis is confirmed, refer the patient to the TB service, which offers specialized care for such patients.

First-line treatment for TB will depend on the likelihood of a drug-resistant strain and the longer-term results of culture and sensitivities. However, the initial approach (as per the National Institute for Health and Clinical Excellence (NICE) guidelines on TB) is with a long-term regimen of four antibiotics: rifampicin and isoniazid for the first 4 months, pyrazinamide and ethambutol for the first 2 months.

Note that long treatment leads to poor compliance. This is a problem that is leading to multidrug-resistant TB, and explains why in some jurisidictions (e.g. New York City, USA) social workers may come and check that patients are taking their medications.

8

Mr Frick is a 28-year-old gentleman who is attending the Respiratory Clinic at his hospital. He has recently had several episodes of haemoptysis. He is well known to the respiratory physicians, who have managed him since he was a child. He has chronic rhinitis and has suffered for most of his life from a rattly cough which is frequently productive of green sputum. He suffered from many episodes of serous otitis media as a child. He still suffers from frequent episodes of sinusitis and has recently been referred to a fertility clinic by his GP because he and his wife have not been able to conceive a child after 18 months of trying. A recent chest CT showed dilated bronchi with thick walls extending to the peripheries of both lungs.

What diagnosis could explain the constellation of symptoms that Mr Frick has suffered during his life? How would you confirm such a diagnosis? How do you think Mr Frick is being managed?

Mr Frick has a history of recurrent cough productive of green sputum and occasional haemoptysis that is highly suggestive of bronchiectasis (*bronchos* = airway; *ektasis* = stretched out). His chest CT does indeed reveal dilated bronchi. In bronchiectasis, the bronchi are chronically inflamed as the lungs struggle to clear irritant mucus for any of a variety of reasons, e.g. obstruction, thickened mucus, poor ciliary function of the epithelia. The consequence of chronic inflammation is the laying down of scar tissue in the interstitial tissue. Remember that scars shrink, therefore the airway walls are pulled back and the airways expand. The mucus is often green due to the constant presence of neutrophils and macrophages fighting pathogens growing in the retained mucus. As neutrophils and macrophages die, they release an enzyme called myeloperoxidase which is green (and closely related to enzymes which give the spicy *wasabi* sauce favoured in Japanese cuisine its green colour). In addition, Mr Frick has suffered from many episodes of sinusitis and serous otitis media (glue ear), both of which suggest an inability to clear mucus.

The inability to clear mucus in various organs of the body is highly suggestive of **primary ciliary dyskinesia (PCD)**. This is an autosomal recessive disorder that affects the protein machinery used by epithelial cells to rhythmically beat their cilia and by spermatozoa to rhythmically beat their tails. The typical consequences of PCD are:

* Bronchiectasis, due to an inability to clear mucus from the lungs.

* Rhinitis and sinusitis, due to an inability to clear mucus from the nasal sinuses.

* Otitis media (both secretory and acutely infective) due to an inability to clear mucus from the middle ear, down the Eustachian tube.

* Male infertility, due to sperm immotility. Females are usually fertile because passage of the oocyte along the Fallopian tubes is more dependent on peristalsis of the Fallopian tubes than on the movement of the ciliae that line these tubes.

* Situs inversus. The rhythmical beating of cilia is thought to play an important part in setting up the usual pattern of body asymmetry during embryogenesis. Many patients with PCD have their organs on the 'other side' (e.g. dextrocardia).

Patients with PCD who show the clinical triad of bronchiectasis, sinusitis, and situs inversus may be said to have Kartagener's syndrome or Kartagener's triad.

Investigation of suspected PCD involves a biopsy of the nasal mucosa and examination under a microscope, looking for abnormal beating of the ciliated epithelia. Microscopy of spermatozoa of PCD males often reveals immobile spermatozoa.

Management of PCD involves:

- Regular physiotherapy, to help clear the lungs of mucus.
- Regular or prophylactic antibiotics, to prevent recurrent chest infections and sinusitis.
- Mucolytics can help clear mucus in the lungs and sinuses more easily in some patients.

It is worth knowing that patients with PCD tend to show an improvement of symptoms by their early thirties and that many patients lead near normal adult lives.

Miss Bonprat is a 31-year-old primary school teacher referred to the medical admissions unit of her local hospital because of sudden haemoptysis. She describes feeling unwell and lethargic for the past few weeks and thinking she had 'caught something off the children'. She developed a cough that morning but was alarmed when she noticed she had coughed up some specks of blood onto her handkerchief. She smokes a pack of 'light cigarettes' every day and has not travelled abroad recently. Systems enquiry is unrevealing. Her past medical history is remarkable for hypothyroidism, for which she takes levothyroxine every day.

Examination of Miss Bonprat reveals only that her blood pressure is 160/110 mmHg and that her urinalysis is positive for protein (+) and blood (+++). A mid-stream urine sample is sent off to the laboratories, who later that day confirm the presence of red cell casts on urine microscopy.

What diagnosis should you be concerned about?

Miss Bonprat has presented with haemoptysis. She also has hypertension, haematuria, and proteinuria on urinalysis suggesting inflammation of her kidneys (glomerulonephritis) that is manifesting as a nephritic syndrome. The presence of red cell casts (clumps of red cells that have squeezed through the glomeruli) is indicative of glomerular damage. The combination of haemoptysis and glomerulonephritis should alert you to the possibility of a **pulmonary–renal syndrome**.

8

Viva questions

Name several causes of clubbing.

There are many of these and you should structure it somehow – for example by physiological system:

- Cardiovascular
  - Infective endocarditis (subacute bacterial endocarditis)
  - Congenital cyanotic heart disease
  - Atrial myxoma
  - Axillary artery aneurysm
  - Brachial arteriovenous fistula
- Respiratory
  - Pulmonary fibrosis
  - Suppurative lung diseases: abscess, empyema, cystic fibrosis, bronchiectasis
  - Bronchial carcinoma, mesothelioma
  - TB
- Gastrointestinal
  - Inflammatory bowel disease
  - Cirrhosis
  - Malabsorption, e.g. coeliac disease
  - Gastric lymphoma
  - Liver abscess
  - Liver or bowel cancer
- Other
  - Congenital clubbing
  - Thyroid acropachy

In the context of a pleural diffusion, what is the difference between a transudate and an exudate? What are the causes of each?

The fluid from a pleural effusion can be defined as a transudate or an exudate depending on the protein content.

- A transudate is defined as having <25 g/L of protein. Transudates are low in protein because they are the result of fluid alone squeezing into the pleural space, either due to increased hydrostatic pressure in the lung vasculature (heart failure, fluid overload, constrictive pericarditis) or due to reduction in the oncotic pressure which usually keeps fluid in the vasculature (reduced serum protein due to liver failure, malabsorption/malnutrition, nephrotic syndrome).

- An exudate is defined as having >35 g/L of protein. Exudates are rich in protein because they are the result of cells in the pleural space: either pathogens (infection), inflammatory cells, or malignant cells.

- If the pleural fluid protein is between 25 and 35 g/L, Light's criteria should be used to differentiate exudates from transudates. These state that the fluid is an exudate if any of the following applies:
  - Pleural fluid protein divided by serum protein >0.5
  - Pleural fluid lactate dehydrogenase (LDH) divided by serum LDH >0.6
  - Pleural fluid LDH more than two-thirds the upper limit of normal serum LDH

How are lung neoplasms classified? How do they respond to treatment?

As for all neoplasms, lung neoplasms can at first be divided into benign and malignant. Malignant tumours in turn can be classified as primary or secondary. Broadly speaking, the primary malignant lung cancers are then classified in two groups based on histology:

1) **Non-small cell lung cancer** (NSCLC, 80%)
   - Subdivided into **adenocarcinoma** (30–40%), **squamous** (20–30%), **large cell carcinoma** (10%), and others (5%)
   - If localized, attempt to remove surgically or treat with radiotherapy
   - Otherwise responds poorly to chemotherapy and has poor prognosis if disseminated
2) **Small cell lung cancer** (SCLC, 20%)
   - Responsive to chemotherapy, although rapid relapse is common. Chemotherapy is given mainly because it improves symptoms rather than mortality
   - Early metastasis therefore surgery is not the therapy of choice

Haemoptysis is more common in squamous cell carcinoma, which usually affects lung tissue closer to the hilar region and thus the blood has relatively little distance to travel before being coughed up.

Which cancers most commonly metastasize to the lungs?

Secondary lung cancers are most commonly the result of metastasis from the following primary cancers:

- Colorectal
- Breast
- Renal
- Female genital tract: cervix, ovary

Note that metastatic lung cancer rarely cause haemoptysis as they are spreading haematogenously and therefore tend to be deep in the interstitium rather than endobronchial.

What ectopic endocrine secretions are associated with which lung cancers? What symptoms do they cause?

Small cell lung carcinomas are derived from endocrine cells in the lung and therefore have the potential to synthesize and secrete hormones or hormone-like substances. The substances secreted by small cell lung cancers are **antidiuretic hormone (ADH)**, resulting in hyponatraemia, and **ACTH**, resulting in Cushing's syndrome.

Squamous cell carcinomas may not have the cell machinery to produce cholesterol-based steroids, but they can produce peptides including **PTHrP**. This causes hypercalcaemia.

8

What extra-pulmonary sites does TB most commonly affect? What does it cause in each?

TB can affect virtually any organ. Some of the more common manifestations include:

- Bone: osteomyelitis, septic arthritis, Pott's disease (in the spine)
- Neurological: meningitis, intracranial granulomas
- Renal: granuloma

TB less commonly affects the heart, skeletal muscles, pancreas, thyroid, or adrenals (causing Addison's disease). Indeed, TB was found on autopsy in 70–90% of Dr Addison's patients in his original description of the eponymous syndrome (this figure is in fact lower in larger, more recent studies).

Give a differential for a solitary coin lesion on a chest radiograph.

A coin lesion could be:

- Parenchymal tumour: benign, primary lung cancer, secondary lung cancer
- Lymph node: lymphoma
- Granuloma: TB, sarcoidosis
- Abscess
- Hamartoma
- Foreign object

What is the doctrine of double effect? How is this relevant to a lung cancer patient being treated with opiates for pain relief?

The doctrine of double effect applies when a treatment has two (or more) effects. The primary (intended) effect is to relieve the symptoms. But a secondary effect, which is foreseen but *not* intended, in some way hastens death. In legal terms, although the treatment is bringing about mortality, as its primary (intended) effect is beneficial it is viewed as distinct from euthanasia.

   This applies directly to the lung cancer patient being treated with opiates. As well as providing analgesia and suppressing the cough reflex (and hence the likelihood of haemoptysis), opiates can cause respiratory depression if given in sufficiently large doses. However, the benefits are considered to outweigh the drawbacks, particularly given that the doses are usually insufficient to cause respiratory depression (making this a somewhat theoretical point). Thus, opiates are commonly used in terminally ill patients suffering with chronic pain.

For a range of Single Best Answer questions related to the topic of this chapter go to
www.oxfordtextbooks.co.uk/orc/ocms/

Chest pain

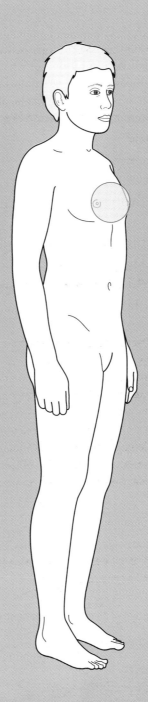

Core case

Core case

! *Read through the sections in red, covering up the sections in white that follow so that you don't see the answer. At the end of each red section, try to answer the question before reading on.*

Mr Shepherd is a 67-year-old man who was referred to accident and emergency (A&E) by his general practitioner (GP) after a 2-hour history of severe chest pain.

What are the most common causes of acute chest pain in an individual of this age?

A good way to come up with a list of causes is to visualize the anatomy of the affected area and think of what could go wrong. Thus, in chest pain, there may be pathology of the heart, aorta, lungs, pulmonary vessels, oesophagus, stomach (upper areas), thoracic nerves, or thoracic muscles.

Common causes of acute chest pain in an individual aged over 60 include:

> Acute coronary syndrome
> Stable angina
> Pulmonary embolism (PE)
> Pleurisy (secondary to infection)
> Musculoskeletal[†]
> Oesophagitis (secondary to gastro-oesophageal reflux disease or hiatus hernia)
> Anxiety
> Oesophageal spasm
> Peptic ulcer disease
> Pneumothorax
> Myopericarditis
> Aortic dissection
> Aortic aneurysm
> Coronary spasm (e.g. secondary to cocaine)
> Boerhaave's perforation of the oesophagus
> Cholecystitis
> Pancreatitis

[†] Most commonly this will be muscle strain, but other causes include Cocksackie B infection (Bornholm's disease), idiopathic costochondritis (Tietze's syndrome), and *Varicella zoster* infection.

How would your differential change if the patient were a 20-year-old woman on the combined oral contraceptive pill?

A younger patient is less likely to be suffering from diseases of old age, such as:

* Acute coronary syndrome
* Stable angina
* Myopericarditis (usually post-infarction)
* Aortic dissection
* Aortic aneurysm

A younger female patient on the combined oral contraceptive pill is more likely to be suffering from:

* PE (the combined oral contraceptive pill is thrombogenic)
* Pneumothorax (especially if tall and thin)
* Cocaine-induced coronary spasm (still rare, but particularly unusual in the elderly!)

> When a patient arrives with chest pain, you need to be thinking about the conditions that present with chest pain that are potentially fatal and require immediate management.
>
> Which diagnoses fall into this category? What features are going to alert you to these conditions?

The following diagnoses require immediate management and should be kept in mind:

* **Acute coronary syndrome** (unstable angina, or myocardial infarction (MI))
* **Aortic dissection**
* **Pneumothorax**
* **PE**
* **Boerhaave's perforation**

The key features of each are listed below.

1) **Features of acute coronary syndrome**:
   - History of sudden-onset, central crushing chest pain radiating to either/both arms and neck, especially in someone with a previous history of angina on exertion or MI and/or cardiovascular risk factors (smoking, hypertension, hypercholesterolaemia, diabetes, family history).
   - Signs of hypercholesterolaemia: cholesterol deposits in small skin lumps on the tendons of the back of the hand or bony prominences like elbows (xanthomata), in creamy spots around the eyes (xanthelasma), or a creamy ring around the cornea (arcus). Note that arcus is a normal finding in the elderly.
   - Signs of systemic atherosclerotic vascular disease: weak pulses, peripheral cyanosis, atrophic skin, ulcers, bruits on auscultation of carotids.
   - Signs of anaemia. Anaemia can cause or exacerbate ischaemic heart disease. You can look for the following signs of anaemia, and should do in an exam, but they are either unreliable or very rare in developed countries: conjunctival pallor (unreliable), glossitis, angular stomatitis, or koilonychia (all very rare).

- Signs of arrhythmia. If a patient has underlying ischaemic heart disease and develops poor cardiac output due to an arrhythmia, it is likely that they will develop chest pain because their poorly perfused heart will become ischaemic. Thus, check for an irregularly irregular pulse (atrial fibrillation, atrial flutter with variable heart block, or frequent ectopics), a slow pulse (heart block), or a very fast pulse (atrial fibrillation/flutter-induced tachycardia, re-entry tachycardias, ventricular tachycardia). Also, atrial fibrillation is commonly due to previous ischaemic damage and therefore offers a clue as to what might be wrong with the patient.

2) **Features of aortic dissection**:
   - History of sudden-onset tearing chest pain radiating to the back.
   - Absent pulse in one arm.
   - Hypertension (in about 50% of cases) or hypotension (in about 25% of cases).
   - A difference in blood pressure between arms >20 mmHg (about a third of cases).
   - New-onset aortic regurgitation. This is caused by the new lumen tracking down to the valve and making it incompetent.
   - Pleural effusion, usually on the left. This is due to irritation of the pleura by the dissecting aorta.

3) **Features of pneumothorax:**
   - History of sudden-onset pleuritic chest pain with breathlessness – but beware, it may present as painless breathlessness.
   - A hyperinflated chest wall with impaired expansion. Normally the lack of air in the pleural space creates a vacuum that holds the lungs to the chest wall. If air gets into the pleural space, unopposed elastic recoil of the chest wall will cause it to pop out, whilst at the same time the lungs will shrivel up. (Note this is different from lung collapse, in which a bronchus is obstructed and the air trapped distally in that segment is gradually absorbed into the blood.)
   - Hyper-resonant percussion over the affected area.
   - Absent breath sounds over the affected area. The crumpled up area of lung will not have any air getting in or out.
   - Tracheal deviation. In *tension pneumothorax*, a flap of pleural membrane acts as a valve so that the pleural space gets increasingly inflated with air. It eventually starts to deviate the mediastinum, and can compress the heart leading to cardiopulmonary arrest. Therefore, a trachea that deviates away from a suspected pneumothorax is an emergency requiring urgent insertion of a large-bore cannula in the mid-clavicular line just above the third rib to allow the air trapped in the pleural space to escape.

4) **Features of PE** (due to **deep vein thrombosis (DVT)**):
   - This is a diagnosis of exclusion as its presentation can be very varied and it is therefore difficult to diagnose clinically.
   - History of sudden-onset shortness of breath and/or haemoptysis and/or pleuritic chest pain in someone with an inflamed limb and/or risk factors for blood clots (e.g. recent surgery, recent stasis, or hypercoagulable blood due to the oral contraceptive pill or malignancy).

- Signs of hypoxia. The patient may appear pale, have cold peripheries, feel lethargic and/or be drowsy or confused, depending on the degree of hypoxia.
- Right heart strain evidenced by a raised jugular venous pressure (JVP).
- You should refer to the Wells' criteria (see viva questions) for diagnosis of PE if you suspect this.

5) **Features of Boerhaave's perforation**: note that this is very rare, but it is associated with a high mortality and hence is included.
   - History of sudden-onset severe chest pain immediately following an episode of vomiting. Shortness of breath and pleuritic pain may develop shortly afterwards due to subsequent pleurisy and effusion.
   - Signs of a pleural effusion after some hours – dullness to percussion, absent breath sounds, decreased vocal resonance.
   - Subcutaneous emphysema is present in a minority of cases.
   - Abdominal rigidity, sweating, fever, tachycardia, and hypotension may be present as the illness progresses but are non-specific.

Bearing in mind the above, you take a history from Mr Shepherd. You find that he localizes the pain to his sternum. He says it came on 2 hours earlier in the afternoon as he was gardening and has been there since. He describes it as like 'wearing a shirt two sizes too small' and says it has not moved since it came on. The pain was not exacerbated by breathing, and was not position dependent. He does not have a cough but his pain improved minutes after he was given a glyceryl trinitrate (GTN) spray sublingually in the ambulance, going from 8/10 severity to 3/10 now.

He is a smoker with a 40-pack-year history, has hypertension that is managed with a calcium-channel blocker and hypercholesterolaemia for which he takes a statin. His father died of stroke in his 70s and his mother of 'old age' in her late 80s. He is not known to be diabetic.

On examination, Mr Shepherd appears relatively comfortable (on pain relief), with arcus but no other peripheral signs of cardiovascular disease. His pulse and blood pressure are taken in both arms and found to be equally regular, 84 bpm and 145/90 mmHg. His oxygen saturation is 98% on room air. Both heart sounds are audible with no added sounds and palpation of the chest does not bring on pain. Carotid bruits can be heard bilaterally on auscultation. His lungs have normal resonance to percussion, good air entry, and no abnormal sounds on auscultation. His trachea is central. His limbs show no signs of inflammation and he is not febrile.

In light of Mr Shepherd's history, risk factors, and examination, a certain diagnosis for his chest pain appears increasingly likely.

What investigations would you like to request? Think particularly of how you can confirm your expected diagnosis and how you can rule out the 'must exclude' diagnoses listed above.

9

Electrocardiogram (ECG)

Perform ECGs on anyone with suspected cardiac disease, either two ECGs 30 minutes apart or, if the patient has continuing chest pain, every 10–15 minutes until the diagnosis is made. If the patient is admitted, ECGs should be performed daily for 3 days thereafter, as changes may take 24 hours or more to develop. In the context of chest pain, you are particularly looking for signs of ischaemia and arrhythmias (causing a drop in cardiac output and thus decreasing coronary perfusion). These signs are explained in detail in any guide to reading ECGs. Note that it is particularly important to look for signs of ST segment elevation or new onset LBBB, as the management protocol for individuals with an ST elevation myocardial infarction (STEMI) differs from that for suspected non-ST elevation myocardial infarction (NSTEMI).

Blood tests

- **Troponin:** this should be measured on admission and at 12 hours from the onset of pain. Troponin levels are extremely useful because of their high sensitivity and specificity for damage to cardiac muscle. The drawback is the minimum 8-hour delay in increased troponin levels. An alternative is **CK-MB**, an isotype of the enzyme creatinine kinase, which is released more rapidly following damage but which is less specific for cardiac damage. CK-MB levels fall back to normal within 2–3 days whereas troponin levels remain high for >7 days. Thus, CK-MB levels that are elevated >4 days after an MI suggest that there has been a re-infarction. *Note: troponin levels are specific for cardiac damage but not 100% specific for acute coronary syndrome – you need to consider the context. Other conditions causing a raised troponin include: coronary artery spasm (e.g. from cocaine) or aortic dissection causing ischaemia, myopericarditis, severe heart failure, cardiac trauma from surgery or road traffic accident, and PE.*

- **Serum cholesterol:** hypercholesterolaemia is another risk factor for cardiovascular disease that is often undiagnosed and that can be treated. It is worth noting that an MI will result in a decrease in total cholesterol, low-density lipoprotein (LDL), and high-density lipoprotein (HDL) within about 24 hours of the infarct, and that levels will not return to normal (for that patient) for 2–3 months post-infarct. Thus, cholesterol levels should be measured as soon as possible if they are to guide future therapy.

- **Full blood count (FBC):** anaemia from any cause is common and will exacerbate any deficiency in cardiac perfusion, resulting in ischaemic heart disease.

- **Urea and electrolytes (U&Es):** pay particular attention to the potassium, as this may be the cause of an arrhythmia.

- **Inflammatory markers:** C-reactive protein (CRP), erythrocyte sedimentation rate (ESR), and the white cell count (WCC) from the FBC are all measures of inflammation. Accordingly these are elevated in inflammatory processes such as pericarditis and Bornholm's disease (inflammation of intercostal muscles due to Coxsackie B virus infection), but will also be elevated following aortic dissection and MI, which cause inflammation of the affected tissues.

- **Capillary glucose:** there is a significant increase in the risk of cardiovascular disease with diabetes mellitus, particularly if untreated. Type 2 diabetics typically suffer from the complications of diabetes prior to becoming symptomatic for the diabetes itself, and as many as 50% may be undiagnosed. Critically, diabetics are more likely to present with 'silent infarcts' – that is, an MI in the absence of chest pain.

Imaging

Erect chest radiograph: this should be done to help exclude a pneumothorax and aortic pathology (aneurysm or dissection, giving a wide mediastinum). Note that it is possible to have a normal chest radiograph in aortic dissection. If Boerhaave's perforation of the oesophagus is suspected, a chest radiograph will typically show air around the heart shadow (pneumomediastinum), a pleural effusion, and/or a pneumothorax.

Second line

D-dimer levels: elevated D-dimers are simply symptomatic of breakdown of a fibrin clot due to any cause such as recent surgery or trauma, and are therefore *not* diagnostic of DVT or PE specifically. However, low D-dimer levels can help *rule out* a DVT or PE as these are unlikely to occur without any fibrin breaking down. These are not done as standard in chest pain but to exclude PE.

Mr Shepherd's ECG is shown in Fig. 9.1. Comment on any abnormalities.

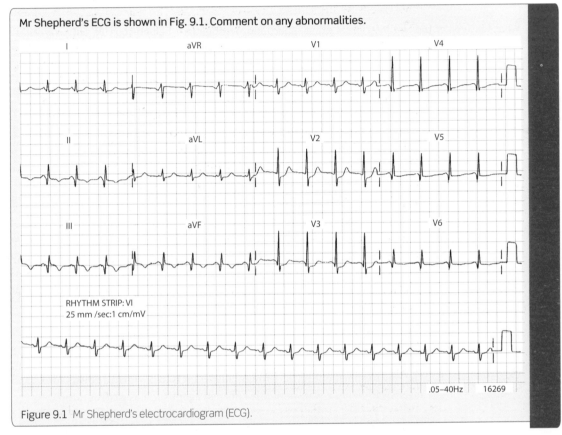

Figure 9.1 Mr Shepherd's electrocardiogram (ECG).

Mr Shepherd's ECG shows ST depression and prominent R waves in V_1–V_3 but no signs of ST elevation.

He begins to complain of pain once the analgesia wears off. His troponin is 6 ng/mL on admission, (normal range given by the lab <0.4 ng/mL). His chest radiograph is normal.

In light of the history, examination, and investigations, what is the diagnosis? How else might this condition present?

Mr Shepherd is a 40-pack-year smoker with hypertension and hypercholesterolaemia who has presented with central crushing chest pain. This picture is typical for **MI**. He has elevation of cardiac troponin levels, suggesting MI.

His ECG shows ST depression in leads V_1–V_3 which would be consistent with an **anterior NSTEMI**. Remember that transmural infarctions normally result in ST elevation on an ECG and are hence referred to as ST elevation myocardial infarctions (STEMIs). However, in the case of posterior wall transmural infarctions, the fact that the ECG chest leads are on the opposite side of the chest wall results in ST depression in leads V_1–V_3 rather than ST elevation. Thus, this could also represent a **posterior infarct**, which are treated like STEMIs despite the lack of ST elevation.

MIs present in many different ways and you should have a low threshold for suspecting it in anyone with cardiac risk factors. Ultimately, diagnosis depends on an elevated 12-hour troponin. Chest pain is not always a feature, particularly in the elderly and long-standing diabetics who frequently have neuropathy and dulled pain sensation. ECG readings are also non-diagnostic, as changes may not be present in infarction.

> **What features of the history, clinical examination, and investigations helped you rule out your other 'must exclude' diagnoses?**

- **Aortic dissection?** Mr Shepherd's pain was not tearing and did not radiate to his back. His pulse and blood pressure were equal in both arms and chest radiography did not suggest a wide mediastinum. Ultimately, the way to rule out aortic dissection if you strongly suspect it is to do CT angiography of the chest or transoesophageal echo, looking for a false lumen.

- **Pneumothorax?** Mr Shepherd did not have areas of the chest that were expanded and hyper-resonant, with decreased air entry. His trachea was not displaced and his chest radiograph is normal.

- **PE?** Remember that this is a diagnosis of exclusion, so you have not strictly speaking ruled it out. However, the normal oxygen saturations (98% on room air), the ST depression on ECG, and the large rise in troponin make this unlikely (a small rise in troponin may be seen in PE). A D-dimer level was not requested but may in any case have been raised as a result of his infarction.

- **Boerhaave's perforation of the oesophagus?** Mr Shepherd did not give a history of vomiting before the onset of his pain. A perforated oesophagus is a very rare diagnosis and even less likely without previous vomiting. Ultimately, the way to rule it out if you strongly suspect it is to perform a chest radiograph after swallowing a water-soluble contrast agent such as gastrograffin.

> **How will the medical team manage Mr Shepherd acutely? How does the management differ between full-thickness infarcts (STEMI and posterior infarcts) and partial-thickness infarcts (NSTEMI)?**

Having assessed the need for resuscitation (airways, breathing, and circulation, ABC), you should consider Mr Shepherd's immediate management. Given that your differential includes life-threatening conditions, treatment should be started in tandem with your diagnostic screen. The longer-term management should consider secondary prevention of further cardiovascular events.

Acutely, all patients with any acute coronary syndrome (STEMI, posterior infarcts, NSTEMI, unstable angina) are started on a cocktail of drugs that can be remembered by the mnemonic MONABASH:

Morphine, for analgesia, and an anti-emetic such as metoclopramide (although there is some evidence that for patients with no gastrointestinal (GI) disturbance there is no benefit in giving an anti-emetic)

Oxygen

N itrates (e.g. GTN, isosorbide mononitrate infusion), for vasodilation

A ntiplatelets: aspirin, clopidogrel, and glycoprotein IIb/IIIa antagonists, to prevent further coronary thrombosis

B eta-blockers, to reduce myocardial oxygen demand. These are contraindicated if the patient is in heart block, has asthma, or has any signs of acute heart failure

A CE inhibitors, for multiple reasons including attenuation of post-infarct ventricular remodelling that can cause arrhythmias, reduction of angiotensin II-induced vasoconstriction improving cardiac blood flow and reducing after-load, and beneficial effects on endothelial function

S tatins, which in addition to reducing cholesterol levels are thought to improve endothelial function, modulate inflammatory responses (e.g. reduce CRP), maintain atherosclerotic plaque stability, and prevent thrombus formation; there is evidence to support their use in the acute setting

H eparin (low-molecular weight heparin, LMWH), to prevent coronary thrombosis

STEMI patients (including posterior infarcts) should also receive either **primary angioplasty** or **thrombolysis** within 12 hours of the onset of pain, the sooner the better, and ideally within 2 hours of the onset of symptoms. Thrombolysis carries significant risks and therefore there are clear indications and contraindications with which you should familiarize yourself before referring a patient for thrombolysis. Angioplasty is superior to thrombolysis if both are equally available, but rapid treatment is even more important so you should not delay thrombolysis if angioplasty is not likely to be achieved within 2 hours of the onset of the symptoms.

NSTEMI patients do not receive thrombolysis, as this does not appear to be effective in them. However, NSTEMI patients are candidates for early angioplasty if their TIMI risk score is ≥3 (see Table 9.1):

Table 9.1 TIMI score for NSTEMI unstable angina

Age >65 years	1 point
≥3 risk factors for coronary artery disease	1 point
Known coronary artery stenosis >50%	1 point
Aspirin use in the last 7 days	1 point
≥2 symptoms of severe angina in last 24 h	1 point
Raised cardiac markers (e.g. troponins)	1 point
ST segment deviation of ≥0.5 mm	1 point

Mr Shepherd's consultant decided that the prominent R waves on the ECG were more likely to represent a posterior infarct than an anterior NSTEMI. A right-sided ECG confirmed this and Mr Shepherd received primary angioplasty.

What advice and medications should Mr Shepherd be discharged on?

Secondary prevention is important in patients with ischaemic heart disease. Mr Shepherd should be given the following advice and medication (lifelong):

- **Lifestyle changes:** smoking cessation, low-salt diet, exercise, and weight loss.
- **Risk factor control with medications:**
  - Blood pressure control: ACE inhibitors if the patient is <55 years and Caucasian, calcium-channel blockers or diuretic thiazides if the patient is >55 years or non-Caucasian. A mixture of these three classes of drug may be prescribed if the blood pressure cannot be controlled with one drug alone.
  - Cholesterol reduction: statins, or fibrates if statins are contraindicated.
  - Diabetic control: tight sugar control is important for cardiovascular risk, although far less important than blood pressure control in diabetics as shown by the United Kingdom Prospective Diabetes Study (UKPDS) trial.
- **Reduced thromboembolic risk:** low-dose aspirin for life and clopidogrel for a period of 1 year.

If there is severe left ventricular dysfunction, i.e. an ejection fraction <30% on echocardiogram, there is an increased risk of ventricular arrhythmias and death. Such patients are therefore candidates for implantable cardioversion devices (ICD), which detect the onset of ventricular arrhythmias and shock the heart to stop the arrhythmia.

9

Short cases

> Mr Shepherd undergoes angioplasty to an occluded circumflex artery and is discharged. Four weeks later he presents again with chest pain. However, he says it is different from his previous pain. This time it radiates to his left shoulder, is worse on deep inspiration, and is aggravated by lying down. You note that he has a fever.
>
> **What are the complications of an MI, and what has probably happened to Mr Shepherd? How should Mr Shepherd be managed on this admission?**

The common complications of MI are covered in the mnemonic DARTH VADER:

Death (probably not a complication to mention if asked!)

Arrhythmia

Rupture (either of the septum or the outer walls)

Tamponade

Heart failure

Valve disease

Aneurysm

Dressler's syndrome (autoimmune pericarditis 2–10 weeks after MI; note that simple post-MI pericarditis is more common than Dressler's syndrome, presenting within 2–4 days)

Embolism

Re-infarction

Given the timing, fever, and pleuritic and positional aspects of the pain, Mr Shepherd has most likely presented with **Dressler's syndrome.**

As in the management of any patient, you should first assess Mr Shepherd's need for resuscitation (ABC), then confirm his diagnosis. A FBC will show leucocytosis and an ECG may show diffuse saddle-shaped ST elevation across a number of leads without reciprocal ST depression, and may also show PR depression. An echocardiogram may show a pericardial effusion; this may also be visible on chest radiograph. The ECG and chest radiograph will additionally help exclude a re-infarction or pulmonary pathology, respectively. Twelve-hour troponin levels should also be measured on this admission for the same reason.

Having ordered the relevant investigations, Mr Shepherd should immediately be started on analgesia. Large doses of aspirin and other non-steroidal anti-inflammatory drugs (NSAIDs) may be given and are usually sufficient. If there is a significant effusion, it can be aspirated (pericardiocentesis) to relieve pressure on the heart.

Mrs Thompson is a 62-year-old woman with known angina who has been referred by her GP following increasing frequency in her episodes of chest tightness. She says she usually suffers from angina two or three times a month, but that over the last 2 months her attacks have become more frequent. Some of these episodes are now occurring at rest, often following meals. They are partly alleviated by the GTN spray she has been using for her angina. She is a heavy smoker, blood pressure 163/94 mmHg, and cholesterol 6.5 mM. She had an angiogram 2 years earlier showing mild stenosis of the left circumflex artery. Her other medical history includes reflux disease, but no other conditions. Notably she has no history of gallstone disease and reports no change in stool or urine. On admission her examination and investigations are normal, including the ECG, 12-hour troponin levels, and temperature. The team has a high suspicion of a worsening of her angina and perform a repeat angiography, which is unchanged from her previous angiogram.

What diagnoses should you be considering? Which investigations will help you determine the correct one?

Attacks of chest pain of increasing frequency and at rest should trigger alarm bells for the progression of her angina from stable to unstable. At the same time, the fact that her angiogram is unchanged should arouse your suspicion of another diagnosis. The insidious course rules out acute conditions such as infarction or pericarditis. The important diagnoses to exclude are oesophageal spasm, cholecystitis, and acute pancreatitis. Both oesophageal spasm and cholecystitis are consistent with the history of pain after meals, although a lack of known gallstone disease, unchanged urine and stool, and apyrexia argue against cholecystitis.

Oesophageal spasm may be detected by barium swallow and oesophageal manometry, although a normal result does not exclude it. Ultimately the diagnosis may come down to a therapeutic trial. Mrs Thompson was prescribed a proton-pump inhibitor for presumptive **oesophageal spasm** secondary to reflux. She responded positively, confirming the diagnosis.

If all else had been excluded, you may have considered a diagnosis of coronary artery spasm (sometimes called variant or Prinzmetal angina) or coronary syndrome X. These are diagnoses of exclusion; they are extremely hard to demonstrate and are, in any case, rare in the absence of underlying coronary artery disease. It is best to avoid such 'dustbin diagnoses' until all other causes have been excluded.

9

Mr Heyward is a 38-year-old man with increasingly severe chest pain that began during an evening in the pub. The pain has not radiated, and was not alleviated by GTN administered in the ambulance. He has a strong family history with both his father and brother suffering heart attacks in their fifties, and is a heavy smoker with a 50 pack year history. He is not known to have diabetes, hypertension, or high cholesterol. He has no other significant medical history, although you note that he had what sounds like a viral upper respiratory tract infection 3–4 days ago. On examination of his cardiovascular system you find no abnormalities. An ECG taken at the hospital is shown in Fig. 9.2. His other investigations were normal apart from mildly elevated inflammatory markers.

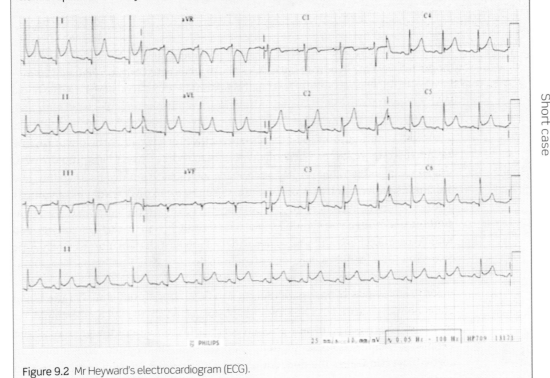

Figure 9.2 Mr Heyward's electrocardiogram (ECG).
With kind permission from Dr J. Dwight.

What does the ECG show? What is the most likely diagnosis?

9

The ECG shows ST elevation in leads I, II, aVL, V_1–V_5, i.e. throughout most leads, and slight PR segment depression. Acute coronary syndromes typically respond to vasodilators such as GTN. In addition, MI causes ECG changes which are reciprocal (i.e. ST elevation in some leads, ST depression in opposite anatomical leads). This is therefore unlikely to be an acute coronary syndrome, although troponin levels 12 hours after the onset of pain should be checked for confirmation.

Pericarditis is the most likely diagnosis despite the atypical sounding pain and lack of a pericardial friction rub, which can be intermittent. A therapeutic trial of NSAIDs was prescribed which diminished the pain. The patient was treated with analgesia as an inpatient for a few days and was discharged once pain free.

Mr Bromley is a 28-year-old, tall, thin man with a sudden onset of severe chest pain. He has recently been on a flight from Egypt and had knee surgery 1 month ago. Otherwise he says he has been fit and well, with no previous medical history. He is not known to have Marfan's syndrome, although it has not been investigated, and there is no family history of note. He is a non-smoker with no risk factors for cardio-vascular disease. On examination he is pale, sweaty, and breathless. His pulse is weak and thready, but otherwise his examination is normal.

What diagnoses are most likely? Which first-line investigations will help you determine the correct one?

In a tall, thin, young individual you should immediately be thinking of pneumo-thorax or Marfan's syndrome predisposing to a dissected aortic aneurysm or aortic dissection. His recent air travel, although only a short trip, and surgery should alert you to the possibility of a PE. All of these conditions are associated with high mortality and so you must act fast. In your assessment of his ABC you should pay particular attention to his blood pressure – patients with an aortic aneurysm are often hypertensive but can become hypotensive if they dissect back into the peri-cardial space and develop cardiac tamponade (along with muffled heart sounds and distended neck veins). If they rupture into the chest cavity they tend to exsanguinate before they make it to hospital. An urgent chest radiograph will rule out a pneu-mothorax (although you should have detected this when palpating, percussing, and auscultating his chest) and will show a widened mediastinum in most cases of aortic dissection (~80%). PE is a diagnosis of exclusion, although CT pulmonary angiogra-phy (CTPA) can be helpful in making the diagnosis.

Mr Bromley was hypotensive (80/46) but there was no difference in the blood pressure in each arm. His chest radiograph suggested a widened mediastinum. As he was not haemodynamically stable it was felt he should not undergo a CT and a transoesophageal echocardiogram was ordered at the bedside. This showed an **aortic dissection** near the aortic root and a pericardial effusion. Any dissection involving the ascending aorta, such as this one, is classed as a Stanford type A and is a surgical emergency. Dissections of the descending aorta, with no involvement of the ascending aorta, are called type B and are managed medically. However, surgery in type B is indicated if medical treatment fails and complications develop.

Mr Perkins is a 32-year-old investment banker who presents with chest pain. It came on while he was at a party in a bar with friends. He has a family history of cardiovascular disease but no other cardiovascular risk factors. He is normally fit and well, although he says he has had a cold and fever for the past couple of days. His ECG shows >2 mm ST elevation in leads V_1–V_4 and, as he is at a hospital with the necessary resources, he is scheduled for primary angioplasty. However, no coronary artery occlusion was seen on his angiogram.

What is the most likely diagnosis? Which question(s) in particular should you ask on the history?

Chest pain and fever suggest an acute inflammation due to, for example, myocarditis/pericarditis but the ECG does not support this (it would classically show saddle-shaped ST elevation in a number of leads not conforming to the territory of a single coronary artery). Normal angiography ruled out coronary artery disease. The most likely diagnosis is **coronary spasm due to cocaine usage**. You should specifically ask about recreational drugs in order to investigate this possibility.

9

Mr Daniels is a 52-year-old man who presents to A&E with a 4-hour history of chest pain associated with nausea and vomiting. His cardiac risk factors include a 15-pack-year history of smoking, although he quit 10 years ago, and a father and brother who had heart attacks in their fifties. He has no other medical history of note and reports no symptoms of reflux disease, but drinks 20 units of alcohol a week. On examination he appears uncomfortable and dyspnoeic. The rest of his examination is unremarkable except for mild consolidation at his left lung base. His ECG and troponin on admission are normal. A chest radiograph confirms a small effusion on the left.

What are the most likely diagnoses? If his 12-hour troponin levels are normal, does this change your differential? What complications should you be particularly wary of?

Nausea and vomiting are commonly associated with inferior MIs. However, the small unilateral pleural effusion should alert you to the possibility of **Boerhaave's syndrome** – a perforation in the oesophagus. This was indeed the case with this patient, whose 12-hour troponin levels proved to be normal. Note that the vomiting should precede the onset of pain in Boerhaave's: contrast this with MI (pain precedes vomiting), as it is the vomiting that causes the perforation (whereas in infarction, it is the post-infarct inflammation that irritates the diaphragm). Not unusually, this patient was not a particularly good historian and could not recall which came first.

Patients with Boerhaave's are prone to develop a pleural effusion, pneumomediastinum and/or pneumothorax, perhaps followed by infection with gastrointestinal flora (mediastinitis and sepsis). Treatment consists of prompt antibiotic therapy and surgical repair of the oesophagus with mediastinal washout. Prognosis is grim, with a 30% mortality if surgical intervention is initiated within 24 hours, rising to 50–65% if surgery is delayed beyond 24 hours. Whilst it is a rare diagnosis it is important to be aware of it as early diagnosis is critical in increasing the chances of survival.

Mrs Peacock is a 74-year-old woman 2 days post-op (carotid endarterectomy following an ischaemic stroke) who has been referred to the medical team for an episode of chest pain that began half an hour ago. She is a type 2 diabetic, for which she takes metformin and gliclazide. She is also treated for hypertension and hypercholesterolaemia, but has never smoked and has no family history of cardiovascular disease. She usually takes warfarin for atrial fibrillation, but this was stopped prior to her operation. She says the pain is always there but is not severe. On examination she appears unwell lying at 30 degrees in bed, with shallow and rapid breathing. Her lung fields are clear on auscultation. Her pulse is weak and irregularly irregular, but her heart sounds are normal, and her examination is otherwise unremarkable. Her oxygen saturation is 91% on room air. The chest radiograph is normal. Her ECG shows atrial fibrillation but no ST elevation or other abnormalities. Her 12-hour troponin levels are not elevated.

What is the most likely diagnosis? What investigation would you order next to investigate this?

Mrs Peacock is presenting with an episode of chest pain and breathlessness, on a background of cardiovascular risk factors. Left heart failure secondary to myocardial ischaemia is a possibility, particularly given her risk factors (atrial fibrillation and recent stroke), with the breathlessness due to pulmonary oedema. However, if that were the case you would expect bibasal crackles on auscultation of her lungs. The chest radiograph, ECG, and troponin levels also fail to show signs of left heart failure or myocardial ischaemia.

Her recent surgery and reduced mobility following her stroke are both risk factors for a **PE**, which would explain her breathlessness and reduced oxygen saturation. PE is a diagnosis of exclusion. However, the advent of CTPA has made it possible to see the embolus in a large number of cases. Mrs Peacock was indeed sent for CTPA and found to have multiple small clots in both lungs. She was started on low-molecular-weight heparin and made a good recovery.

9

Viva questions

Why do some but not all patients with acute MIs get nausea and vomiting?

This is called the Betzhold–Jarisch reflex. Infarction of the inferior myocardium irritates the diaphragm, resulting in vomiting. It is not uncommon for this to happen during angiography (and worth warning patients undergoing angiography about!). Patients with infarcts in other territories will not irritate their diaphragm.

How might occlusion of the different coronary vessels be distinguished on ECG?

There are four main patterns of infarction, resulting from occlusion of each of the main coronary arteries

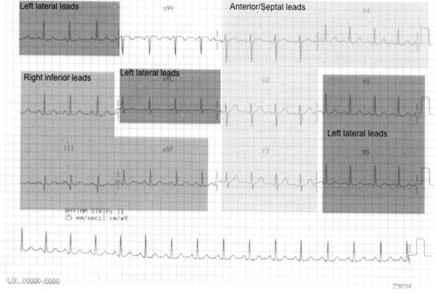

Figure 9.3 Electrocardiogram (ECG) showing the coronary artery territories. The 'Anterior/Septal leads' correspond to the portion of the heart supplied by the left anterior descending artery. The 'Right inferior leads' correspond to the portion of the heart supplied by the right coronary artery. The 'Left lateral leads' correspond to the lateral wall of the left ventricle, supplied by both the left anterior descending and the circumflex arteries.

- **Anterior infarct:** ST elevation in leads V_2, V_3, and V_4 indicates infarction of the anterior surface of the left ventricle, supplied by the left anterior descending artery (LAD).

- **Right/inferior infarct:** ST elevation in leads II, III, and aVF indicates infarction of the inferior surface, supplied by the right coronary artery (RCA).

- **Lateral infarct:** ST elevation in leads V_5 and V_6 indicates infarction of the lateral surface of the left ventricle and may be involved in a circumflex (Cx) or LAD lesion.

- **Posterior infarct:** ST depression in V_1–V_3 with tall R waves is indicative of circumflex occlusion, i.e. a true posterior infarct. This can be difficult to distinguish from LAD territory ischaemia: look particularly for a dominant R wave in V_1 and inferior lead ST elevation in infarction.

What are the earliest biochemical changes in MI? Why do we use troponin levels if they are only reliable after 8 hours?

Troponin levels are used because they have a very high specificity and sensitivity for cardiac damage. Other biochemical markers rise earlier, specifically myoglobin and CK-MB, one of the isomers of the enzyme creatinine kinase. However, these are far less specific for cardiac damage.

Compare the mechanism of action of aspirin, clopidogrel, and abciximab/tirofiban.

All of these are antiplatelet agents with different mechanisms of action:

- **Aspirin** is an irreversible inhibitor of the enzyme cyclooxygenase (COX), which synthesizes inflammatory mediators including the platelet aggregator thromboxane A2. Platelets have no nuclei so cannot synthesize new COX enzymes to compensate for this irreversible inhibition. Aspirin's action is reversed on synthesis of new platelets.
- **Clopidogrel** irreversibly blocks the adenosine diphosphate (ADP) receptor on platelet cell membranes that prevents them binding to fibrinogen and hence inhibits platelet aggregation.
- **Abciximab** and **tirofiban** reversibly block fibrinogen binding to the glycoprotein IIb/IIIa receptors on platelet cell membranes that mediate platelet aggregation (abciximab is a monoclonal antibody, tirofiban a small molecule).

9

A patient attends A&E with central crushing chest pain. Investigations reveal a normal ECG and normal troponins. All other investigations and examinations are normal, and a presumptive diagnosis of new-onset angina is made.

What investigations should you request for a patient such as this presenting with new onset angina?

Exercise tolerance test. An exercise tolerance test may be performed to investigate the possibility of coronary artery disease and therefore the potential benefit to be derived from angioplasty. A patient's ECG and blood pressure are monitored during increasing amounts of exercise (e.g. on a treadmill). ST depression of ≥2 mm, typical symptoms of exertional angina, or ST elevation ≥1 mm usually indicate stenosis of the coronary arteries. A fall in blood pressure during the test is a poor prognostic sign. It is worth noting that this test only has an 80% sensitivity and 70% specificity for detecting ischaemic heart disease (i.e. 30% of positive results will be false positives).

Stress echocardiogram. Some patients cannot perform an exercise tolerance test, for example due to an inability to walk from severe arthritis, severe peripheral vascular disease, or COPD. In these cases a stress echocardiogram can be conducted. The patient is given dobutamine to simulate 'stress' while their cardiac function is assessed by echocardiogram. A normal heart shows increased motility when stressed, whereas ischaemic myocardium is hypokinetic.

Myoview scan. This is an alternative to the tests above and provides a way of looking directly at blood flow within the heart muscle either during exercise (e.g. on an exercise bike) or under medically induced stress. Patients are injected with a radioactive contrast agent (thallium) and a picture taken with a gamma camera.

Pictures at rest and immediately after exercise/stress are compared. Areas of the myocardium with good perfusion appear as 'warm' spots on the scan.

Angiography/angioplasty. If any of the tests above are positive, the patient is suitable for angiography to identify if there is stenosis of a coronary artery. If significant coronary artery disease were found, most centres would undertake coronary angioplasty.

What ECG abnormalities would you expect in a patient who suffered a full thickness inferior MI 2 years previously? What is the basis for these changes?

Old infarcts are visible on ECGs as the infarcted tissue no longer conducts electrical impulses. If they are full thickness, they can be thought of as a window. Thus an electrode positioned next to an area of full-thickness infarct will look through the window of infarcted tissue and pick up the electrical impulses passing through the myocardium on the other side of the heart. This is evident in the ECG in the form of deep, so-called pathological, Q waves (>2 mm deep).

Describe the progression of ECG changes you would expect to see over 7 days in a patient presenting with acute STEMI.

Classically you see the following changes:

1) Tented T waves in the affected leads within minutes of the occlusion (due to localized hyperkalaemia following myocyte ischaemia)
2) ST elevation in the affected leads with ST depression in the reciprocal leads, lasting 24–48 hours
3) T wave inversion, developing in 1–2 days and persisting for weeks or months
4) Q waves, developing within days and remaining permanently

What are the Wells' criteria for PE?

The Wells' criteria establish the pre-test probability of someone having a PE based on several factors:

Clinical symptoms and signs of DVT	3 points
PE is the most likely diagnosis	3 points
Heart rate >100 bpm	1.5 points
Immobilization >3 days or surgery in the last 4 weeks	1.5 points
Previously diagnosed DVT or PE	1.5 points
Haemoptysis	1 point
Malignancy diagnosed in the last 6 months	1 point

Score ≤4 = Low probability of PE. If D-dimer <500 ng/mL, start LMWH, do CTPA to check for PE and treat accordingly.

Score >4 = High probability of PE. Start LMWH, do CTPA to check for PE and treat accordingly.

Treatment for a CTPA verified PE is to continue with LMWH and start warfarin therapy, stopping the LMWH once the INR is stable in the range 2-3. How long to continue with warfarin depends on local protocols, but will usually be 4 weeks to 12 months.

9

For a range of Single Best Answer questions related to the topic of this chapter go to
www.oxfordtextbooks.co.uk/orc/ocms/

Shortness of breath

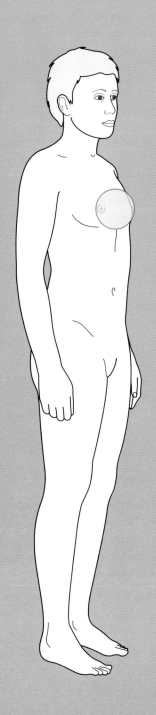

Core case

! *Read through the sections in red, covering up the sections in white that follow so that you don't see the answer. At the end of each red section, try to answer the question before reading on.*

Mrs Finnegan is a 78-year-old widow who presents to your clinic complaining of increasing shortness of breath. She describes that for the past 4 months she has gradually become increasingly short of breath when she walks back up the hill to her bungalow after going to the shops. She is finally seeking medical help because she now finds herself short of breath when she does her gardening. Her sister (a lifelong smoker) died of lung cancer aged 73, and given that Mrs Finnegan used to smoke, she is especially concerned that she may have lung cancer.

In broad terms, what pathological processes could cause shortness of breath?

Shortness of breath essentially means either that not enough oxygen is getting around the body or that there is a cause for increased respiratory drive. This could be due to:

1) **Insufficient oxygen getting into the lungs:**
   - Obstructed airways (obstructive lung disease impairing airflow, e.g. asthma, chronic obstructive pulmonary disease (COPD), lung cancer, or upper airway obstruction, e.g. anaphylaxis)
   - Decreased lung compliance (restrictive lung disease limiting inspiratory volumes, e.g. pulmonary fibrosis)
   - Decreased lung space (e.g. pneumothorax, lung collapse)
   - Weak diaphragm (e.g. Guillain–Barré syndrome, myasthenia gravis)
   - Chest wall that cannot inflate properly (e.g. obesity, kyphoscoliotic spine)

2) **Insufficient oxygen getting from the air into the blood (ventilation–perfusion mismatch):**
   - Pulmonary oedema (e.g. heart failure, liver failure, nephrotic syndrome)
   - Pneumonia
   - Pulmonary embolism (PE; area of lung is not perfused, so no exchange can occur)
   - Pulmonary fibrosis

3) **Insufficient oxygen getting around the body:**
   - Reduced cardiac output (e.g. heart failure, aortic stenosis)
   - Anaemia
   - Shock (i.e. blood pressure <90/60 mmHg from any cause, e.g. sepsis, haemorrhage)

4) **Increased respiratory drive *per se*:**
   - Hysterical hyperventilation
   - Acidaemia (e.g. diabetic ketoacidosis)

> Good history-taking begins with listening to whatever the patient has to tell you, followed by open questions to avoid leading the patient's answers. You can then move on to specific questions that can help narrow your differential diagnosis.
>
> **What specific questions might you ask someone who presents with shortness of breath?**

About the shortness of breath

- **Timing of onset?** This is crucial because vascular (e.g. PE) and mechanical (e.g. pneumothorax, foreign body) pathologies typically present suddenly. At the other end of the spectrum, it may take weeks or months before diseases such as lung cancer or pulmonary fibrosis cause noticeable dyspnoea.

- **Alleviating or exacerbating factors?** Most shortness of breath will be worse on exertion. However, heart failure will also be worse on lying flat; asthma will usually be worse at certain times of the year (e.g. due to pollen allergy), in certain places (e.g. in dusty environments, or when the pets are around), during intense cardiovascular exercise (e.g. running), or in the early hours of the morning. Psychogenic hyperventilation will be worse at times of anxiety and stress.

Risk factors

- **Smoking?** Never forget to ask about smoking and to quantify this in terms of 'pack years' smoked (1 pack = 20 cigarettes; 20 cigarettes a day for a year = 1 pack year).

- **Pets?** The patient may be allergic to pets, especially new ones.

- **Occupational history?** Ask about jobs – there are still lots of people who have been exposed to asbestos, silica dust, and coal particulates in past jobs and who are at risk of pneumoconioses.

- **Medications?** Certain drugs can cause pulmonary fibrosis, e.g. amiodarone, methotrexate, cyclophosphamide, bleomycin, hydralazine, busulphan.

- **Nutritional status?** Even in today's Western societies, some patients present with malnourishment – typically elderly patients who live alone on a 'tea and toast' diet or homeless people with alcoholism who fail to maintain an adequate diet. Such patients are at risk of anaemia and thus shortness of breath.

Associated symptoms

- **Cough?** A cough points strongly towards a respiratory pathology. The nature of the cough is important: *Is it productive? What colour is the sputum? Is there any blood? When does the cough occur? What does the cough sound like?* A persistent, productive cough over the last few days suggests pneumonia; a persistent, productive cough on most days of the past 3 months and spanning years suggests chronic bronchitis; a dry cough present mainly during the episodes of shortness of breath or at night suggests asthma, but may also be a feature of left ventricular failure; blood-stained sputum may suggest a PE, lung cancer, or a cavitating pneumonia. Certain pathologies are associated with characteristic-sounding coughs – for those of you with a veterinary bent, croup is said to sound like a barking seal, whereas recurrent laryngeal nerve palsy (sometimes associated with lung cancer) can produce a bovine cough.

10

- **Chest pain?** If there is chest pain, is it pleuritic? Pleuritic chest pain can suggest pneumonia, a PE, or a pneumothorax, because these often involve the parietal pleura. Non-pleuritic chest pain could indicate a cardiovascular pathology.

- **Muscular weakness or fatigue?** Neuromuscular diseases (e.g. Guillain–Barré syndrome, myasthenia gravis, Lambert–Eaton syndrome, polymyositis, motor neuron disease) will usually be accompanied by muscular weakness or fatigueability.

- **Tender limbs?** Pulmonary emboli can originate from anywhere in the venous system. Patients usually only notice deep vein thrombosis (DVT) if it occurs in a limb as this will usually cause inflammation – a swollen red, tender, warm, shiny looking limb. It is often stated that clots forming below the knee pose less risk of embolizing to the lungs, but autopsy studies have shown that approximately 35% of fatal PEs originate from calf DVTs.

- **Weight loss? Night sweats? Loss of appetite?** These are 'red flag' signs that suggest that a highly metabolic, systemic inflammatory process is going on – often a cancer. Always ask these questions, regardless of the presentation.

- **Loss of blood?** Anaemia can cause or exacerbate shortness of breath, so always ask about heavy menstrual bleeding (in women) and melaena.

> How would the speed of onset influence your differential diagnosis? Think of which pathologies present over seconds to minutes, hours to days, and weeks to months.
>
> Which of these conditions must you exclude, due to their need for urgent treatment or poor prognosis?

Shortness of breath can present over various timescales. Table 10.1 shows the diagnoses that you must exclude in red. Rare diagnoses are in a smaller font.

Table 10.1 Differential diagnosis of shortness of breath

Seconds to minutes	Hours to days	Weeks to months
Acute asthma attack	Pneumonia	COPD
Anaphylaxis	Bronchitis	Chronic asthma
Laryngeal oedema (secondary to burns or chemical irritation)	Heart failure	Heart failure
PE	Pleural effusion	Pulmonary fibrosis
Pneumothorax	Post-operative atelectasis	Anaemia
Flash pulmonary oedema	Chronic, multiple pulmonary emboli	Bronchiectasis
Laryngotracheobronchitis (croup)	Altitude sickness	Physical deconditioning
Hysterical hyperventilation	Guillain–Barré syndrome	Obesity
Inhaled foreign body	Myasthenia gravis	Pulmonary hypertension
Tension pneumothorax	Acute respiratory distress syndrome	Mesothelioma
Acute epiglottitis/ supraglottitis	Lung collapse (e.g. secondary to bronchial carcinoma)	Pulmonary tuberculosis
		Kyphoscoliosis
		Ankylosing spondylitis
		Motor neuron disease

> We already know that Mrs Finnegan's dyspnoea has developed over several months.
>
> **What key clues on history and examination will help you differentiate between the potential diagnoses?** Try to think of key clues for the most common diagnoses in the 'weeks to months' column above.

- **COPD**
  - Remember that COPD is a bracket term encompassing chronic bronchitis and emphysema.
  - History of chronic bronchitis (a clinical diagnosis, based on the presence of a cough, productive of sputum (~10 mL daily), on most days of 3 months for 2 consecutive years) and permanent, largely irreversible, shortness of breath.
  - Presence of risk factors suggesting a cause for COPD:
    - Smoking (usually more than 20 pack years)
    - Occupational exposure to lung irritants, e.g. in coal miners, tunnel workers
    - α_1-Antitrypsin deficiency (liver failure, family history).
  - Signs of COPD:
    - Hyperexpanded chest
    - Breathing through pursed lips
    - Reduced air entry/chest expansion
    - Hyper-resonant percussion note (particularly resonance over the heart and liver).

- **Chronic asthma**
  - History of transient, reversible cough, wheeze and shortness of breath – often worse at night, during exercise, or when exposed to allergens or cold
  - Presence of associated atopic conditions personally or in family members (eczema, hayfever, allergies, nasal polyps)
  - Symptoms may be exacerbated by drugs such as non-steroidal anti-inflammatory drugs (NSAIDs), aspirin, β-blockers (including those in eye drops used for glaucoma)
  - Wheeze on auscultation of the lungs.

- **Pulmonary fibrosis**
  - History of exposure to asbestos, silica, or coal (pneumoconioses causing fibrosis), exposure to drugs (e.g. methotrexate)
  - Signs on examination include:
    - Clubbing (in usual interstitial pneumonitis)
    - Reduced air entry/chest expansion
    - Late inspiratory, fine crackles (often heard throughout the chest rather than just the lung bases as in pulmonary oedema).

- **Heart failure**
  - History of shortness of breath on exertion, orthopnoea (breathless when lying flat), paroxysmal nocturnal dyspnoea (waking up short of breath)
  - Presence of risk factors suggesting a cause for heart failure:
    - Ischaemic heart disease (smoking, diabetes mellitus, hypercholesterolaemia, hypertension, South Asian descent, strong family history)
    - Other atherosclerotic disease (e.g. stroke, transient ischaemic attack (TIA), limb claudication)

- Hypertension (can cause heart failure by itself, in the absence of ischaemic heart disease)
  - Valvular disease (e.g. rheumatic fever, endocarditis, Marfan's syndrome)
  - Cardiomyopathy
- Signs on examination include:
  - Displaced apex beat
  - Third and fourth heart sounds
  - Crackles in both lung bases
  - Raised jugular venous pressure (JVP), hepatomegaly, peripheral oedema (ankles, sacrum).

* **Anaemia**
  - History of bleeding (menorrhagia, melaena, haematochezia) or malnutrition ('tea and toast' diet in elderly, poor diet of homeless). Fatigue as well as shortness of breath on exertion
  - Signs of peripheral (fingers) or central (tongue) cyanosis. Specific signs such as koilonychia, glossitis, and angular stomatitis (all rare). Checking for conjunctival pallor is routinely done but is unreliable.

* **Bronchiectasis** would be suggested by a history of productive cough and recurrent chest infections, or a history of cystic fibrosis.

* **Obesity, kyphoscoliosis, ankylosing spondylitis** can be excluded on inspection.

* **Physical deconditioning** is a diagnosis of exclusion.

10

Your history-taking reveals that Mrs Finnegan is a retired office worker who is diabetic and takes 'aspirin, a pill for the diabetes, and a water tablet for blood pressure'. Her past medical history is significant for an anterior myocardial infarction (MI) 5 years ago, after which she received a single vessel coronary artery bypass graft (CABG). Her parents 'died of old age' and her only sister died of lung cancer. She smoked about 10 cigarettes a day from her early 20s until her late 60s. She has slept propped up with several pillows for the last few years as this is 'more comfortable'. She becomes short of breath when gardening or walking uphill, but feels much better if she stops to catch her breath for a minute. She has not had any cough, chest pain, or dark or bloody faeces or urine. She has not lost any weight, had any night sweats, or noticed any change in appetite. However, she is worried that she may have lung cancer like her sister and was hoping you might be able to do some test to rule that out.

On examination, there are no signs of cyanosis or anaemia. Her blood pressure is 155/80 mmHg and her heart rate is 85 bpm and regular. There is no cervical lymphadenopathy. Her JVP is elevated to 6 cm above the angle of Louis and her apex is most prominent lateral of the mid-clavicular line, in the sixth intercostal space. There is a median sternotomy scar from her CABG 5 years ago. There are no heaves or thrills, and auscultation reveals no murmurs. Chest expansion is symmetrical and resonant to percussion. The trachea is central and breath sounds are heard throughout both lungs, albeit with crackles in both lung bases. Her liver is not enlarged or tender but there is pitting oedema in both ankles. Abdominal examination is normal. Neurological examination is also normal.

Mrs Finnegan's history and examination are consistent with a particular diagnosis for her shortness of breath, but this should be confirmed or refuted with basic investigations.

Given the history and examination, what is the most likely cause of Mrs Finnegan's shortness of breath?

Mrs Finnegan is an elderly lady with shortness of breath and significant risk factors for both cardiovascular disease (ex-smoker, hypertension, diabetes mellitus, previous MI) and respiratory disease (>20 pack years of smoking). However, she gives a clear history of predictable shortness of breath on exercise that is relieved by rest. She has orthopnoea, and has a displaced apex beat, bilateral pulmonary oedema, and ankle oedema. Put together, this all suggests that Mrs Finnegan likely has **congestive heart failure** that is causing reduced cardiac output, pulmonary oedema, and peripheral oedema.

What investigations would you like to arrange?

Bloods

- **Full blood count (FBC):** looking for anaemia.
- **Blood cholesterol, glucose, and HbA1c:** abnormal cholesterol levels (total >5 mM, low-density lipoprotein (LDL) >3 mM or high-density lipoprotein (HDL) <1 mM) and abnormal glucose levels (random >11.1 mM or fasting >7 mM) will give clues about risk factors for ischaemic heart disease, the main cause of heart failure. Mrs Finnegan is a known diabetic, so her HbA1c level will be useful as this is a measure of her glucose control over the preceding 60 days (non-diabetic HbA1c <6.5%).
- **Thyroid function tests (TFTs):** hyperthyroidism can cause a tachyarrhythmia and high-output cardiac failure.
- **Urea and electrolytes (U&Es):** if you think the patient might have excess fluid and therefore there is a chance you might start diuretics to offload some fluid, you need a baseline of electrolyte levels and renal function. It is best to take all the bloods now, both to avoid putting a needle in the patient twice and because an earlier baseline is better.

Imaging

- **Chest radiograph:** looking for signs of heart failure, pneumonia, bronchiectasis, or fibrosis (pneumothorax and collapse are unlikely given the examination findings).
- **Electrocardiogram (ECG):** the ECG is nearly always abnormal in patients with heart failure (indeed, an entirely normal ECG has a negative predictive value for heart failure of about 98%). An important cause of heart failure is necrosis to areas of the heart caused by MI. Diabetics often have 'silent infarcts', which are not noticed by the patient. The presence of pathological Q-waves or a bundle branch block on the ECG would suggest a previous, full-thickness MI.

Other

If the history were suggestive of lung pathology (rather than cardiac pathology) as the cause of breathlessness, you might consider performing:

- **Peak expiratory flow rate (PEFR).** This can be used to stratify the severity of an asthma attack in chronic asthma.

- **Spirometry.** This is used to distinguish between obstructive and restrictive lung disease. In obstructive airways disease (e.g. asthma, COPD, bronchiectasis), the bronchi are narrowed by mucus such that less air can be forcibly exhaled during a single second (forced expiratory volume in 1 second; FEV_1 <70% of predicted), but the total lung capacity is not reduced (forced vital capacity; FVC >70%). In restrictive airways disease (e.g. pulmonary fibrosis), the total lung volume is reduced (FVC <70%) but the amount of air that can be exhaled in the first second remains the same (FEV_1 >70%).

Mrs Finnegan's chest radiograph is shown in Fig. 10.1.

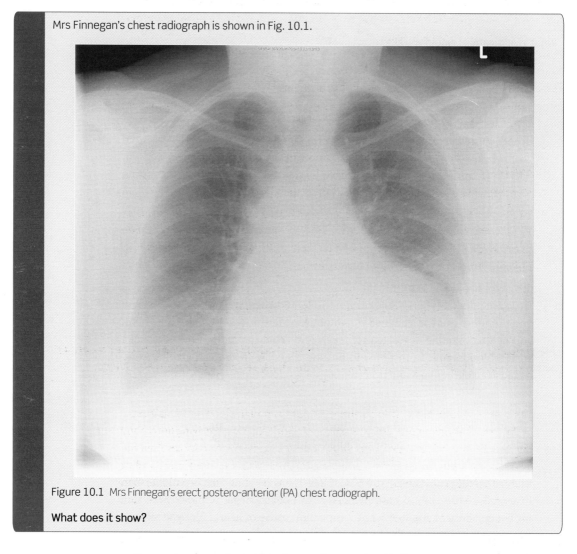

Figure 10.1 Mrs Finnegan's erect postero-anterior (PA) chest radiograph.

What does it show?

Remember to go through radiographs systematically.

- Check the patient details are correct: none are shown here for confidentiality.
- Check the radiograph is technically adequate: full coverage, good penetration, not rotated, adequate inspiration. This radiograph is rotated to the right.
- Present your findings logically. Mrs Finnegan's radiograph shows a reticular pattern of opacification throughout both lung fields, which is much denser in the lower zones bilaterally. There is upper lobe diversion of the pulmonary veins in both lung fields. The heart shadow is significantly enlarged. There are faintly visible sternal sutures (from her CABG) and a small amount of fluid in the transverse fissure.

10

Mrs Finnegan's ECG shows pathological Q waves in leads V_1–V_4. Her FBC is normal. Her glucose is 6.2 mM and her HbA1c is 6.8%. Her total cholesterol = 6.2 mM, LDL = 3.1 mM and HDL = 1.1 mM.

What is the diagnosis for Mrs Finnegan? Can you identify any risk factors for this diagnosis in her history and investigations?

Mrs Finnegan is probably suffering from **congestive cardiac failure** as she has signs of both left ventricular failure (bibasal crackles suggestive of pulmonary oedema, and a displaced apex beat as well as a chest radiograph showing bilateral pulmonary oedema) and right ventricular failure (peripheral oedema and a raised JVP).

Heart failure is a syndrome, not a true pathological diagnosis. Mrs Finnegan's heart failure could be due to any number of causes (e.g. hypertension, valvular disease, alcohol-induced cardiomyopathy) but it is important to remember that the most common cause of heart failure is ischaemic heart disease and that this patient has significant risk factors for this pathology:

- She smoked 10 cigarettes (half a pack) every day for 40 years = 20 pack years.
- She has diabetes mellitus.
- Her total cholesterol (6.2 mM) and LDL (3.1 mM) are elevated.
- Her hypertension is not well controlled (155/80 mmHg). National Institute for Health and Clinical Excellence (NICE) guidelines recommend a target blood pressure of <140/85 mmHg for most people, <130/80 mmHg for diabetics or <125/75 mmHg for patients with proteinuria.

The absence of angina in Mrs Finnegan does not exclude ischaemic heart disease since patients with diabetes mellitus may have 'silent' ischaemia.

How does Mrs Finnegan's diagnosis explain her symptoms (shortness of breath on exertion, orthopnoea) and signs (displaced apex beat, crackles in the lungs, peripheral oedema, raised JVP)?

- **Shortness of breath.** The failing heart can't pump enough blood out. This is especially true if venous return to the heart is increased (e.g. exercise, lying down) and the heart is forced to work harder (e.g. exercise). Back pressure forces fluid out from the pulmonary vasculature into the alveoli, causing 'wet lungs' and a feeling of shortness of breath (some patients will say it feels like drowning). A combination of decreased lung compliance, decreased gas exchange, and airways obstruction are the important drivers of dyspnoea in most left ventricular failure patients.

- **Orthopnoea.** Lying down increases venous return to the heart, which is already struggling to pump out all the blood reaching it. This makes congestion of blood in the pulmonary vessels even worse, forcing more fluid out into the lungs and therefore causing shortness of breath. This is why patients with heart failure often sleep propped up with pillows.

- **Displaced apex beat.** The failing heart can't pump out all of the blood reaching it, so it gradually but inexorably dilates, leading to a displaced (and weak) apex beat. This can be thought of as a volume-overloaded heart. Do not confuse this with hypertrophy, which is caused by hypertension or aortic stenosis. Here, the heart has to pump harder and thus grows concentrically, leading to

10

an undisplaced but forceful or heaving apex beat. This can be thought of as a pressure-overloaded heart. Ultimately, a pressure-overloaded heart can also dilate and fail, but this occurs later in the disease process.

- **Crackles in the lungs.** The build-up of blood in the pulmonary vessels forces fluid out of the vasculature into the alveoli. The alveoli are usually kept open by surfactant, but the interstitial fluid dilutes this and results in increased alveolar surface tension, leading to collapse of the alveoli. As the patient breathes in deeply, the alveoli eventually 'pop open' – the crackles you can hear with the stethoscope.

- **Peripheral oedema.** This is caused mainly because the failing heart cannot pump all of the blood reaching it (venous return), so one gets back pressure in the venous system. This is further compounded by salt and water retention due to activation of the renin–angiotensin–aldosterone system by a low cardiac output. The resultant pressure in the venous system often manifests as a raised JVP and/or a tender, enlarged liver. The increased blood pressure in the venous system also forces fluid out into the surrounding tissues, particularly in places where the venous pressure is highest, i.e. the dependent parts of the body (ankles in someone who has been standing, sacrum in someone who has been in bed). A raised JVP and hepatomegaly are not always clinically apparent.

What second-line investigations should be arranged for Mrs Finnegan?

- **Echocardiography** to assess ventricular function and confirm low cardiac output and heart failure, assess valve patency, and look for areas of dyskinesia.
- **Coronary angiography** if you suspect this lady's heart is failing because of coronary artery disease. This is quite likely in Mrs Finnegan's case given her history of previous MI and risk factors for atherosclerotic disease.

Mrs Finnegan went for echocardiography. This showed anterior akinesia and a left ventricular ejection fraction of 36%. Coronary angiography showed patent graft vessels but an occluded left anterior descending artery, plus severe stenosis of the right coronary and circumflex arteries. Based on this, it is fair to proceed based on a working diagnosis of congestive heart failure secondary to ischaemic heart disease.

What drug treatments would you offer this lady? Don't worry about specific drugs. Try to think what types of drug might help with: (1) her symptoms (too much fluid in lungs and limbs), (2) the pathological mechanism involved in heart failure, and (3) the underlying cause of the problem (atherosclerosis, in her case).

1) **Symptomatic relief**: her symptoms are largely due to her left ventricular failure (pulmonary oedema). You should treat this as follows:
   - In those patients presenting with acute pulmonary oedema (i.e. not our patient) – sit upright, give oxygen, and reduce cardiac pre-load with **vasodilators** such as morphine, nitrates, and furosemide.
   - Chronically – with a loop **diuretic** such as furosemide, which may be combined with the potassium-sparing diuretic spironolactone.

2) **Pathophysiological mechanism**: reduced cardiac output activates two physiological systems that actually worsen the situation in heart failure: the

sympathetic and the renin–angiotensin systems. Greater sympathetic activation increases heart rate and contractility via β-adrenergic receptors. This increases the heart's oxygen demand, which may already be compromised in heart failure (particularly if secondary to ischaemic heart disease), and at higher heart rates filling time and therefore cardiac output may be further reduced. Activation of the renin–angiotensin system results in increased water retention, leading to fluid overload. Logically, therefore, addressing the unhelpful response of these two systems is associated with improved mortality:

- **Reduce the oxygen demand of the heart**: heart failure is usually due to not enough blood reaching the hard-working myocytes, which start to die. One way of treating this is to use a β-**blocker** which slows the heart beat, although β-blockers must never be used if patient is in acute LVF. The patient won't like it (as a slower beating heart will make them feel tired and lethargic) but the many double-blinded, randomized controlled trials have shown that the patient will live longer. The trick is to start with a small dose of β-blocker and increase it very slowly.

- **Inhibit the renin–angiotensin–aldosterone system**: angiotensin-converting enzyme (ACE) inhibitors limit activation of the renin–angiotensin–aldosterone pathway, thus reducing reabsorption of sodium and water from the kidneys. Several double-blinded, randomized controlled trials have now shown that ACE inhibitors reduce mortality in heart failure. Angiotensin II receptor blockers (ARBs) may be used as an alternative to ACE inhibitors. NICE guidelines suggest that aldosterone antagonists such as spironolactone can also be used.

3) **Underlying cause**: the most common cause of heart failure is **atherosclerosis** of the coronary arteries and you should consider addressing this. There are various ways of preventing atherosclerosis getting worse (and maybe even helping the body start to reverse it): **statins** to reduce cholesterol levels and prevent progression of the atheroma; **aspirin** to reduce the risk of thrombosis leading to heart ischaemia or infarction; and **medication for diabetes mellitus** if the patient is diabetic, as uncontrolled diabetes leads to hyperglycaemia which accelerates atherosclerosis.

In advanced heart failure, treatments can include digoxin, cardiac resynchronization therapy (biventricular pacemakers), implantable cardioversion devices (ICDs), mechanical assist devices, or heart transplantation.

Also, in addition to drug treatments, your management should include conservative measures, such as advice to adopt a healthy (low-salt) diet, minimizing alcohol intake, and taking regular exercise.

Mrs Finnegan told you that she was concerned she may have lung cancer, because she used to smoke and her sister died of lung cancer.

Can you reassure Mrs Finnegan that she does not have lung cancer?

It is important to address a patient's concerns and expectations. If these issues are not addressed, patients will go away unsatisfied and worried. This is not only unethical, as you could prevent the unnecessary agitation, but potentially uneconomical, as they may seek a second opinion.

Mrs Finnegan does not give a history suggesting any warning signs for lung cancer (dry cough, haemoptysis, hoarse voice, loss of weight, poor appetite, night sweats). Head and neck examination revealed no lymphadenopathy or Horner's syndrome. Her chest radiograph showed no 'coin lesions' that could indicate a tumour. But despite all this, it would be unwise to categorically inform the patient that 'she does not have lung cancer' because one cannot be 100% sure that she doesn't have a small tumour which we simply haven't picked up. Given her 20-pack-year smoking history, it is probably wiser to explain that although she is at an increased risk of lung cancer because of her previous smoking, you could not see any tumours on her current chest radiograph nor were there any signs in her history or examination that are suggestive of cancer. Explain that you cannot rule out cancer 100% with any tests, but that you have found no evidence of it at the moment and her current symptoms are much more likely to be due to heart failure.

10

Short cases

> Mr Humbolt is a 52-year-old gentleman who underwent a partial hepatectomy for primary hepatic carcinoma 24 hours ago. On the ward round, Mr Humbolt complains of a 'painful, rattling cough'. His pulse is 105 bpm regular, blood pressure 125/75 mmHg, respiratory rate 18/min and temperature 37.1°C. Chest expansion is reduced bilaterally and there are crackles in both lung bases. The base of the right lung is dull to percussion and has reduced breath sounds on auscultation.
>
> **What reasons can you think of for this patient's breathlessness? What is the most likely diagnosis in this patient?**

There are many reasons for breathlessness post-operatively:

- **Atelectasis (alveolar collapse).** Pain sometimes prevents patients from breathing adequately and expectorating any mucus in their lungs. The mucus eventually plugs the bronchioles, preventing air entry, and areas of lung collapse as the trapped air is gradually absorbed into the surrounding tissues. In some countries this is prevented by having post-operative patients blow bubbles though a straw placed in a bottle of water, which encourages forceful expiration.

- **Pneumonia.** This is fairly common post-operatively for a combination of factors: poor clearance of mucus due to pain, aspiration of gastric contents, infection from operative intubation, and a somewhat weakened immune response from the physiological stress of surgery.

- **Pulmonary oedema.** This can be due to heart failure and/or excessive fluids peri-operatively.

- **PE.** DVT is very common after surgery due to the combination of trauma and immobility, and classically occurs 10 days post-operation. Large DVTs can be prevented by using compression stockings on the legs, mobilizing patients as early as possible, and using low-molecular weight heparin.

- **Anaemia.** Patients may be anaemic if there was significant blood loss during surgery.

- **Pneumothorax.** This should always be considered if the patient has had any interventions near the chest either during the surgery or around the time of surgery (e.g. insertion of central venous line, intercostal anaesthetic block).

The 'rattling cough' is highly suggestive of mucus trapped in the lungs. The reduced chest expansion, crackles, and dull percussion all suggest a collapse of a segment of lung, most notably on the right. This picture would fit with **post-operative atelectasis**, caused by the patient not breathing out deeply enough to clear his lungs of mucus. This can be prevented with adequate analgesia. Nonetheless, it is important to confirm this diagnosis and exclude the others listed above so this patient would require a chest radiograph (looking for collapse, consolidation from pneumonia, oedema, or a pneumothorax), FBC (looking for anaemia or a raised white cell count (WCC) from infection such as pneumonia), and C-reactive protein (CRP) levels (which will be raised in infection or tissue damage but is useful to monitor as a sign of improvement or deterioration). The most important treatment for post-operative atelectasis is physiotherapy, analgesia and oxygen.

10

Maggie is a 16-year-old student referred to the respiratory physicians for her recurrent shortness of breath. She describes how she has found herself getting short of breath over the last few months. This mainly occurs in the evenings, and is often associated with a dry cough. In between these episodes, she describes herself as being fine, although she admits that she feels 'a bit unfit because I'm breathless when I go for even a gentle run with my dad'. She denies any weight loss, fevers, dark faeces, or changes in menstruation. She thinks her father suffers with eczema, and is sure that her brother and father have mild hayfever, as does she. She lives at home with her family, none of whom smoke, and a pet dog.

What is the most likely cause of shortness of breath in Maggie? How can this be confirmed? What long-term management will Maggie require?

Maggie has intermittent episodes of shortness of breath that are worse in the evenings and on exercising. Some episodes are associated with a dry cough but in between episodes she is apparently fine. She also has a family history of atopic individuals, with several members including herself having hayfever and/or eczema. The picture of reversible, intermittent shortness of breath and cough in someone with a family history of atopy is strongly suggestive of **asthma**.

Asthma is a disease caused by a hypersensitive immune reaction in the bronchi, which leads to excessive mucus production and bronchoconstriction. The combination leads to an **obstructive airways disease** which can be **confirmed on spirometry**. This should show a relatively normal FVC but a significantly reduced forced expiratory ratio (FER) – as the problem is not lung capacity but obstruction affecting the speed at which air can get out of the lungs. (For the precise diagnostic criteria see Chapter 7.)

Management of asthma is based on three different mechanisms:

1) **Avoidance of trigger(s)**. These can include smoke, allergens (e.g. dust mites, pollen, pets), or exercising in cold air, but often no obvious trigger is known.

2) **Bronchodilation**. Dilatation of the bronchi can be achieved by either increasing sympathetic stimulation to the lungs (e.g. β_2-agonists or phosphodiesterase inhibitors = theophyllines) or decreasing parasympathetic stimulation to the lungs (e.g. antimuscarinics). These compounds can be inhaled in short-acting forms for acute attacks, or in long-acting forms for prophylaxis. β_2-Agonists can also be given intravenously (IV) if needed.

3) **Reduction of immune response in lungs**. This can be achieved using inhaled or, in severe cases, oral corticosteroids.

Mr Marley is a 67-year-old retired musician. He has been referred to the respiratory physicians by his GP because of persistent shortness of breath and recurrent chest infections. You enter the room to find him standing, with his arms propped against the edge of the table. His breathing is laboured and he has a rattling cough. He finally sits down and explains that he always feels short of breath, and his wife has noticed that he often wheezes. He coughs up phlegm every day, and says he has been doing so for at least 2 years almost non-stop, although it is worse in winter. He knows this is all because of his lifetime habit of smoking – he has smoked about 30 cigarettes a day for over 40 years.

On examination, you find there is peripheral and central cyanosis. His breathing is laboured, with intercostal recession and an audible wheeze. His chest appears slightly hyperinflated and chest percussion fails to reveal the usual dullness over the liver and heart. The rest of the examination is normal.

Spirometry in the clinic reveals FVC = 70% of expected and FER = 60% of expected.

What is the likely diagnosis? How should this be managed?

Mr Marley is a patient with >20 pack years of smoking who has had a productive cough every day for >3 consecutive months a year for at least 2 years (chronic bronchitis) and hyperinflated lungs (suggesting emphysema). The combination of chronic bronchitis and emphysema in a lifelong smoker is highly suggestive of **COPD**. This is a disease caused by the persistent toxicity of smoke, which leads to goblet cell hyperplasia (and thus excessive mucus production), damaged ciliated epithelial cells (which usually clear mucus), and inhibition of α_1-antitrypsin (and thus active trypsin, which degrades the interstitial matrix proteins, leading to loss of elasticity of the lungs and alveoli merging into bullae). The result is lungs with decreased compliance (hence the decreased FER), less surface area (hence the decreased FVC), and lots of mucus that cannot be cleared. As a consequence, patients suffer chronically from poor gas exchange in their lungs and recurrent infections.

According to British Thoracic Society (BTS) guidelines, COPD can only be diagnosed if spirometry shows FEV_1 <80% predicted and FEV_1:FVC (FER) ratio <70% predicted. Notice that spirometry in COPD patients often shows both a reduced FER (due to obstructed airways) and a reduced FVC (although the lungs are hyperinflated, their lack of elasticity means they shift a smaller volume of air as much remains trapped in the lungs). This is not the case in asthma, where usually only the FER is affected. Notice also that the shortness of breath in COPD is persistent and largely irreversible. Again, this is not the case in asthma, where patients are not short of breath between attacks.

The management of COPD (as per the NICE 2004 guidelines) involves:

- **Smoking cessation.** This is the single most important factor in limiting the progression of the disease.

- **Effective inhaled therapy.** As in asthma, short- and long-acting β_2-agonists and/or antimuscarinics can be used to control symptoms and improve exercise tolerance in patients. Inhaled corticosteroids should be added to long-acting bronchodilators to decrease exacerbation frequency in patients with an FEV_1 less than or equal to 50% predicted who have had two or more exacerbations requiring treatment with antibiotics or oral corticosteroids in a 12-month period.

- **Pulmonary rehabilitation** (for all patients who need it). A programme of physiotherapy, exercise, education, etc. This increases exercise tolerance and quality of life.

10

- **Non-invasive ventilation (NIV).** This is the treatment of choice when medical therapy fails to control persistent hypercapnic ventilatory failure during exacerbations.

- **Long-term oxygen.** Patients who are hypoxic with an arterial partial pressure of oxygen (P_aO_2) <7.3 kPa on air, or <8.0 kPa and pulmonary hypertension, should use long-term oxygen for 15 hours each day. This prevents progression to cor pulmonale but does not improve symptoms. Ambulatory oxygen can be given to those who desaturate whilst walking, whilst short-burst oxygen is for psychological benefit only.

- **Manage exacerbations.** Appropriate use of inhaled steroids, bronchodilators, and vaccines should be used to reduce the incidence of exacerbations. The impact of exacerbations should be minimized by:
    - Giving self-management advice on responding promptly to the symptoms of an exacerbation
    - Starting appropriate treatment with oral corticosteroids and/or antibiotics
    - Use of non-invasive ventilation when indicated
    - Use of hospital-at-home or assisted-discharge schemes.

10

Mr Marley (from the previous case) is admitted to hospital 5 months after he is diagnosed with COPD by the respiratory physicians. He has become very short of breath, confused, and unable to complete full sentences. His daughter explains that he has been deteriorating gradually over the past week and was due to see the respiratory physicians again next week. He is immediately given high-flow 100% oxygen. An arterial blood gas (ABG) is performed and shows P_aO_2 = 6.2 kPa, P_aCO_2 = 7.3 kPa, pH = 7.28, bicarbonate = 33 mM, base excess = −1 (on 15 L of O_2). The emergency physicians request a chest radiograph, which shows no signs of consolidation (pneumonia) or pulmonary oedema. His ECG, FBC, and serum biochemistry are normal.

What is the problem? How would you proceed?

Mr Marley's arterial blood gas shows **type II respiratory failure** (P_aO_2 <8 kPa and P_aCO_2 >6.5 kPa). With his history and ABG results (indicating a degree of metabolic compensation but with an acute acidosis), this is an acute-on-chronic picture.

Type II respiratory failure is **a medical emergency.** Untreated, the rising CO_2 will narcose the patient, who will fall into an irreversible coma and die. Treatment involves:

1) **Controlled oxygen therapy**. The high CO_2 that defines type II respiratory failure often means that patients no longer rely on CO_2 levels to stimulate breathing. If you give 100% oxygen, you risk causing a respiratory arrest so this must be stopped in Mr Marley's case. Instead, give controlled oxygen (24–28% using a special connector on the oxygen mask) aiming for oxygen saturations of 80–90%. Perform repeated arterial blood gases, looking for a drop in P_aCO_2.

2) **Improve ventilation**. If the CO_2 does not drop with controlled oxygen therapy, ensure the airway is fully patent and involve the intensive therapy unit (ITU) physicians as the patient will need assisted ventilation (e.g. non-invasive ventilation) and/or respiratory stimulants (e.g. doxapram).

3) **Treat the underlying cause**. Assess for reversible causes of reduced gas exchange (e.g. pneumothorax, pneumonia, pulmonary oedema, PE) and reversible causes of reduced ventilation (e.g. airway obstruction due to reduced consciousness, opiate medication).

10

Miss Chanda is a 27-year-old factory worker from Zambia who has been referred to the medical admissions unit of her hospital because of severe shortness of breath, which has been present for the last few days. She finds she is always breathless but it is worse with even mild exertion such as walking. She has felt very weak for the last few days and has had a dry cough and fever. On hindsight, she thinks she has probably been losing weight for the past few months. Her past medical history is unremarkable and she takes no regular medications.

On examination, Miss Chanda has a temperature of 37.6°C and a respiratory rate of 25/min. Her JVP is not raised, there is no peripheral oedema, and both heart sounds are present without any added sounds. There are fine crackles heard over the entirety of both lung fields. The rest of the examination is entirely normal. Her oxygen saturations are 90% on air but the attending nurse comments that when Miss Chanda came back from walking to the toilet, her saturations had dropped to 82%. A chest radiograph shows diffuse interstitial shadowing throughout both lung fields.

What is the likely diagnosis? What tests will you arrange?

The clinical picture of dry cough, shortness of breath, low oxygen saturation/desaturation on exercise, and diffuse interstitial shadowing throughout the lungs on a chest radiograph in a young patient from Africa should always make you suspicious of ***Pneumocystis jiroveci* pneumonia** (previously known as *Pneumocystis carinii* pneumonia, or PCP). *Pneumocystis* is an opportunistic organism that rarely causes problems in healthy adults but commonly causes pneumonia in immunosuppressed patients. Indeed, *Pneumocystis* pneumonia is a common complication of patients with AIDS. It is diagnosed by performing microscopy (+ silver staining) and culture on sputum and broncho-alveolar lavage samples.

If you suspect *Pneumocystis* pneumonia, you should arrange to test for two other infections:

- **HIV testing.** Offer Miss Chanda an HIV test. If this is positive, you will need to check her CD4+ lymphocyte levels, as these dictate the need for antiretroviral therapy.

- **Tuberculosis testing,** as this is a frequent cause of pulmonary pathology in HIV-positive patients. Testing is by microscopy (+ Ziehl–Neelsen staining) and culture of sputum and broncho-alveolar lavage samples.

Mrs Betty is a 48-year-old magistrate who attends your clinic complaining of persistent breathlessness that has been getting worse over the last year. It is worst when she takes her dog for a brisk walk, but is always present, even at rest. She denies any cough, weight loss, or night sweats. She smokes 'the odd cigarette' at social events, but never more than five cigarettes a month. A recent blood test ordered by her referring GP shows:

RBC	4.7×10^{12} cells/L
WCC	8×10^9 cells/L
Hb	11.5 g/dL
ESR	72 mm/h
HbA1c	5%
Blood glucose	4.8 mM
Total cholesterol	4.3 mM
LDL	2.2 mM
HDL	2.1 mM

(Hb, haemoglobin; ESR, erythrocyte sedimentation rate)

Her past medical history includes rheumatoid arthritis, for which she takes methotrexate.

On examination, you notice swelling of the metacarpophalangeal joints (MCPJs) and ulnar deviation of her fingers on both hands. Her pulse is 80 bpm and regular, her blood pressure is 120/80 mmHg and she is apyrexial. There are no signs of peripheral or central cyanosis, anaemia, or lymphadenopathy. Her trachea is central and her apex beat undisplaced. Heart sounds I and II are present with no added sounds, and no carotid bruits. Her lungs expand symmetrically and show normal resonance to percussion. However, very fine crackles can be heard all over her lung fields. She has no peripheral oedema and her abdominal and neurological examinations are entirely normal.

Flow spirometry reveals FVC = 65% and FEV_1 = 88%. An ECG shows sinus rhythm with no abnormalities.

What is the most likely cause of Mrs Betty's shortness of breath? How would you confirm this?

Mrs Betty does not have any features that are strongly suggestive of the 'most likely' or 'must exclude' diagnoses listed in Table 10.1. Her flow spirometry suggests a *restrictive lung pathology* as her expiratory rate is normal (FEV_1 >70%) but her lung capacity is reduced (FVC <70% predicted value) – in other words, the problem is not getting air out but how much air her lungs can hold. The fine crackles heard all over her lungs, combined with her flow spirometry and absence of another obvious diagnosis, suggest that Mrs Betty has **pulmonary fibrosis.** Pulmonary fibrosis can be caused by congenital diseases (e.g. neurofibromatosis, Gaucher disease), systemic inflammatory diseases (e.g. rheumatoid arthritis, ankylosing spondylitis, sarcoidosis), chemical irritation (e.g. silica, asbestos, coal dust, chlorine), drugs (e.g. methotrexate, amiodarone), allergic reations (e.g. bird-funcier's lung), radiation, or the cause may not be known (e.g. cryptogenic fibrosing alveolitis/usual interstitial pneumonitis).

The best way to confirm Mrs Betty's postulated diagnosis of pulmonary fibrosis is a high-resolution chest computed tomography (CT) scan. Radiologists can diagnose pulmonary fibrosis with high sensitivity and specificity by looking for characteristic linear reticular opacities and a ground-glass appearance of the lung.

Mrs Betty should switch from methotrexate to another immunosuppresive agent in order to control her rheumatoid arthritis. Whilst this is unlikely to improve her condition significantly, it will at least prevent further deterioration, particularly if the fibrosis was mainly due to the methotrexate rather than the rheumatoid arthritis (which explains her elevated ESR).

10

Claire is a 15-year-old student who presents to her GP complaining of general fatigue and shortness of breath when she exercises. She has recently found herself feeling unusually tired towards the end of the day and complains that she is more breathless than usual during her netball training. She does not smoke, denies any cough, and is never woken at night feeling short of breath. She has never travelled further than Italy, and is otherwise fit and well. She has no family history of respiratory disease. When specifically asked, she reveals with some embarrassment that her periods are 'a bit heavy' but she denies her faeces ever being dark or bloody. Physical examination is unremarkable. Spirometry reveals an FVC = 90% and FER = 88%.

What tests should the GP arrange? What is the most likely diagnosis?

This patient does not have any features of heart failure (no clinical features and a bit young), aortic stenosis (no murmur), asthma (no cough, no wheeze, normal spirometry), COPD (young with no family history to suggest α_1-antitrypsin, non-smoker, no cough), Guillain–Barré syndrome (no recent infection, normal spirometry), lung collapse (no physical signs), or pneumothorax (no physical signs). However, she does complain of fatigue and admits to having menorrhagia (heavy menstrual periods). It is therefore very likely that this patient is **anaemic**, as the most common cause for anaemia in menstruating women is menorrhagia. The GP should order an FBC (which will probably reveal a microcytic hypochromic anaemia, compatible with an iron-deficiency anaemia) and clotting studies (to rule out a clotting disorder that may be causing or exacerbating her menorrhagia). If a gynaecologist referral does not reveal any abnormality causing the menorrhagia, the patient will probably benefit from pharmacological treatment. NICE guidelines recommend a levonorgestrel-releasing intrauterine device (LNG-IUD) or the combined oral contraceptive pill.

10

Mr Andreyov is a 42-year-old investment banker who presents to your clinic complaining of shortness of breath. He says the sensation of breathlessness is always present. He doesn't think it is connected, but mentions that he has found it increasingly difficult to type at his computer recently and he has noticed some twitching of his thighs that he initially put down to stress. He has no relevant past medical history and is not on any medication. He has never smoked and drinks approximately 10 units of wine a week with evening meals. He sleeps well and has not noticed any change in his appetite nor any bloody or dark faeces or urine. He is worried he may be developing heart problems because he admits his diet is not very healthy and he doesn't exercise enough.

Cardiovascular, respiratory, and abdominal examination is unremarkable. Neurological examination reveals that the first dorsal interossei on both hands are wasted. In addition, you note fasciculations over both his thighs, reduced power (4/5) on knee flexion, and an upgoing plantar reflex. Flow spirometry reveals FVC = 60% and FER = 80%.

What important diagnosis should you consider in this patient?

10

Mr Andreyov has presented with shortness of breath and a history suggestive of weakness/poor coordination in distal muscle groups of his upper limbs. He has wasting of his hand muscles (suggesting a lower motor neuron or muscular pathology). He also has fasciculations in his right leg (suggesting a lower motor neuron pathology) but an upgoing plantar reflex (suggesting an upper motor neuron pathology). The combination of upper and lower motor neuron pathology signs in any patient should always arouse the suspicion of **motor neuron disease** and warrants referral to a neurologist. The shortness of breath is likely to be due to diaphragmatic weakness, usually a late sign of this disease.

Mr O'Hara is a 62-year-old retired paratrooper who presents to your clinic complaining of shortness of breath. He first noticed this a month ago when he was jogging, but says he now feels breathless with minimal exertion. He has not had a cough and has never smoked. He drinks a few pints of ale every weekend. His only past medical history is a fractured right tibia 20 years ago and hypertension for which he takes a thiazide diuretic and an ACE inhibitor. He has not noticed any changes in his bowel habit or urine, but admits that he has probably lost weight over the past few months.

On examination, you can feel several enlarged lymph nodes in the right anterior cervical chain of his neck. His right lung shows decreased expansion and is dull to percussion in the bases. Vocal fremitus is markedly reduced on the right. His cardiovascular, abdominal, and neurological examinations are all normal.

What diagnosis should you consider for Mr O'Hara? What are your next steps?

Mr O'Hara gives a history of worsening shortness of breath and weight loss. His respiratory examination reveals lymphadenopathy of the neck and signs consistent with a right-sided **pleural effusion**. The combination of weight loss, lymphadenopathy, and pleural effusion should make you think of a **malignant pleural effusion** caused by infiltration of the pleural space by metastatic cancer cells.

Your next step should be to arrange a **chest radiograph**. If this confirms a right-sided pleural effusion, the effusion should be sampled (**thoracocentesis**) to determine if the fluid in the pleural space is due to changes in osmotic forces (*transudate*, with protein <25 g/L) or due to infiltration of the pleural space by metastatic cancer cells, infectious agents or inflammatory proteins (*exudate*, with protein >35 g/L). A finding of protein between 25 and 35 g/L is considered indeterminate and you should then use Light's criteria (see Chapter 8).

You should also arrange for a **lymph node fine needle aspiration (FNA)**, as Mr O'Hara's history of weight loss should alert you to the possibility of a malignancy.

Mr O'Hara's chest radiograph showed a massive pleural effusion in his right lung. Thoracocentesis showed it to be an exudate, with low glucose and abnormal-looking lymphocytes. A lymph node biopsy confirmed the presence of binucleated lymphocytes (Reed–Sternberg cells), which are diagnostic of Hodgkin's lymphoma.

10

Viva questions

The notes of a patient you are asked to see state that his past medical history is of 'asthma/COPD'. Is such a diagnosis possible?

It is obviously possible to have both COPD and asthma at the same time, but it is much more likely that a clear diagnosis has simply not been made. Asthma and COPD are very different diseases and should not be confused:

- Asthma is a *reversible* and *transient* obstruction of the airways caused by excessive mucus production, airway inflammation, and constriction of the bronchi. Flow spirometry shows only obstructive changes (i.e. drop in FEV_1 <70% but normal FVC, that is, a reduced rate of air flow but a normal lung capacity). It is usually accompanied by a cough and is often worse at night. It is often linked to triggers such as pollen, dust mites, or cold air and is common in patients who are atopic (i.e. who suffer from multiple diseases caused by excessive IgE-mediated hypersensitivity, such as eczema, hayfever, or urticaria).

- COPD is an *irreversible* and *progressive* obstruction of the airways. There is a history of chronic bronchitis and/or emphysema. Flow spirometry shows obstructive changes (i.e. drop in FEV_1 <70%) but often also a degree of restrictive change (i.e. FVC <70%). Patients are usually older and have a smoking history of >20 pack years.

Which different classes of inhaled drugs are used in obstructive airways disease (asthma and/or COPD)? What is the mechanism of action of each drug?

1) Short-acting bronchodilators
   - Salbutamol (UK: blue, 'Ventolin'): selective β_2-agonist. Acts on a G-protein-coupled receptor, activating adenylate cyclase and increasing the formation of cAMP, leading to relaxation of the smooth muscle lining the airways.
   - Ipratropium (UK: white + green, 'Atrovent'): antimuscarinic/cholinergic. Antagonizes muscarinic acetylcholine receptors in the airways, preventing parasympathetic-mediated smooth muscle contraction. Often used in COPD, but less often in asthma.
   - Salbutamol + ipratropium (UK: white + orange, 'Combivent').

2) Inhaled steroids
   - For example beclometasone, budesonide (UK: brown inhalers), fluticasone (UK: orange inhaler). Work by affecting intracellular transcription of various proteins to reduce inflammation in the airways. Used in asthma and COPD as second-line treatment.

3) Long-acting bronchodilators
   - Salmeterol, formoterol: long-acting β_2-agonist (LABA). Mechanism like the short-acting variant.
   - Tiotropium: long-acting anticholinergic (LACA). Mechanism like the short-acting variant. Used in COPD but not asthma.
   - Long-acting bronchodilators can also be combined with inhaled steroids, e.g. budesonide + formoterol (UK: red, 'Symbicort') or fluticasone + salmeterol (UK: purple, 'Seretide').

4) **Oxygen**. Don't forget that this is a drug! It may be given acutely, e.g. in an ambulance or in hospital, or long-term, e.g. in severe COPD.

Oral drugs are also sometimes used, including oral steroids, xanthine derivatives (theophylline, aminophylline), leukotriene antagonists (montelukast), and cromones (sodium cromoglycate, nedocromil sodium).

What is the difference between bronchitis and pneumonia, and between broncho- and lobar pneumonia?

Both are lower respiratory tract illnesses, but bronchitis is a disease of the airways whereas pneumonia is a disease of the alveoli. In bronchitis, airways inflammation leads to excess mucus production and partial airway obstruction. In pneumonia, pus accumulates in the alveoli impairing gas exchange and appearing as consolidation on a chest radiograph.

Pneumonia can be classified by the pattern of anatomical involvement. In bronchopneumonia, focal areas are affected in a patchy distribution that may involve one or more lobes. Lobar pneumonia, as the name suggests, involves most or all of a single lobe.

Why do we get short of breath at altitude? What is the pharmacological mechanism of action of the altitude sickness drug acetazolamide ('Diamox')? How might this influence breathlessness at altitude?

At altitude, there is a lower partial pressure of oxygen in the environment. Thus there is a smaller concentration gradient driving oxygen from air in the alveoli into the blood. As a result there is a reduction in gas exchange, leading to hypoxia. This causes breathlessness and compensatory hyperventilation to correct the hypoxia. The hyperventilation causes a respiratory alkalosis, which makes one feel lightheaded. One either feels breathless (from hypoxia) or dizzy (from hyperventilation).

Acetazolamide inhibits carbonic anhydrase, an enzyme that catalyses the conversion of CO_2 and H_2O into HCO_3^- and H^+. There are two theories as to how this might alleviate breathlessness. The first suggests the inhibition of carbonic anhydrase leads to a build-up of CO_2, stimulating the respiratory centre and increasing the ventilatory drive. The other theory suggests that the inhibition of carbonic anhydrase in the kidneys leads to a bicarbonaturia and hence a metabolic acidosis, which offsets the respiratory alkalosis due to hyperventilation at altitude. The acidosis caused by acetazolamide enables one to hyperventilate at altitude (thus reducing hypoxia and shortness of breath) without becoming lightheaded from the alkalosis that would otherwise result from hyperventilating.

There has been a large decrease in the incidence of epiglottitis in recent years, particularly in children. How can you explain this?

Historically, epiglottitis primarily affected children and was a severe, sometimes fatal, condition. It is nearly always due to bacterial infection by *Haemophilus influenzae* B (HiB). The development and introduction of a HiB vaccine into the UK vaccination schedule in the mid-1990s has led to a decrease in both meningitis (another condition often caused by HiB) and epiglottitis.

10

What is the difference between type I and type II respiratory failure? What are some of the causes?

Respiratory failure is defined as impairment of pulmonary gas exchange sufficient to result in hypoxaemia (P_aO_2 <8 kPa or 60 mmHg) and/or hypercapnia (P_aCO_2 >6 kPa or 45 mmHg). It is divided into two types depending on whether CO_2 is expelled (and therefore normal or low) or retained (and therefore raised):

Type I respiratory failure

- Pathology: this is a problem with *one* gas (oxygen), i.e. **hypoxaemic respiratory failure**. It is caused by a **ventilation–perfusion mismatch** in the lungs, with ventilation of the unaffected alveoli normal. Compensatory hyperventilation increases CO_2 removal but not O_2 saturation as blood leaving the unaffected alveoli is already saturated.
- Causes: any lung disease, e.g. asthma, COPD, pneumonia, pulmonary fibrosis, pulmonary oedema.

Type II respiratory failure

- Pathology: this is a problem with *two* gases (oxygen and carbon dioxide), i.e. **hypercapnic respiratory failure** (low P_aO_2 and a raised P_aCO_2). This is caused by **ventilatory failure**, i.e. impairment of the respiratory 'bellows', resulting in alveolar hypoventilation.
- Causes:
  - Decreased respiratory drive, e.g. opiates, central neurological damage (stroke, head trauma)
  - Impaired lung movements, e.g. chest wall deformity (as in Duchenne's muscular dystrophy for example), neuromuscular impairment (as in motor neuron disease)
  - Lung pathology, e.g. long-standing COPD, pulmonary fibrosis.

What is the difference between a 'pink puffer' and a 'blue bloater'?

Note that these terms are not synonymous with type I and type II respiratory failure! They are outdated terms but still used on the wards sometimes to describe two distinct clinical pictures that arise in chronic lung disease (e.g. COPD), although this is of course a simplification and every patient will be different:

- 'Pink puffers' respond to hypercapnia and hypoxaemia by increasing their respiratory rate, resulting in normal P_aO_2 levels and a 'pink' appearance. As a result of the hard work to maintain their oxygenation, they often have a barrel-shaped, hyperinflated chest and may breathe through pursed lips. They nonetheless complain of shortness of breath on mild exertion. Broadly speaking, their prognosis is better than that of 'blue bloaters'.

- In 'blue bloaters' the presence of chronically high P_aCO_2 levels results in desensitization of the respiratory centre to P_aCO_2 and chronic cyanosis, giving them a 'blue' appearance. They are chronic CO_2 retainers, becoming reliant on their hypoxic (rather than hypercapnic) drive. They are often bloated because of widespread peripheral oedema caused by right heart failure secondary to the lung problems (cor pulmonale). In general, their prognosis is poor.

10

What is Eisenmenger's syndrome?

Eisenmenger's syndrome describes the situation where a left to right cardiac shunt becomes a right to left (or bidirectional) shunt. It follows a sequence of events beginning with a left to right cardiac shunt, due to, for example, a ventricular and/or atrial septal defect, patent ductus arteriosus. Over time this causes progressive pulmonary hypertension as the delicate pulmonary vasculature is subjected to blood emerging from the left ventricle, via the shunt, at greater pressures than normal pulmonary pressures. Eventually the pulmonary hypertension provides enough resistance to reverse the direction of the shunt.

Ultimately it leads to heart failure and can only be cured by heart–lung transplant. Women of childbearing age must be warned about the increased mortality in pregnancy (over 50%) and strongly advised against it. This condition has become relatively rare in the UK due to early surgical correction of cardiac defects (indeed this is the rationale behind early correction of such defects).

Which muscles are responsible for inspiration and expiration: (a) at rest and (b) during exercise or respiratory distress?

Table 10.2 Muscles responsible for inspiration and expiration

	Inspiration	Expiration
(a) At rest	Diaphragm External intercostals	(Passive – natural elastic recoil of lung)
(b) During exercise/ respiratory distress	Diaphragm External intercostals Scalene Sternocleidomastoids	Natural elastic recoil of lung PLUS: Internal intercostals Abdominal muscles (rectus and transversus abdominus, internal and external obliques)

10

What is the differential diagnosis for bibasal crepitations? Which features in the history and examination will help you to distinguish them?

Table 10.3 Differential diagnosis for bibasal crepitations

Cause of crepitations	Key clue
Pulmonary oedema	Displaced apex, raised JVP, ankle oedema
Pulmonary fibrosis	Reduced expansion, clubbing, crepitations that do not vary with cough
Bronchiectasis	Chronic productive cough, wheeze, and crepitations that vary with cough, clubbing
Pneumonia	Acute productive cough, fever, chest pain, bronchial breathing, dull percussion

What is your differential diagnosis for shortness of breath in a post-operative patient? What key clues will help you identify the most likely cause? How will you manage each cause?

Table 10.4 Common causes of post-operative dyspnoea

Cause	Key clue	Management
Pulmonary oedema	Displaced apex, raised JVP, ankle oedema, frothy sputum ± evidence of MI on ECG or biochemically (troponins)	Sit patient up, furosemide, oxygen, morphine, nitrates
PE	Fever, tachycardia, signs of DVT in leg. Onset typically 10 days after surgery	LMWH, start warfarin, TED (anti-embolism) stockings to prevent more DVTs
Atelectasis	Crepitations, mild fever, fruity and painful cough. Onset typically during first 48 h after surgery	Analgesia, oxygen, and lung physiotherapy
Pneumonia	Productive cough, fever, chest pain, bronchial breathing, dull percussion, increased vocal resonance, consolidation on chest radiograph	Antibiotics
Pneumothorax	Area of lung with decreased air entry, hyper-resonance and air in pleural space on chest radiograph	Chest drain

LMWH, low-molecular weight heparin.

Once a patient has been diagnosed with chronic heart failure, there are several medications that can help reduce their mortality. What are the key trials demonstrating mortality benefit in chronic heart failure?

- **ACE inhibitors**: the **SAVE**[1] and **SOLVD**[2] trials both showed that ACE inhibitors can significantly reduce mortality from chronic heart failure, from 8–28% depending on how symptomatic the patient is (more symptomatic patients gain more benefit). In patients who cannot tolerate ACE inhibitors because of their side-effects (e.g. cough), the **ELITE II**[3] study and **Valsartan Heart Failure Trial**[4] have shown that **angiotensin II receptor blockers** (A2RB) are as effective as ACE inhibitors in reducing mortality. However, a third trial (**RESOLVD**[5]) had to be stopped because of increased mortality in the group receiving the A2RB.

- **β-Blockers**: Several trials[6] including **CIBIS-II**[7] and **MERIT-HF**[8] have shown that β-blockers reduce mortality from chronic heart failure by about 25%.

- **Spironolactone**: the **RALES**[9] trial found that the aldosterone receptor spironolactone reduced mortality from chronic heart failure by about 30%.

[1] Pfeffer MA, Braunwald E, Moye LA, Basta L, Brown EJJ, Cuddy TE *et al.* (1992). Effect of captopril on mortality and morbidity in patients with left ventricular dysfunction after myocardial infarction. Results of the survival and ventricular enlargement trial. The SAVE Investigators. *New Engl J Med*, **327**: 669–677.

[2] SOLVD Investigators (1991). Effect of enalapril on survival in patients with reduced left ventricular ejection fractions and congestive heart failure. The SOLVD Investigators. *New Engl J Med*, **325**: 293–302.

[3] Pitt, B, Poole-Wilson PA, Segal R, Martinez FA, Dickstein K, Camm AJ *et al.* (2000). Effect of losartan compared with captopril on mortality in patients with symptomatic heart failure: randomised trial – the Losartan Heart Failure Survival Study ELITE II. *Lancet*, **3551**: 1582–1587.

[4] Cohn JN, Tognoni G (2001). A randomized trial of the angiotensin-receptor blocker valsartan in chronic heart failure. *New Engl J Med*, **345**: 1667–1675.

[5] Tsuyuki RT, Yusuf S, Rouleau JL, Maggioni AP, McKelvie RS, Wiecek EM *et al.* (1997). Combination neurohormonal blockade with ACE inhibitors, angiotensin II antagonists and beta-blockers in patients with congestive heart failure: design of the Randomized Evaluation of Strategies for Left Ventricular Dysfunction (RESOLVD) Pilot Study. *Can J Cardiol*, **13**: 1166–1174.

[6] Doughty RN, Rodgers A, Sharpe N, MacMahon S (1997). Effects of beta-blocker therapy on mortality in patients with heart failure. A systematic overview of randomized controlled trials. *Eur Heart J*, **18**: 560–565.

[7] CIBIS-II Investigators (1999). The Cardiac Insufficiency Bisoprolol Study II (CIBIS-II): a randomised trial. *Lancet*, **353**: 9–13.

[8] Hjalmarson A, Goldstein S, Fagerberg B, Wedel H, Waagstein F, Kjekshus J *et al.* (2000). Effects of controlled-release metoprolol on total mortality, hospitalizations, and well-being in patients with heart failure: the Metoprolol CR/XL Randomized Intervention Trial in Congestive Heart Failure (MERIT-HF). MERIT-HF Study Group. *J Am Med Assoc*, **283**: 1295–1302.

[9] Pitt, B, Zannad F, Remme WJ, Cody R, Castaigne A, Perez A *et al.* (1999). The effect of spironolactone on morbidity and mortality in patients with severe heart failure. Randomized Aldactone Evaluation Study Investigators. *New Engl J Med*, **341**: 709–717.

10

 For a range of Single Best Answer questions related to the topic of this chapter, and hyperlinks to a selection of keypapers go to **www.oxfordtextbooks.co.uk/orc/ocms/**

Breast lump

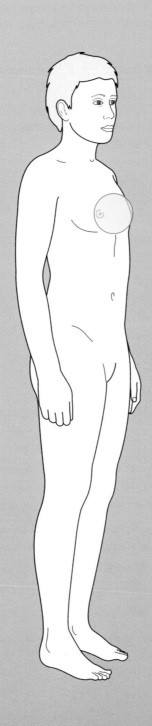

Core case

> **!**
> •
> *Read through the sections in red, covering up the sections in white that follow so that you don't see the answer. At the end of each red section, try to answer the question before reading on.*

> Miss Collins is a 28-year-old teacher who presents to her general practitioner (GP) because she has noticed a lump in her breast.
>
> **What is your differential diagnosis for a breast lump?** Consider which diagnoses are more or less likely, and try to stratify your differential according to the age of the patient.

The four most common diagnoses for a breast lump are:

> Benign cystic change (also known as fibrocystic change, fibroadenosis, or benign breast change)
> Fibroadenoma
> Cyst
> Carcinoma

If we consider women of all ages, there are a number of other potential diagnoses:

> Fat necrosis
> Periductal mastitis
> Abscess
> Galactocele
> Phyllodes tumour
> Sarcoma
> Duct papilloma
> 'Non-breast' lumps, e.g. lipoma, sebaceous cyst

The age of the patient is one of the most useful pieces of information for narrowing the differential (see Fig. 11.1). As an approximate guide, the most common diagnoses in the following age groups are:

- <30 years: physiologically normal lumpy breast; benign cystic change; fibroadenoma; abscess (if breast-feeding); galactocele (if breast-feeding)
- 30–45 years: benign cystic change; cyst; abscess (especially smokers); carcinoma
- 45–60 years: cyst; abscess (smokers); carcinoma
- >60 years: carcinoma

Note: It is worth emphasizing that **breast cancer is possible in all ages, is common, and is potentially very serious.** Therefore you **must exclude it in any**

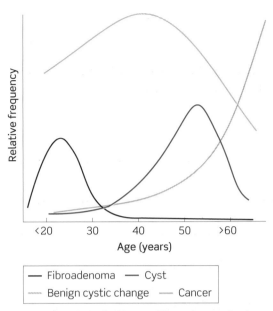

Figure 11.1 Relative incidence of fibroadenoma, benign cystic change, cyst, and carcinoma by age.

presentation of breast lump, regardless of how benign it seems. Failure to diagnose breast cancer is the most common malpractice claim in the USA!

> **Are there any diagnoses that you would only encounter in breast-feeding women?**

Galactoceles may occur during or shortly after the cessation of lactation. They may present as a firm mass (often subareolar) and are caused by the obstruction of a lactiferous duct. The duct gradually becomes more distended with milk and epithelial cells, and may rarely be complicated by a secondary infection leading to abscess formation. Clinically, a galactocele is very similar to a cyst on examination.

In addition, lactating women are predisposed to **mastitis** (whether or not they have a galactocele). The causative organisms are usually skin commensals such as *Staphylococcus aureus* or *Staphylococcus epidermidis* – this is in contrast to the periductal mastitis and abscess formation seen in older women, in whom anaerobic bacteria may also be implicated.

> The vast majority of women who present with a breast lump will be concerned that they have breast cancer. As part of a thorough history-taking it is obviously important to enquire about risk factors.
>
> **What are the main risk factors for breast cancer?**

Two of the greatest risk factors for breast cancer are being female and of advanced years. Otherwise, the following are recognized as important factors:

* **Previous breast cancer**
* **Family history of breast cancer.**[†] Suspicions should be raised if:
  - Three close blood relatives (on the same side of the family) develop breast cancer at any age

- Two close blood relatives develop breast cancer before the age of 60
- One close blood relative develops breast cancer before the age of 40
- One male close blood relative develops breast cancer
- One close blood relative develops bilateral breast cancer

♦ **Previous ovarian, endometrial, or bowel cancer**

♦ **Irradiation to the chest wall** (such as mantle irradiation for Hodgkin's lymphoma)

♦ **Increased exposure to oestrogens,** especially cyclical stimulation:
  - Early menarche (<13 years)
  - Late menopause (>51 years)
  - Nulliparity
  - Having a first child after the age of about 30 years
  - Not breast-feeding
  - Hormone replacement therapy (HRT)[†]
  - Use of combined oral contraceptive pill (COCP)
  - Obesity

[†] Remember that the vast majority of women presenting with a breast lump will be concerned that they have cancer – even if they do not voice these concerns explicitly. As such, a frank but sensitive discussion of any familial cases of breast cancer serves to illustrate your familiarity with these concerns and expectations. Although many patients will consider that breast cancer in their 82-year-old grandmother constitutes a significant family history, this is not the case. Whilst it is important to establish how many family members have been affected by breast cancer, it is also informative to ascertain how many women in the family have *not* had breast cancer. For example, a history of an aunt and a sister with breast cancer becomes less significant if the patient is one of 10 sisters and has 7 aunts.

[†] Not only does HRT usage increase the risk of breast carcinoma, but it also extends the normal age range of benign cystic disease and cysts – which are not normally seen in post-menopausal women. Combined HRT (oestrogen and a progestogen) increases the risk of breast cancer more than oestrogen-only HRT.

The first stage is to take a history from Miss Collins.

What are the relevant pieces of information to obtain from the history?

While addressing the history of the presenting complaint, you will need to establish:

♦ **How long has the lump been there? Why was it first noticed?** An abscess or cyst can appear very rapidly, whereas tumours such as fibroadenomas or carcinomas typically grow more slowly. Of course, it is perfectly possible for a mass such as a carcinoma to be present for a long time before it is noticed. It may be that a lump was noticed during routine self-examination, or by a partner, or because of associated skin changes, or perhaps due to pain.

♦ **Has there been any breast trauma?** Trauma, whether accidental (such as a seat-belt injury) or iatrogenic (e.g. aspiration of a cyst), predisposes to fat necrosis and infective sequelae such as an abscess.

♦ **Has the lump got bigger, smaller, or stayed the same size? Are changes related to the menses?** Just as an abscess or cyst can appear 'almost overnight', they can also undergo rapid increases in size. Lumps that undergo cyclical changes in size or character (for example, becoming more tender) are far more likely to represent benign cystic breast disease than a more sinister condition such as carcinoma.

* **Is the lump painful?** Benign cystic change, acute mastitis, and abscesses classically cause breast pain and tenderness. Benign cystic change may, however, be painless. Simple cysts may or may not be tender. While it is perfectly possible for a carcinoma to be painful, it is more common for carcinoma to present as a non-tender lump.

* **Has she noticed any skin changes on her breasts?** Warm erythematous skin should raise your suspicions of an infective or inflammatory process such as mastitis or an abscess, or perhaps an inflammatory breast carcinoma (rare). The patient may have noticed puckering of the overlying skin ('peau d'orange'), and this suggests carcinoma until proven otherwise.

* **Has she noticed any changes to her nipples?** Some women will naturally have inverted nipples, but any recent distortion of the nipple also hints at carcinoma.

* **Has she noticed any discharge from her nipples?** A nipple discharge in the context of a breast mass is suggestive of carcinoma (bloody discharge), intraductal papilloma (serous or serosanguinous discharge), periductal mastitis arising from duct ectasia (green, brown, or yellow discharge), or a galactocele (milky discharge).

* **Is the patient otherwise fit and well?** The majority of patients presenting with a breast lump will have no other symptoms. Patients with mastitis or an abscess may be febrile. Breast carcinoma rarely presents with generalized systemic symptoms – such as weight loss, night sweats, and fevers – that are sometimes seen with other forms of malignancy. They may, however, present with signs of metastasis, such as back pain (spinal metastases).

* **Does the patient have any of the risk factors mentioned earlier?**

11

Miss Collins reports that she noticed the lump in her right breast two days ago while she was showering. The lump has not changed in size or location since she first noticed it. It is non-tender. There is no reported history of breast trauma and she is otherwise fit and well. She is a non-smoker and is taking no medications. She started having periods when she was 13 years old, but has no children and has no significant gynaecological history. Her stepmother was diagnosed with ovarian cancer at the age of 52, and her paternal grandmother died of breast cancer aged 79.

You perform a breast examination.

What will you look for on *inspection* of the breasts?

The key features to look for are:

* **Asymmetry:** many women will have one breast that is larger than the other, but any new change is significant.

* **Contours:** any disruption to the normally smooth curvature of the breast is suspicious, although it could simply be due to fibrocystic change or naturally lumpy breasts.

- **Skin changes:** look for erythema, ulceration, dimpling, peau d'orange. Radio-therapy tattoos (small black/blue dots) may be visible in patients who have had previous treatment.
- **Nipple changes or discharge:** note any new inversion of the nipple, and the colour of any discharge.

Miss Collins' breasts appear normal on gross inspection. There is no asymmetry, skin abnormality, or nipple inversion. Having inspected Miss Collins' breasts, the GP moves on to palpation. Having palpated the normal breast, axillary tail, and axilla, she then asks Miss Collins to point to the lump in her right breast. As with any lump, it is important to characterize the site, size, shape, surface, borders, and consistency.

Which of these features are most useful for distinguishing between a carcinoma, fibroadenoma, cyst, and benign cystic disease? What other information should the GP hope to gain from the examination?

The four most common presentations of a breast lump (across all age groups) classically differ, in the ways listed in Table 11.1.

Table 11.1 The four most common presentations of a breast lump

Lump	Surface	Borders	Consistency	Mobility	Fixity[†]	Lymphadenopathy
Solitary cyst	Smooth	Distinct	Firm to lax	No	No	No
Fibroadenoma	Smooth	Distinct	Rubbery	Yes	No	No
Benign cystic change	Irregular	Indistinct	Mixed	No	No	No
Carcinoma[‡]	Irregular	Indistinct	Hard	No	Maybe	Maybe

[†] Fixity or tethering to skin or underlying muscle. It will not be possible to move intradermal masses such as sebaceous cysts independently of the overlying skin. If a deeper mass shows the same fixity to skin and/or underlying pectoralis muscle (assessed by asking the woman to push her hands into her hips, hence contracting the muscle) it is highly suggestive of a malignancy. Fixation of a deeper mass to skin is almost diagnostic of cancer – the only conditions that may mimic this are fat necrosis or a pointing abscess.

[‡] Please bear in mind that this is a classical presentation of breast carcinoma – but not all carcinomas have read the books. You MUST retain a high index of suspicion for any solid breast lump, particularly those presenting in older women.

Miss Collins has an oblong-shaped lump in the upper inner quadrant of her right breast. The lump is approximately 2 cm × 1 cm. It has a smooth surface, clearly defined margins, a rubbery consistency, and is highly mobile.

What diagnosis is most likely? What features of history and examination make other common diagnoses in a 28-year-old woman less likely?

It is most likely that Miss Collins has a **fibroadenoma**. Fibroadenomas are aberrations of normal breast development that contain both stromal and epithelial elements. As many as 7–13% of young women will have a fibroadenoma at some stage during their teens or twenties.

The most common breast lumps in women of Miss Collins' age are fibroadenomas, benign cystic change, normally lumpy breasts, and lactation-related abscesses. As Miss Collins is not lactating, and has no breast tenderness, warmth, or erythema, we can effectively rule out an abscess. The fact that her lump is very clearly delineated points us away from diffuse benign cystic disease, and the fact that she has recently noticed a new lump argues against this being part of normally lumpy breasts.

We should at least consider a cyst or carcinoma, even though they are rare in women of this age. The clearly defined borders of this lump are consistent with those of a cyst, but the rubbery nature of the lump is not cyst-like (cysts are either firm or lax, according to the pressure of fluid within them). Furthermore, cysts are not highly mobile lumps. Miss Collins has no risk factors for breast carcinoma (her family history is non-significant) and malignant breast lumps are typically hard with irregular margins – although it is often hard to differentiate the characteristics of a lump on clinical examination.

What should the GP do next?

11

All women with a palpable breast lump should be referred to a surgical breast clinic, even if you are fairly certain from your history and examination that the lump is benign – the risk of misdiagnosis is simply too high. As Miss Collins is less than 30 years old and has a lump which does not appear to be growing in size, and which is not hard or fixed to the skin (in other words, there are no alarming features of the lump or history) she should be sent as a **non-urgent** referral.

How are all solid lumps investigated in the breast clinic?

Breast lumps undergo **triple assessment**, the components of which are:

1) **Clinical examination.**

2) **Radiological examination:**
   - Ultrasound if <35 years old. The breast tissue in younger women is too dense to evaluate by radiography (mammography).
   - Two-view mammogram (± ultrasound) if >35 years old. Cancer is suggested by increased density, irregular margins, spiculation (like shards of glass), and accompanying clustered irregular microcalcifications.

3) **Fine needle aspiration** (FNA) or **core biopsy**. FNA will only provide information on the type of cells (and whether they are dysplastic or not) whereas core biopsy will additionally provide information on local architecture (e.g. invasion of surrounding structures).

Miss Collins was referred to the breast clinic and was seen 1 month later. She underwent triple assessment which revealed that the lump was a fibroadenoma.

What treatment options are available to Miss Collins?

There are two treatment options. The majority of fibroadenomas will resolve over several years and pose no increased risk of malignancy. As such, it is often appropriate to adopt a conservative stance and **reassure** the patient that this is a benign lesion.

The second option is to remove the fibroadenoma by **excisional biopsy**. Indications for this include patient preference, a lump that is increasing in size (either clinically or as measured by ultrasound), or a lump that is causing discomfort.

11

Short cases

Mrs Sowerby is a 78-year-old lady who presents to her GP with a lump in her right breast. She reports that the lump has been there for some time, but that she didn't want to bother the doctor unnecessarily. She has had two breast cysts aspirated in the past – one in her early fifties and one in her early sixties. Her delay in presentation to the GP was because she thought that this was another cyst and, as she remembers being told that cysts are harmless, she wanted to see if it would go away of its own accord. However, this lump now feels different from her previous cysts and she is keen for the doctor to take a look.

The lump has gradually got bigger over the past few months, but she reports that it is not painful. She is not aware of any trauma to her breast. When specifically asked about any changes to her nipples, or any nipple discharge, she says that the right nipple is now quite flat whereas it used to be prominent. She has not, however, noticed any discharge.

Mrs Sowerby has one daughter, aged 55, whom she breast-fed. She started having periods 'at the same time as everyone else', and underwent the menopause aged 50. She did not use HRT. She wears a ring pessary for vaginal prolapse but has no other significant gynaecological history.

When asked about any family history of breast cancer, she says that her daughter was told she had a 'breast mouse' when she was younger, but she is unaware of any other breast disease in the family. Her husband died of prostate cancer aged 81.

She is otherwise fit and well. She takes a thiazide and angiotensin-converting enzyme (ACE) inhibitor for hypertension.

On examination, Mrs Sowerby has an obvious lump in the upper outer quadrant of her right breast. The lump extends towards her nipple, which is observed to be inverted. There is skin tethering over the superior portion of the lump. Palpation of the mass reveals a hard irregular lump approximately 5 cm × 4 cm. The edges are irregular and poorly defined. The mass is non-mobile and appears fixed to the overlying skin. Several lymph nodes are palpable in the right axilla. The left breast and axilla appears normal.

What is the most likely diagnosis? What is the next step for Mrs Sowerby?

The long history of a progressively enlarging non-tender lump, together with skin and nipple changes, and examination findings of an irregular, hard, fixed mass with local lymphadenopathy are highly suggestive of breast **carcinoma**.

Mrs Sowerby should be **urgently referred** to the breast surgeons for triple assessment.

Mrs Sowerby was seen by the surgeons within a fortnight. She underwent triple assessment. Core biopsy revealed a poorly differentiated ductal carcinoma.

Where are the most likely sites of metastasis and how should these potential sites be investigated if there is any suggestion of metastasis?

Breast carcinoma most commonly metastasizes to lungs, liver, bone, and brain. As such, appropriate staging investigations include:

- **Lungs:** chest radiograph.
- **Liver:** abdominal palpation; liver enzymes; liver ultrasound.

- **Bone:** palpation for sites of bony tenderness; serum calcium and phosphate; isotope bone scan (or magnetic resonance imaging, MRI).
- **Brain:** a computed tomography (CT) head scan may be conducted if there are symptoms or signs suggestive of brain metastases, such as fitting or early morning headache and nausea.

Staging investigations were all negative for Mrs Sowerby.

In broad terms, what treatment options are available to her?

Treatment options include:

- **Local treatments:** surgery, radiotherapy
- **Systemic treatments:** chemotherapy, hormonal therapy, monoclonal antibodies (e.g. herceptin)

The precise treatment will depend upon size, stage, and grade of the tumour, nodal status, receptor status, suitability for surgery, and other comorbidities.

Hormonal therapy is usually given to all women who have tumours expressing oestrogen receptors ('ER positive') and/or progesterone receptors ('PR positive'). Such therapy decreases oestrogen synthesis (aromatase inhibitors) or selectively blocks oestrogen receptors (e.g. tamoxifen).

11

Mrs Regan is a 55-year-old housewife who presents to her GP with a lump in her left breast. She first noticed the lump as a painful swelling above her nipple 2 days ago. The lump has increased in size slightly during that time. She says that the overlying skin is quite red and tender, but that there have been no nipple changes. She has felt a bit feverish for the past day or so but is otherwise well.

She underwent the menarche aged 13 and the menopause aged 52. She has four children, all of whom are in their thirties, and all of whom were breast-fed. She has been taking HRT for the last 3 years. She is not aware of any previous breast disease and has had no gynaecological operations. There is no family history of breast cancer.

She smokes cigarettes and has a 21-pack-year history. She drinks 12–15 units of white wine per week. She reports that she is otherwise fit and well, and only occasionally takes sumatriptan for migraines.

On examination, there is peri-areolar erythema of the left breast. The reddened skin is warm to the touch. An irregular firm mass, approximately 1.5 cm in diameter is palpable medial to the nipple, within the boundaries of the erythema. There is skin tethering. Two lymph nodes are palpable in the left axilla. The right breast and axilla appear normal. Mrs Regan is febrile.

What is the likely diagnosis? How should Mrs Regan be managed?

The sudden appearance of a painful lump in the breast of a middle-aged smoker, combined with examination findings of fever, skin erythema, and tethering, make it highly likely that this is a **breast abscess**.

Mrs Regan should be started on appropriate antibiotics that give anaerobic cover. She will also need referring to the surgeons to either have the abscess drained surgically or aspirated. Any residual solid mass that remains after drainage and antibiotic treatment will need triple assessment.

11

Mrs Dean is a 42-year-old lady who presents to her GP because she noticed a tender lump in her right breast 2 days previously. She first noticed the lump while examining her breasts in the bathroom mirror (she does this each month). She says that she has not had any previous breast lumps. She feels well.

She started having periods aged 13, and is pre-menopausal. She has no children. She uses the combined oral contraceptive pill. There is no family history of breast cancer. She does not smoke or drink alcohol, and takes no regular medications.

Her breasts appear normal on gross inspection. Palpation of the right breast reveals a well-circumscribed tender mass in the lower inner quadrant. The lump is approximately 2 cm in diameter, has a smooth surface, and is firm to the touch. It is non-mobile and is not fixed or tethered to the overlying skin. Both axillae and the left breast appear normal.

The GP refers Mrs Dean for triple assessment. Ultrasound reveals a well-defined hypoechoic mass in the left lower inner quadrant.

What is the most likely diagnosis? How should Mrs Dean be managed?

The history and examination findings are most consistent with a **cyst**. The well-circumscribed nature of the lump, combined with the smooth surface and firm texture, could possibly be confused for a fibroadenoma, but fibroadenomas are not typically painful and would be unusual in a woman of this age. Furthermore, the ultrasound scan indicates a cystic mass (a solid mass will be hyperechoic on ultrasound, whereas a fluid-filled cyst will be hypoechoic).

The diagnosis can be confirmed by aspirating the cyst. Most cysts contain fluid that is a shade of green (ranging to almost black), brown, or yellow. If the aspirate is blood-stained it should be sent for cytology. The breast should be re-examined after the cyst has been aspirated to dryness. If there is not complete resolution of the lump it will require triple assessment as carcinoma may occur within a cyst.

Miss Pennyweather is a 34-year-old lady who presents to her GP because her left breast is 'lumpy' and tender. She says that she first noticed that her breast felt tender 3 months ago. She has not noticed any skin or nipple changes and has not had any nipple discharge. When asked directly about any relationship to her menstrual cycle, Miss Pennyweather describes how her left breast is more tender in the build-up to her period. Her breast also feels more 'lumpy' during this time, but the lumpiness appears to fade once her period has begun.

She started having periods when she was 13 years old, and has no children. She uses the combined oral contraceptive pill. She was referred to the surgeons with a lump in her left breast when she was 21 years old. This was diagnosed as a fibroadenoma and was managed conservatively. Her mother was diagnosed with breast cancer aged 61 and had a mastectomy.

She has no significant past medical or gynaecological history, and takes no medications. She enjoys the odd social cigarette, but does not drink alcohol.

On examination, Miss Pennyweather's breasts appear normal on gross inspection. Palpation reveals an indistinct area of tender nodularity in the upper outer quadrant of the left breast. The nodularity spans an area of approximately 10 cm in diameter. Discernible lumps within the nodularity have a rubbery texture. The right breast and both axillae appear normal.

What is the most likely diagnosis and how should Miss Pennyweather be managed?

This diffuse nodularity, which shows cyclical variation in both prominence and tenderness, is most likely **benign cystic change** (fibrocystic change, fibroadenosis, or benign breast change). As there are areas of discrete nodularity within the breast these will require triple assessment, and reassurance if no abnormality is detected.

Mr John is a 50-year-old wine merchant. He presents to his GP because he is concerned that he is developing what he refers to as 'moobs'. He has recently started playing rugby for a local veterans team and says that he has become the butt of incessant jokes about his prominent breasts. He says that he has had prominent breast tissue for a few years but would now like to know what is causing it and whether anything can be done about it.

Mr John is not aware of any recent change in the size of his breasts. He says that they are occasionally tender however. There is no family history of breast cancer.

Mr John had a cholecystectomy when he was 43 years old. He takes allopurinol for gout, and a thiazide and ACE inhibitor for hypertension. He smokes a dozen cigars each week, and is not quite sure how much alcohol he actually drinks each week, but estimates that it is approximately three bottles of wine.

On inspection, Mr John has a feminine contour to both breasts, with bilateral areolar prominence. There are no skin changes. The swelling is tender to palpation, but is of uniform consistency. There are no areas of nodularity and both axillae are normal.

What is the most likely diagnosis? What can cause this condition?

11

This generalized enlargement of the male breasts is almost certainly **gynaecomastia**. Although 1% of breast cancer does occur in men, this would be a very unusual presentation as male breast cancer is typically unilateral, non-tender, with an irregular surface, indistinct margins, and a hard consistency (just as in women).

Palpable breast tissue is present in almost a third of adult men and two-thirds of pubertal boys, but is more prominent in some men than others. The majority (two-thirds) of gynaecomastia is 'physiological', and occurs at times of hormonal fluctuation, such as during the neonatal period, puberty, and old age. Pathological causes include:

- Liver disease
- Drugs (e.g. cimetidine, spironolactone, phenothiazines, finasteride, anabolic steroids)
- Primary testicular failure (e.g. anorchia, bilateral cryptorchidism)
- Acquired testicular failure (e.g. mumps orchitis)
- Secondary testicular failure (e.g. panhypopituitarism)
- Endocrine tumours (e.g. testicle, adrenal, pituitary)
- Non-endocrine tumours (e.g. bronchial carcinoma)

Viva questions

What factors determine the prognosis with breast carcinoma?

The principal determinants of prognosis are tumour stage (which reflects the spread of the cancer and therefore incorporates tumour size, nodal status, and presence of metastasis), tumour grade (which reflects the loss of differentiation of the cancerous cells and therefore incorporates their histopathological appearance), hormone receptor status (oestrogen, progestogen, and human epidermal growth factor receptor 2 (HER2)), tumour type (such as lobular or ductal), patient age, and treatment type.

There are various scoring systems, such as the Nottingham Prognostic Index, which incorporate some or all of the factors above to produce an estimate of survival.

What is peau d'orange and what causes it?

Peau d'orange ('orange peel') refers to the skin changes that may occur with an infiltrating carcinoma of the breast. The skin has a dimpled appearance – much like the skin of an orange. Blockage of the dermal lymphatics by a tumour, surgery, or radiotherapy results in cutaneous oedema. Sweat ducts and hair follicles tether the skin, thus resulting in dimples within the oedematous areas.

What is the difference between skin fixity and skin tethering?

If a lesion is fixed to the skin, it cannot be moved independently of the overlying skin. A lesion that is tethered to the skin can be moved independently of the skin to some extent. However, if you imagine that the lesion is tethered to the skin as if by a length of string, it will only move independently of the skin within the limits of the length of string. If you try to move the lesion beyond those limits it will distort and dimple the overlying skin.

Contrast the roles of adjuvant and neo-adjuvant chemotherapy.

Adjuvant chemotherapy is used after surgery and thus the main aim is to treat any micrometastases which remain following surgical excision of the primary. By contrast, neo-adjuvant chemotherapy is delivered before surgery and aims to shrink the primary tumour (thus making it operable, or more amenable to surgical removal) as well as minimizing the metastatic tumour burden. The main advantage of neo-adjuvant chemotherapy is that tumour size can be assessed for response to therapy (which is obviously not possible after surgical resection), and non-response can lead to second-line treatments. Patients selected for neo-adjuvant chemotherapy are typically those at highest risk of micrometastases – young patients, those with large tumours, and those with palpable lymph nodes.

When is mastectomy preferred over breast-conserving surgery?

Breast conserving surgery by wide local excision (WLE) followed by radiotherapy has been shown to produce equal long-term survival to mastectomy, with only a slight increase in the rates of local recurrence. However, not all patients will have cancer that is suitable for WLE. Mastectomy may be necessary to achieve tumour clearance if the tumour is of a large size relative to the breast (i.e. a large tumour, small breast, or both), a tumour that occupies a central position within the breast, multifocal tumours, recurrent tumours, or if the patient prefers this to a WLE. Mastectomy is also indicated for the treatment of male breast cancer.

Although WLE has the theoretical advantage that it may produce better cosmesis, the patient will need to be counselled about the requirement for adjuvant radiotherapy, and perhaps further surgery if there are positive surgical margins or local recurrence. By contrast, mastectomy may obviate the need for further surgery or radiotherapy. Mastectomy may also produce an acceptable cosmetic result if combined with reconstructive procedures such as a latissimus dorsi or transverse rectus abdominis myocutaneous (TRAM) flap.

What are the advantages and disadvantages of FNA over core biopsy?

11

FNA:

- Advantages
  - Quick
  - Minimally invasive
  - Low risk of bruising or local complications
  - Adequate for assessing the hormone receptor status of the cancerous cells.

- Disadvantages
  - May have poor sensitivity (inadequate specimens)
  - *In situ* and invasive disease cannot be differentiated as local architecture is lost during the aspiration (you end up with a solution of floating cells).

Core biopsy:

- Advantages:
  - *In situ* and invasive disease can be differentiated as local architecture is preserved during the biopsy.

- Disadvantages:
  - Higher risk of local complications and bruising than FNA
  - Results are not immediate (compared with FNA)
  - Requires local anaesthesia
  - More invasive and time consuming than FNA.

What methods exist for axillary staging of breast cancer?

There are three main techniques for axillary staging of breast cancer:

1) **Axillary clearance**: removal of all local lymph nodes. Three levels of clearance (I, II, and III) refer to removal of increasing numbers of lymph nodes lateral, posterior, and medial to pectoralis minor.

2) **Axillary sampling**: a minimal dissection of the axilla is undertaken and a selection of at least four nodes is removed from the low axilla for histological analysis.

3) **Sentinel lymph node biopsy**: aims to identify the first node which drains the breast (and is thus the most likely site of metastasis). Blue dye and/or radio-isotope is injected into the peri-areolar tissue in the same breast quadrant as the cancerous tissue. The sentinel node will take up this dye and/or radio-isotope and is identified intraoperatively as 'hot', 'blue', or 'hot and blue'. This single sentinel node can then be removed and sent for histology. The sentinel node is located in the low axilla in >90% of cases. The main advantage of the technique is a considerable increase in sensitivity of lymph node analysis, and avoidance of the high morbidity associated with axillary clearance.

A woman is discussed during a multidisciplinary team (MDT) meeting as having a P4R4C4B5 breast lump. What does this mean?

There are two components to this scoring system. The letters refer to triple assessment:

P = physical examination
R= radiological examination
C = cytology (FNA)
B = biopsy (core)

Each aspect of the triple assessment is then given a score out of 5:

1 = normal (in the context of examination, radiology, biopsy) or inadequate sample (cytology)
2 = benign
3 = probably benign
4 = probably malignant
5 = malignant

Hence a P4R4C4B5 lump had a high probability of being malignant that has been confirmed by biopsy. The overall sensitivity of triple assessment in most UK units is >99.5%.

What is ANDI?

ANDI refers to Aberrations of Normal Development and Involution. These aberrations include fibroadenomas, benign cystic changes (fibroadenosis), intraductal papillomas, duct ectasia, and cysts.

A 40-year-old lady comes to see you, her GP, because she is concerned that two of her younger sisters have developed breast cancer in their thirties. She has not had any genetic testing but has heard about *BRCA* genes on the news. She is convinced that she must be *BRCA*-positive and would like to be referred to a breast surgeon for a prophylactic bilateral mastectomy. How would you approach such a consultation?

It is of course perfectly understandable that this lady is anxious about her chances of developing breast cancer, and it is vital that her concerns are addressed in a sensitive manner. The notion of 'risk' is open to a huge amount of personal interpretation, and part of the challenge in such a consultation is to establish the

11

patient's frame of reference. While it may be all too easy for medics to talk about absolute and relative risk as definable entities, such values will be skewed by socioeconomic and cultural factors and by the patient's personal experience. It is also of paramount importance to use language which the patient understands – some patients may be very familiar with terms such as heritability and dominant traits, whereas for other patients it may be more appropriate to talk about familial or inherited conditions.

A consultation such as the one described above will obviously be directed to a large part by the patient's questions. However, as the GP you may wish to address the following points – if the patient wishes to hear them:

- What does she know about breast cancer, its risk factors, and potential genetic predisposition?

- What is her frame of reference? What where the circumstances surrounding the diagnosis in her two sisters? What was the outcome for her sisters?

- What constitutes a significant family history of breast cancer? (see earlier in this chapter.)

- What proportion of breast cancer is familial? It is important to explain that only a minority (~5%) of breast cancer is familial. This patient, however, is likely to be in that minority as she has two sisters who have been diagnosed before the age of 40.

- What would genetic counselling and genetic testing involve? Many patients are under the false impression that testing will give an immediate result, and are unaware that affected relatives will need to give blood and that test results may take weeks.

- If testing reveals that she is positive for *BRCA1* or *BRCA2*, does this imply that she will definitely develop breast cancer? Does it have implications for the risk of developing other cancers such as ovarian cancer, malignant melanoma, or prostate cancer (in male relatives)? What does a positive result imply for any other of the patient's siblings or children?[†]

- She has mentioned prophylactic bilateral mastectomy, but is she aware of any other options? What about annual mammogram screening? Is she aware that bilateral mastectomy does not entirely eliminate breast cancer risk? Is she aware that some women will also request prophylactic oophorectomy as this reduces risks of both breast and ovarian carcinoma?

- Has she considered any potential effect that genetic testing may have on insurance premiums? – this may sound rather callous, but is a real concern for some patients.

- Is she aware of patient support websites such as http://www.breastcancercare.org.uk/ or http://www.breastcancergenetics.co.uk/?

[†] There are three main genes (*BRCA1*, *BRCA2*, and *TP53*) that are known to carry an increased risk of breast cancer. Possession of one of these mutations significantly increases the risk of developing breast cancer, but does not imply that breast cancer is inevitable. It is, however, important to remember that the *BRCA* mutations also predispose to other cancers. *BRCA1* is associated with an increased risk of ovarian and bowel cancer, while *BRCA2* is associated with an increased risk of ovarian and prostate cancer, male breast cancer, and malignant melanoma.

For a range of Single Best Answer questions related to the topic of this chapter go to
www.oxfordtextbooks.co.uk/orc/ocms/

Epigastric pain

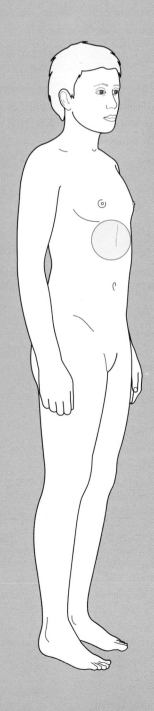

Core case

Mr Simpson is a 60-year-old man who presents to accident and emergency (A&E) with acute epigastric pain.

What is your differential diagnosis for acute epigastric pain? Try to also identify those conditions that you must attempt to exclude at the earliest possible opportunity because they require urgent treatment (surgical or medical).

We have arranged the differential diagnosis in order of likelihood in a man of this age with more likely diagnoses in larger font and less likely diagnoses in smaller font. Pathologies that should be excluded at the earliest possible opportunity are shown in red. Bear in mind that this differential diagnosis refers to epigastric pain as a presentation of 'acute abdomen' and thus differs markedly from epigastric pain presenting as outpatient dyspepsia.

12

> ## Acute pancreatitis
> ## Gastritis/duodenitis
> ## Peptic ulcer disease (gastric or duodenal)
> ## Perforated peptic ulcer
> ## Biliary colic
> ## Acute cholecystitis
> ### Basal pneumonia
> ### Oesophagitis (due to gastro-oesophageal reflux disease, GORD)
> ### Ruptured abdominal aortic aneurysm (AAA)
> Ascending cholangitis
> Myocardial infarction
> Mesenteric ischaemia
> Acute hepatitis
> Non-ulcer dyspepsia (NUD)[†]
> Chronic pancreatitis
> Incomplete bowel obstruction
> Gastric cancer
> Pancreatic cancer (although cancer in the head of the pancreas is normally painless)
> Boerhaave's perforation
>
> [†] Also known as functional dyspepsia; this is a diagnosis of exclusion, made in approximately 30% of patients who are investigated for dyspepsia whose endoscopy is negative. Patients typically complain of discomfort rather than pain and it is unusual for this to present acutely to hospital.

Note that although we have adopted a standard approach of history, examination, and investigations over the course of the following pages, you should use clinical judgement to deviate from this path if one of the 'must exclude' diagnoses is suspected, or if there is a need for urgent resuscitation. For example, if a 69-year-old male diabetic patient with known unstable angina presents with exercise-induced epigastric pain, you would be wise to perform an electrocardiogram (ECG) and obtain baseline observations at the earliest opportunity.

> The first step when taking the history is to characterize the pain using a system such as SOCRATES.
>
> **What key features of the pain would point you to some of the diagnoses above?**

Various characteristics of the pain will help to narrow our differential diagnosis of epigastric pain:

Site:

- Pain that has spread from the epigastrium to involve the rest of the abdomen may suggest peritonitis.
- Pain that has spread from the epigastrium to involve the chest may be cardiac.
- Biliary disease, although anatomically located in the right upper quadrant, may present with purely epigastric symptoms.

Onset:

- Pain that is of very sudden onset suggests perforation of a viscus (e.g. a perforated duodenal ulcer or Boerhaave's perforation) or myocardial infarction.
- Pain from acute pancreatitis and biliary colic develops maximal intensity over 10–20 minutes.
- Inflammatory processes such as acute cholecystitis, hepatitis, and pneumonia typically take hours to reach their peak.

Character:

- 'Crushing' or 'tightness' qualities are typical of cardiac pathology.
- Sharp, 'burning' pain is typical of peptic ulcers, gastritis, and duodenitis.
- Deep 'boring' pain is typical of pancreatitis.

Radiation:

- Back pain is classically associated with pancreatitis, and sometimes seen with peptic ulcers.
- Shoulder tip pain due to irritation of the phrenic nerve suggests diaphragmatic involvement.
- Jaw, neck, or arm pain suggests cardiac pathology.
- Retrosternal pain suggests oesophagitis.

Attenuating factors:

- Patients with acute pancreatitis may find that sitting forwards relieves their pain.
- Surgical dogma suggests that eating makes the pain of gastric ulcers worse but relieves the pain from duodenal ulcers, but these are unreliable features for distinguishing the two in clinical practice.

12

Timing:

- Biliary colic, peptic ulcer disease, and idiopathic dyspepsia are likely to be self-limiting over timescales of less than 6–8 hours.

- Bear in mind that biliary colic does *not* produce truly colicky pain (where the pain waxes and wanes during a single episode), but rather the pain is relatively constant for the duration of the attack.

- Epigastric pain made worse by exercise must make you consider cardiac pathology.

Exacerbating factors:

- Movement worsens severe pain of intra-abdominal origin and peritonitis.

- Deep breathing (pleuritic pain) can worsen epigastric pain when it is due to basal pneumonia (or, very rarely, to pulmonary embolus, pneumothorax, pericarditis, or any cause of pleural inflammation).

- The triggering of self-limiting pain by fatty meals is highly suggestive of biliary colic.

Severity:

- Uncomplicated peptic ulcer disease, gastritis, duodenitis, and idiopathic dyspepsia are usually not severe (and many patients will not present to hospital).

- Severe pancreatitis, perforated peptic ulcers, and myocardial infarction are typically very painful.

12

Once you have characterized the pain, which other symptoms should you ask about?

- **Nausea and/or vomiting?** While any abdominal inflammatory condition can induce vomiting, this is typically most pronounced with acute pancreatitis. An inferior MI can also cause vomiting by irritation of the diaphragm. Boerhaave's perforation is precipitated by forceful vomiting. Be clear about whether the vomiting immediately preceded the pain or immediately followed it.

- **Fever?** Could suggest an infection (e.g. viral hepatitis, pneumonia) or widespread inflammation in the peritoneum (i.e. peritonitis).

- **Dyspepsia and/or waterbrash?** Patients who describe the constellation of symptoms including heartburn, retrosternal discomfort, and a bitter taste in the mouth are very likely to be suffering from GORD, or sequelae such as oesophagitis.

- **Have they noticed any change in their stool recently?** Pale stools indicate that bile is not reaching the bowel. Foul-smelling, floating stools (steatorrhoea) indicate poor digestion of fat, usually due to pancreatic exocrine insufficiency or long-standing biliary disease (as it implies chronic obstruction).

- **Cough?** In the absence of abdominal symptoms other than epigastric pain, cough and/or productive sputum raises the likelihood of basal pneumonia.

What is the particular relevance of the past medical/surgical history?

There are four diseases or groups of diseases that you should pay particular attention to. However, patients may not have a proven diagnosis and may not have related previous symptoms to a particular disease process. For example, while many patients are adept at recognizing angina, few may recognize the symptoms of biliary colic. Clinical judgement may thus be required to tease out such conditions from the history of the presenting complaint and past medical history.

- **Biliary disease:** patients with a known history of gallstone disease are prone both to recurrence of the biliary disease and to complications such as acute pancreatitis. For example, a patient with known gallstones may present with a repeat episode of biliary colic, but is also at increased risk (relative to the population as a whole) of developing acute cholecystitis, ascending cholangitis, or gallstone-induced acute pancreatitis. Note that even patients who have had a previous cholecystectomy can suffer the effects of gallstones left in the common bile duct.

- **Peptic ulcer disease:** a wise maxim is to regard all patients with known peptic ulcer disease, presenting with sudden-onset severe epigastric pain, as having a perforated ulcer until proven otherwise.

- **GORD:** has a high rate of recurrence.

- **Vascular disease:** patients with widespread arterial disease are at increased risk of both myocardial infarction and mesenteric ischaemia. Mesenteric ischaemia may occur as an acute presentation, or as chronic 'mesenteric angina'. The latter can be regarded in a similar way to cardiac ischaemia in that it may be preceded by work-related pain which, in the case of the gut, is manifested as colicky post-prandial abdominal pain. Risk factors for *chronic* mesenteric ischaemia include smoking, hypertension, diabetes mellitus, hypercholesterolaemia, and a family history of cardiovascular disease. Risk factors for *acute* mesenteria ischaemia reflect potential sources of emboli, and thus include atrial fibrillation, recent myocardial infarction, and cardiac valvular disease.

When asking about drug history, are there any particular medications that would predispose to conditions in our differential diagnosis?

Both peptic ulcer disease and acute pancreatitis can be drug induced, although the link is far stronger for the former. Drugs to consider include:

- **Peptic ulcer disease:** non-steroidal anti-inflammatory drugs (NSAIDs), steroids, bisphosphonates, salicylates. Bear in mind that steroids not only predispose to peptic ulcer disease, but they can also dampen the inflammatory response to any subsequent ulcer perforation and hence partially mask signs of peritonism.

- **Acute pancreatitis:** while many drugs have been linked to acute pancreatitis by way of sporadic case reports, some of the more robust links to be aware of include sodium valproate, steroids, thiazides, and azathioprine.

12

> **Does family history have any relevance to the presentation of acute epigastric pain?**

The most compelling reason to ask about family history in the context of epigastric pain is to establish cardiovascular disease risk. However, there are also some very rare hereditary causes of acute pancreatitis (such as mutations in *PRSS1*, *SPINK1*, and *CFTR*) that may be significant if there is a strong family history.

> **Why is Mr Simpson's social history of particular relevance?**

While you should always ask about smoking and alcohol intake, it is particularly important that you spend some time establishing alcohol intake when faced with a patient complaining of epigastric pain. Acute pancreatitis can be caused both by chronic alcohol consumption (developing in about 10% of chronic alcohol abusers) and by binge drinking. Smoking is a risk factor for both peptic ulcer disease and vascular causes of epigastric pain (e.g. myocardial infarction, mesenteric ischaemia).

Mr Simpson describes his pain as severe and constant. He says it came on suddenly while he was preparing lunch about 5 hours ago. The pain gradually increased in intensity over the first 15 minutes or so. He rates it as 9/10 and says that it radiates to his back. He has been sick several times, including twice since he arrived at the hospital half an hour ago. He says that he is no longer bringing very much up, but feels very nauseated and is retching. He has had no cough, fever, or dyspepsia, and denies any change to his stool. He has lost his appetite.

He has a history of episodes of right upper quadrant pain; most recently a couple of years ago. Mr Simpson did not seek medical help during any of these episodes as he was able to control the pain with paracetamol and the pain resolved within a few hours. He is not aware of any particular triggers for these episodes, but direct questioning reveals that they may have followed meals. He has taken paracetamol today but it has not helped to relieve his pain. He has no other significant medical history, takes no medications, and has no allergies. There is no significant family history. He does not smoke, and states that he drinks perhaps two or three glasses of red wine with meals each week.

What signs should you look for on examination?

First you should check Mr Simpson's need for resuscitation (Airway, Breathing, Circulation, ABC). If his condition is severe, he may have a fever, tachycardia, hypotension, tachypnoea, and low oxygen saturations, and may require transfer to intensive care.

When examining Mr Simpson, particularly focus on:

* **Position:** patients with peritonitis lie completely still and rigid; any movement (e.g. the car ride to the hospital) is exquisitely painful. The pain of pancreatitis is said to be positional, improving when patients sit forward. Patients with severe pancreatitis may, however, lie completely still.

* **Jaundice:** this may be seen with acute hepatitis, or with post-hepatic causes of biliary obstruction such as ascending cholangitis and gallstone-induced acute pancreatitis. Acute pancreatitis can also cause jaundice in the absence of gallstones, because oedema of the head of the pancreas compresses the common bile duct (usually 2–3 days after symptom onset).

- **Cullen's or Grey Turner's signs:** discoloration due to extravasated blood in the retroperitoneum, around the umbilicus, and flank respectively. These may be seen in acute haemorrhagic pancreatitis but are rare, non-specific, and late (>48 hours) signs.

- **Signs of small bowel obstruction:** a distended abdomen (which may be hard to appreciate in a patient with a high body mass index (BMI)) and absent or tinkling bowel sounds.

- **Tenderness and guarding:** there may be localized tenderness, as in the case of acute cholecystitis (Murphy's sign), or mild pancreatitis. Acute mild pancreatitis may produce a degree of local peritonism. If the tenderness is more severe, generalized, and seen in combination with guarding and board-like rigidity, this is likely to be peritonitis.

- **Masses:** check for the presence of a central, laterally expansile, pulsatile mass (AAA). Don't forget to check the inguinal folds and femoral canal for hernias which may be causing bowel obstruction (although epigastric pain would be a slightly unusual presentation of such an obstruction).

- **Respiratory examination:** never forget that pathology of the lung bases may masquerade as abdominal pain. Check for signs of consolidation including decreased expansion, dullness to percussion, decreased breath sounds, and increased vocal resonance.

> Looking at Mr Simpson, you note that he is jaundiced and sitting forward in bed – a position he says he finds more comfortable. On palpation there is mild epigastric tenderness, but no rebound tenderness or guarding. There are no palpable masses, obvious abdominal distension, or discolouration. A digital rectal examination (DRE) is unremarkable. The lung bases are clear.
>
> His observations are as follows: temperature of 38.6°C, heart rate 111 bpm, blood pressure 106/79 mmHg, respiratory rate 17/min, oxygen saturations 97% on room air.
>
> **Which investigations should you request for Mr Simpson?**

12

Bloods

- **Full blood count (FBC):** look for signs of infection or inflammation (elevated white cell count), or blood loss (low haemoglobin), for example due to a bleeding peptic ulcer. Neutrophilia is a prognostic indicator in pancreatitis.

- **C-reactive protein (CRP):** elevated in the case of inflammation or infection, but non-specific as to the cause. Establishing a baseline enables you to monitor progression.

- **Pancreatic amylase or lipase:** slight increases (200 to 600 U/L) in amylase levels are most commonly caused by pancreatitis, but such concentrations are relatively non-specific (see viva questions for other causes). However, very high amylase levels (>1000 U/L) or elevated lipase levels (>300 U/L) are usually regarded as diagnostic of acute pancreatitis, as they are released following autodigestion of the pancreas (exact cut-offs will depend upon your local laboratory protocols). There are a number of points to note regarding the interpretation of pancreatic enzymes. Firstly, if the amylase is not raised you cannot exclude acute pancreatitis. Values should be interpreted in the context of time elapsed since the onset of abdominal pain. Amylase levels usually rise within hours of onset of pancreatitis, but fall back to normal within 3–5 days. Lipase has a longer half-life and thus may be a more suitable marker if the patient presents late (urinary amylase also takes longer to fall than serum amylase). As many as 30% of patients presenting with acute pancreatitis will have a normal amylase level – either because of a late presentation, very severe pancreatitis, or acute-on-chronic pancreatitis (as there is little active pancreas left).

- **Liver enzymes:** look for hepatic pathology. Elevated levels of aspartate amino-transferase (AST) and alanine aminotransferase (ALT) suggest pathology *within the liver* as these are released by damaged hepotocytes. A raised alka-line phosphatase (ALP), bilirubin, and gamma-glutamyl transferase (GGT) suggests pathology *in the biliary tree*, or extrinsic compression of the biliary tree (such as by pancreatic oedema). A rise in ALP in the absence of GGT suggests a source other than the liver (e.g. bone or placenta). An isolated rise in GGT is more likely to reflect alcohol excess (but *not* necessarily alcoholism).

- **Albumin:** this is useful as a prognostic factor if the patient has pancreatitis.

- **Urea and electrolytes (U&Es) and creatinine:** as a baseline prior to fluid resuscitation. Also these may be deranged due to renal hypoperfusion if the patient is in shock, or if the patient has been vomiting.

- **Calcium:** a prognostic indicator in pancreatitis. Hypercalcaemia has been associated with acute pancreatitis, but its causative role in aetiology is unclear.

- **Glucose:** a capillary glucose (BM) will suffice. Hyperglycaemia is a marker of severity of pancreatitis.

- **Arterial blood gas (ABG):** should be requested if the patient is dyspnoeic, as acute respiratory distress syndrome (ARDS) is a complication of acute pan-creatitis. Low Pao_2 is also a poor prognostic indicator in pancreatitis.

- **Troponin:** although myocardial infarction does not usually present with epi-gastric pain, you will not want to miss it. Troponin levels are usually taken on admission and at 8–12 hours from the onset of pain. Use clinical judgement as to whether this test is indicated.

ECG

While Mr Simpson's history is atypical, and he has no known risk factors for cardio-vascular disease, you should still exclude cardiac ischaemia. In higher-risk patients you should perform an ECG at the earliest possible opportunity.

Imaging

- **Abdominal radiograph:**
  - Dilated loops of small bowel (>3 cm) could indicate small bowel obstruc-tion, although dilation of a few 'sentinel loops' (local ileus) could also be a response to local inflammation, for example of the pancreas (typically a duodenal sentinel loop).
  - Signs of pneumoperitoneum may suggest a perforated peptic ulcer, although these signs are much easier to see on an erect chest radiograph.
  - Spots of calcification in the biliary system suggest gallstones, although only 10% of gallstones are radio-opaque.

- Calcification speckled over the pancreas suggests chronic pancreatitis.
- You should check for the outline of each psoas muscle – these can become obscured with a ruptured AAA or severe pancreatitis, although this sign is unreliable.

- **Erect chest radiograph**:
  - Air under the diaphragm may suggest a perforated peptic ulcer.
  - Lower lobe consolidation suggests a basal pneumonia.
  - A pleural effusion can occur in pancreatitis and with a Boerhaave's perforation.

- **Abdominal ultrasound**:
  - Exclude gallstones.
  - Exclude biliary dilation (>6mm common bile duct diameter) secondary to obstruction or inflammation.
  - Exclude an AAA.
  - If there is a clinical suspicion that the patient has gallstone-induced pancreatitis, but no stones are viewed by ultrasound, the patient should either be sent for magnetic resonance cholangiopancreatography (MRCP) or rescanned several days later (as dilated loops of bowel may mask the view in the acute setting).

Should patients presenting with epigastric pain have a computed tomography (CT) scan?

CT is not routinely requested as a first-line investigation. In the acute setting, CT is only useful if the clinical, biochemical, and other radiological findings are inconclusive or if an AAA is suspected clinically or radiographically. In the context of acute pancreatitis, contrast-enhanced CT may be indicated if there is persisting organ failure, signs of sepsis, or a deterioration in clinical status 6–10 days after admission (note that pancreatic necrosis is not visible until 4 days after symptom onset). CT may be diagnostic of acute pancreatitis in situations where clinical and biochemical findings are inconclusive.

12

You request bloods, an erect chest radiograph, abdominal radiograph, and biliary ultrasound. The two radiographs are normal. The ultrasound is yet to be performed. The blood results are shown below:

Hb	13.7 g/dL
RBC	5.1×10^{12} cells/L
WCC	15.3×10^9 cells/L
Platelets	276×10^9 cells/L
MCV	93 fL
CRP	46 mg/L
Total bilirubin	46 μM
Albumin	36 g/L
ALT	97 U/L
AST	41 U/L
ALP	158 U/L
GGT	20 U/L

Serum amylase	1264 U/L
Ca	2.32 mM
Na	137 mM
K	3.9 mM
Urea	9.1 mM
Creatinine	132 μM
BM (capillary glucose)	4 mM

(Hb, haemoglobin; RBC, red blood cell [count]; WCC, white cell count; MCV, mean corpuscular volume).

An ABG shows: pH 7.37, arterial partial pressure of oxygen (P_aO_2) = 12.4, arterial partial pressure of carbon dioxide (P_aCO_2) = 5.6, bicarbonate 35 mM.

Given the history, examination, and investigations, what is the most likely diagnosis?

The most likely diagnosis is **acute pancreatitis**, an inflammatory condition of the pancreas in which activated pancreatic enzymes are released and begin to autodigest the gland. Mr Simpson has sudden-onset epigastric pain, which radiates to the back and is relieved by sitting forward. He has a past medical history suggestive of biliary colic, but minimal alcohol intake – hence making a gallstone aetiology for the pancreatitis most likely. He has minimal abdominal signs (a common finding in mild pancreatitis). His amylase is significantly raised and there are no other obvious causes for such a high level given his history and examination findings.

What are the causes of acute pancreatitis? How will you start investigating the aetiology?

The causes can be remembered with the mnemonic **I GET SMASHED**:

Idiopathic[†] (10–20%)

Gall stones

Ethanol

Trauma

Steroids

Mumps/HIV/Coxsackie infection

Autoimmune

Scorpion bites – vanishingly rare so do not mention this until you have covered common causes first!

Hyperlipidaemia/hypercalcaemia/hypothermia

Endoscopic retrograde cholangiopancreatography (ERCP)

Drugs (e.g. sodium valproate, steroids, thiazides, and azathioprine)

Given that by far the most common causes are gallstones and ethanol, these should be the first you investigate. The exact contribution varies according to geography – for example, gallstones are the most common cause in the UK but alcohol is more common in the USA.

[†] You should be reluctant to label pancreatitis as 'idiopathic' until you have performed a vigorous search for gallstones. Modern use of endoscopic ultrasound and MRCP has shown that many cases of pancreatitis that would have previously been labelled as 'idiopathic' are actually due to microlithiasis (gallstones <3 mm in diameter) or sludge (crystals) in the biliary tree.

12

An ultrasound is requested and indeed reveals gallstones in the gallbladder and dilation of the biliary tree. No mass compressing the common bile duct was obvious on ultrasound, so Mr Simpson then had an MRCP. This did not show any gallstones in the common bile duct nor any masses in the head of the pancreas. In Mr Simpson's case, his probable pre-existing gallstone disease is likely to be the underlying cause, with a stone having blocked the ampulla of Vater and caused retrograde flow of digestive enzymes in the pancreatic duct. The stone had obviously passed by the time of the MRCP.

Do you know of a scoring mechanism used clinically for assessing severity and prognosis of pancreatitis? Using the results above, what is Mr Simpson's score?

There are two scoring scales commonly used in clinical practice – the Ranson scale, developed and more commonly used in the USA, and the Glasgow (or Imrie) scale, developed and more commonly used in the UK. Both include criteria predictive for outcome. They are fairly similar, the Glasgow scale being a little simpler using eight rather than 11 criteria. Both have been validated, although Ranson's was validated in a sample of predominantly alcohol-induced pancreatitis whereas the Glasgow scale has been validated in patients with both alcohol- and gallstone-induced pancreatitis.

The Glasgow scale can be remembered using the mnemonic PANCREAS[†] (it should be based on results within 48 hours of admission):

Pao$_2$ <8 kPa or <60 mmHg

Age >55 years

Neutrophilia >15 × 10^9 cells/L (WCC)

Calcium <2.0 mM

Renal function: urea >16 mM

Enzymes: lactate dehydrogenase (LDH) >600 U/L or AST >200 U/L

Albumin <32 g/L

Sugar >10 mM (in non-diabetics)

[†] Courtesy of Mr Etienne Moore, FRCS.

Each criterion scores a single point, totalling eight. A score of 3 or more is considered severe pancreatitis, requiring more intensive management in an intensive therapy unit (ITU)/high-dependency unit (HDU) setting. Note that pancreatic amylase and lipase levels are *not* prognostic indicators.

Mr Simpson scores 2/8 on the Glasgow scale (elevated white cells, and age over 55). He therefore has **mild pancreatitis** and will require regular observations to intervene promptly if he deteriorates (e.g. rapid development of shock needing fluid resuscitation). Remember that these scoring systems are only a guide and should not be a substitute for regularly checking the patient's clinical condition.

How should Mr Simpson be managed?

First, as always, you must have initially checked Mrs Simpson's need for resuscitation (ABC). Even patients with mild pancreatitis can decompensate rapidly so you must continually reassess:

- Airway.

- Breathing – severe cases may develop ARDS, so you must monitor oxygen saturations and blood gases closely.

- Circulation – patients with severe pancreatitis can become hypotensive due to the so-called 'third space' fluid loss that follows the severe inflammatory response. Decreased intravascular volume may be due to a combination of increased capillary permeability, ascites, and ileus. Fluid leaking through the vasculature into an unusual location such as the peritoneum is referred to as 'third space' fluid loss; the first space is vascular, the second space is the natural reservoirs like the bladder. You must monitor fluid balance very closely. All patients will require large-bore intravenous (IV) access. A urinary catheter will aid monitoring of fluid balance if Mr Simpson's condition deteriorates.

Be prepared for a transfer to ITU/HDU if his condition does suddenly deteriorate.

Having ensured that Mr Simpson is stable, you can begin treating the symptoms and the relevant underlying factors – in this case, gallstones. In the acute setting, Mr Simpson will primarily need supportive care. This includes:

- IV fluids.

- Oxygen.

- Stop oral feeding. In the acute phase Mr Simpson may benefit from resting the pancreas (by not stimulating it with food). Once feeding is reinstated he may require nasogastric feeding if still feeling nauseated. The use of total parenteral nutrition is controversial.

- Analgesia.

- Anti-emetics.

- Deep vein thrombosis (DVT) prophylaxis.

How will you prevent a recurrence of this condition in Mr Simpson?

Most patients will recover without further therapy within a week. If complications develop (see viva questions), for example acidosis or sepsis, these should be treated as appropriate. There is, however, no specific treatment for severe pancreatitis *per se*. There appears to be some evidence for the use of prophylactic antibiotics in severe pancreatitis only, but this is debated by some surgeons.

Unless the underlying gallstone aetiology is dealt with, Mr Simpson is liable to suffer another attack of acute pancreatitis. In the case of *mild* pancreatitis, gallstones are usually identified by biliary ultrasound and a **laparoscopic cholecystectomy** is done within the same hospital admission. In the case of patients with *severe* pancreatitis, the patient should have **ERCP** within 72 hours of the onset of the pain if biliary obstruction, biliary sepsis, or persistent organ dysfunction are present. ERCP is accompanied by sphincterotomy, and is followed by delayed cholecystectomy unless patients are too sick to undergo surgery.

In patients who have alcohol-induced pancreatitis, prevention of recurrence is centred upon cessation of drinking.

Short cases

> Mr Bickerstaff is a 38-year-old accountant who presents to his GP with a 2-week history of epigastric pain. The pain can come on at any time, he says, but typically follows meals. It is a burning pain and does not radiate anywhere. He has not suffered from waterbrash and has not vomited. The symptoms are no worse at night or when Mr Bickerstaff bends forwards. He has tried over-the-counter antacids with no success. He does not take any regular medications, but smokes 20 cigarettes a day, and drinks 25–30 units of alcohol a week.
>
> On examination, Mr Bickerstaff is obese. There are no obvious stigmata of gastrointestinal disease on inspection. He complains a little of tenderness in the epigastric region on deep palpation, but his abdomen is otherwise soft and non-tender, with no masses or organomegaly. Bowel sounds are present and normal.
>
> **What is the most likely diagnosis? How should the patient be managed?**

It is most likely that Mr Bickerstaff is suffering from **peptic ulcer disease** or **NUD**. It is possible that he has **GORD,** but the episodic nature of the pain, inability to re-create the discomfort with a positional change (touching his toes), and lack of history of an acid taste in the mouth make it less likely. His risk factors for peptic ulcer disease include smoking and alcohol. The ineffectiveness of antacids in treating his pain is not unusual; severe dyspepsia often requires stronger medications, such as histamine H_2 receptor antagonists or proton-pump inhibitors (PPIs).

Mr Bickerstaff should initially be given lifestyle advice. In the short term he may derive symptomatic benefit from reducing or eliminating his intake of alcohol, caffeine, chocolate, and fatty foods, and stopping smoking. Weight loss will also help him in the longer term.

If conservative management fails to resolve Mr Bickerstaff's symptoms he should be given a trial of either **full-dose PPIs** for 1 month, or should be offered 'test and treat' therapy for *Helicobacter pylori*. *Helicobacter pylori* is the most common cause of peptic ulcers. If present (as detected by a ^{13}C-urea breath test, anti-*Helicobacter* blood serology or an *H. pylori*-positive endoscopic biopsy), eradicating it with triple therapy should allow the ulcers to heal. There are numerous variations so local guidelines should be checked; NICE guidelines suggest a 7-day, twice-daily course of a full-dose PPI with either metronidazole 400 mg and clarithromycin 250 mg, or amoxicillin 1 g and clarithromycin 500 mg.

There are specific recommendations regarding which patients with dyspepsia should be referred for endoscopy (see viva questions).

12

Mr Singh is a 58-year-old man with epigastric pain who has reluctantly been brought to A&E by his wife. He insists that he only has 'indigestion', as he ate a large meal a couple of hours earlier – around the time that the pain started. His wife confirms that he does suffer from indigestion at times, but is concerned that the pain has not yet subsided and that the over-the-counter antacids she gave him haven't worked. You also discover that her father was recently diagnosed with gastric cancer, which may be a factor in her anxiety.

Mr Singh describes his pain as a burning pain and points to just below the xiphisternum. He says it hasn't radiated or changed in character, and is 8/10 in severity. He has felt nauseated but has not vomited, and has experienced no other symptoms. He has diabetes, for which he takes metformin. He has had no recent health complaints or GP visits, and no previous hospital admissions. He has no risk factors for hepatitis infection or peptic ulcer disease.

On examination, he appears uncomfortable but is haemodynamically stable with a pulse of 87 bpm and blood pressure of 137/88 mmHg.

At this stage, the team managing Mr Singh feel that he is suffering from dyspepsia ('heartburn'). They nonetheless request an ECG and blood tests. His ECG is unremarkable. His blood tests on admission include a haemoglobin of 14.3 mg/dL, white cell count of 6.3×10^9 cells/L, urea of 5 mg/dL, creatinine of 80 μM, and troponin of 6 ng/mL.

What is the most likely diagnosis and why?

Mr Singh has almost certainly had a (partial thickness) **non-ST elevation myocardial infarction** (NSTEMI), based on his elevated troponin. He is in some ways lucky – had his troponin on admission been normal and his symptoms improved, he may have been discharged without waiting for a 12-hour troponin level (and with a normal ECG).

Mistaking myocardial infarction for 'heartburn' or 'indigestion' is common – cases of a missed diagnosis of myocardial infarction account for the most dollars recovered in medical malpractice suits in the USA! An estimated 6% of patients with myocardial infarction are thought to be misdiagnosed in the UK. Prompt treatment is crucial in the prognosis after myocardial infarction, thus the delay caused by a missed diagnosis is very serious. You must therefore keep myocardial infarction in mind in a patient presenting with epigastric pain – if you don't think about it, you won't diagnose it.

12

Mrs Lloyd is a 54-year-old advertising sales manager who was brought into hospital by ambulance with severe epigastric pain. The pain came on spontaneously while she was in a meeting 3 hours ago, and is described as a constant stabbing pain. The pain has not radiated and has not been relieved by ibuprofen. She has felt nauseated but has not vomited or had any other symptoms. She rates the pain as 10/10 in severity. She last opened her bowels first thing in the morning (8 hours ago) and has noticed no recent change in her stool. In her past medical history she suffers from chronic back pain, for which she takes regular over-the-counter NSAIDs (ibuprofen). She has not been diagnosed with gallstone disease nor recalls suffering from right upper quadrant pain. She has never smoked but drinks 'maybe 20 units' a week at social events with clients.

Her initial observations are: heart rate 104 bpm regular; blood pressure 126/81 mmHg; respiratory rate 17/min; saturations of 100% on room air; temperature 36.6°C.

As you are examining her, she complains of worsening pain. She is lying motionless on the bed. There is widespread guarding and percussion tenderness. Bowel sounds are absent. The lung bases are clear.

The results of routine bloods requested on admission come back:

Hb	11.8 g/dL
WCC	13.3 × 10⁹ cells/L
Platelets	243 × 10⁹ cells/L
MCV	102 fL
AST	28 U/L
ALT	31 U/L
ALP	23 U/L
Urea	7 mM
Creatinine	77 μM
Ca	2.43 mM
Amylase	387 U/L
Troponin	<0.2 ng/mL

Her erect chest radiograph and supine abdominal radiograph are shown in Fig. 12.1.

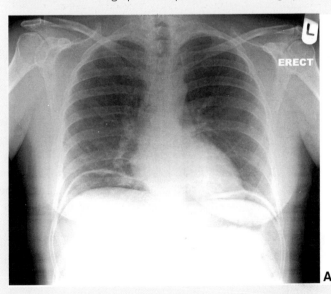

A)

Short case

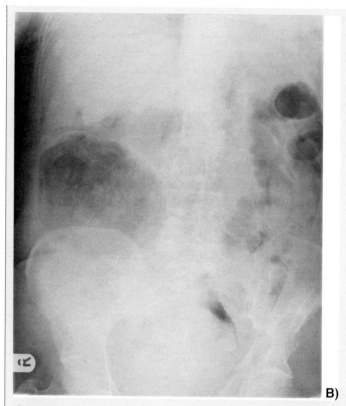

B)

Figure 12.1 Mrs Lloyd's radiographs. A: erect chest radiograph. B: supine abdominal radiograph.

What is the most likely cause of her presenting symptoms? What happened whilst in hospital to make her symptoms worse?

12

The most likely diagnosis is **duodenal perforation**. This is consistent with severe epigastric pain, and in her history she has two risk factors for duodenal ulcers: long-term NSAID use and significant alcohol consumption. She also describes suffering from occasional heartburn. Of the blood results, the amylase is significant: it is not as elevated as is typical in acute pancreatitis (>1000 U/L), but is sufficiently elevated to be consistent with a perforated duodenal ulcer, bowel obstruction, mesenteric ischaemia, mumps, pancreatic carcinoma, or opiate medications. Notice that the erect chest radiograph shows air under the diaphragm (bilaterally, in this case) and that the supine abdominal radiograph shows the 'football sign' (a large bubble of air, in the right side of the abdomen in this case). Air under the diaphragm (pneumoperitoneum) is diagnostic of a perforated gastrointestinal tract, unless the patient has had recent abdominal surgery to explain this presence of air in the peritoneal cavity.

Whilst in hospital she has developed **peritonitis**. This is identified by the triad of a motionless patient, tenderness and guarding on abdominal palpation, and absent bowel sounds.

Her case is a surgical emergency and she should be referred immediately to the surgeons. In the meantime, she should be made **nil by mouth, prescribed IV fluids, analgesia, oxygen,** and **antibiotics**.

Miss O'Riley is a 31-year-old lady referred to your gastrointestinal outpatients clinic for review of her epigastric pain. She has had epigastric pain for the last 12 months, for which she has seen the GP three times and gone to A&E once. The A&E admission was followed by an outpatient biliary ultrasound, which was reported as normal. There are no obvious precipitants to painful episodes. It is a moderately severe (5/10), burning pain that does not radiate. It is not alleviated by food or defecation. She adds that she often feels bloated and uncomfortable after meals. Miss O'Riley has had no other symptoms. She tells you that, so far, no one has been able to find a cause, much to her distress.

She is taking an antidepressant (citalopram), having recently suffered a traumatic relationship break-up, but no other medications. She has no smoking history and drinks modestly, less than 5 units a week.

An abdominal examination is unremarkable. Her GP's letter adds that he has requested an FBC, CRP, U&Es, creatinine, calcium, and liver function tests, and that all were within the normal ranges. The GP says a therapeutic trial of a proton-pump inhibitor for 6 weeks was also unsuccessful in alleviating her symptoms.

You arrange for an oesophagogastroduodenoscopy (OGD) to be performed as an outpatient. Nothing remarkable is seen, and you meet with her for a further consultation.

What is the most likely diagnosis? What will you tell Miss O'Riley?

No organic cause can be found for Miss O'Riley's chronic epigastric pain, as evidenced by normal blood tests, a normal OGD, and normal biliary ultrasound, so the most likely diagnosis is **NUD**. This is a diagnosis of exclusion, albeit a common one accounting for about 30% of cases of investigated dyspepsia.

As with other functional disorders, the doctor–patient relationship is key to management. You must be sensitive to her concerns in your consultation, particularly as she sees you as something of a last resort and you will not want her to feel alienated by the health service. Each individual case should be treated differently, but in your discussion you may wish to:

- Acknowledge that her symptoms are real. Remember that not being able to find an organic cause does not make her symptoms any less real.

- Reassure her that the good news is that the tests have shown no signs of any of the worrying causes of epigastric pain. You may wish to add that her condition is very common.

- Managing her expectations:
  - Take care not to overly investigate her. Excessive investigation (e.g. magnetic resonance imaging, MRI) is not only costly, but runs the risk of identifying asymptomatic 'incidentalomas' which may require invasive and risky testing.
  - Be honest about the limitations of medical treatment. She is likely to be worried about prognosis and so you should address it. Prokinetic agents, H_2-receptor antagonists, and PPIs have been shown to have some beneficial effect in some patients and may all be considered (although a PPI has not worked in this case).
  - You should also be honest about her prognosis. Idiopathic dyspepsia is typically a relapsing condition (60–90% of patients have symptoms 2–3 years after diagnosis). However, diagnosis and the lifestyle and medical therapies available make most patients feel better.

- Suggest that she starts with simple measures such as dietary and lifestyle modification. Some patients benefit from avoiding fatty foods and eating smaller, more frequent meals. It is also sensible to avoid drugs that irritate the lining of the gastrointestinal tract (e.g. NSAIDs), and to stop smoking for the same reason.

- She may be interested in the cause. If she is, you should explain that the causes are poorly understood at present. You can direct her to sources of more information if she is interested.

- Keep the door open. This is partly in case any organic disease manifests itself, but also to protect her relationship with health professionals.

12

Viva questions

What are the indications for endoscopic investigation of dyspepsia?

According to the 2004 National Institute for Health and Clinical Excellence (NICE) guidelines, endoscopic investigation is indicated if any of the following 'red flag' signs are present:

- persistent vomiting
- chronic gastrointestinal bleeding
- weight loss
- progressive dysphagia
- iron-deficiency anaemia
- epigastric mass
- suspicious barium meal
- age ≥55 with unexplained and persistent, recent-onset dyspepsia.

How does the breath test for *H. pylori* work?

The carbon urea breath test works as follows: the patient is given a drink of ^{14}C- or ^{13}C-labelled urea. This is metabolized by the bacteria, if present, into labelled CO_2. A breath test is conducted 15 minutes later, and will detect the labelled CO_2 if *H. pylori* is present.

What are the complications of peptic ulcers?

The five main complications of peptic ulcers are:

- **Haemorrhage.** Is associated with high morbidity, and can be particularly severe in patients on anticoagulant therapy. Cardinal symptoms include haematemesis and/or melaena.
- **Perforation.** Patients taking NSAIDs are most at risk. Perforation usually leads to peritonitis, with the corresponding development of peritonitic signs.
- **Penetration.** This refers to penetration of the ulcer through the bowel wall without leakage into the peritoneum (as in perforation). This may occur into the pancreas, omentum, biliary tract, colon, and vasculature. Patients typically have a chronic history of peptic ulcer disease. They will report a change in symptoms, such that there is no relationship between pain and mealtimes, and it is no longer relieved by antacids. Weight loss and diarrhoea may also be seen.
- **Scarring.** If sufficiently severe, this can cause gastric outlet obstruction. The patient experiences early satiety, bloating, and/or vomiting of partially digested food.
- **Malignancy.** Chronic gastric ulcers are a risk factor for adenocarcinoma of the stomach.

What are the complications of pancreatitis?

The complications of pancreatitis can be divided into local and systemic:

Local

- Pancreatic
  - Necrosis of the pancreas
  - Abscess formation
  - Pseudocyst (accumulation of fluid in the lesser peritoneal sac)
- Other
  - Paralytic ileus
  - Duodenal stress ulceration
  - Fistula formation to colon
  - Obstructive jaundice due to choledocholithiasis or pancreatic oedema

Systemic

- Sepsis
- Shock, due to release of inflammatory mediators and loss of fluid to the peritoneum ('third space loss') or haemorrhage through the pancreas
- Acute renal failure, secondary to hypoperfusion
- Respiratory compromise, due to release of inflammatory mediators and increased permeability of the alveoli. This ranges from mild atelectasis to pleural effusion to ARDS
- Disseminated intravascular coagulation (DIC), triggered by the strong prothombotic stimulus provided by the pancreatic inflammation
- Metabolic
  - Hypocalcaemia due to saponification of fats in the retroperitoneum
  - Hyperglycaemia due to massive release of glucagon (also insulin but this is more than offset by glucagon release)/due to the inability to produce insulin
- Pancreatic encephalopathy, due to cerebral hypoperfusion, ranging from confusion to coma.

What is the role of stool elastase in chronic pancreatitis management? Why?

Stool elastase is a very good marker of pancreatic function as it is:

- Only synthesized in and excreted by the pancreas
- Stable in transit through the gastrointestinal tract, thus there is a direct correlation between elastase in the stool and in pancreatic fluid

A low stool elastase has a high sensitivity for pancreatic compromise (100% for severe and 77% for moderate disease), with a specificity of about 93%. The specificity of stool elastase levels is compromised in patients with diseases of the small bowel such as coeliac disease, Crohn's, and short gut syndrome.

What are Cushing's and Curling's ulcers?

Cushing's and Curling's ulcers are peptic ulcers distinguished by aetiology. Cushing's ulcers arise after brain injury (remember that Harvey Cushing was a neurosurgeon). Curling's ulcers occur after burns.

What is the differential diagnosis of a raised serum amylase level?

An elevated serum amylase level may be due to:

- Pancreatic pathology
  - Pancreatitis
  - Pancreatic trauma
  - Pancreatic carcinoma
- Other intra-abdominal pathology
  - Perforated peptic ulcer
  - Acute appendicitis
  - Acute cholecystitis
  - Ectopic pregnancy
  - Pelvic inflammatory disease
  - Mesenteric ischaemia
  - Leaking AAA
- Decreased amylase clearance
  - Renal failure (amylase is renally excreted)
  - Macroamylasaemia (amylase is bound to immunoglobulin and cannot be renally excreted)
- Miscellaneous conditions
  - Diabetic ketoacidosis
  - Head injury

12

For a range of Single Best Answer questions related to the topic of this chapter go to
www.oxfordtextbooks.co.uk/orc/ocms/

Nausea and vomiting

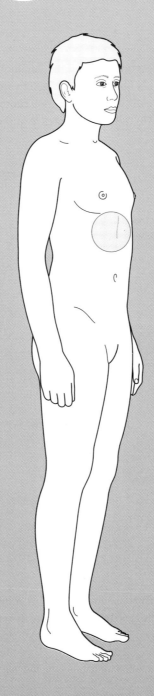

Core case

Mr Price is a 47-year-old electrician who presents to his local emergency department complaining of nausea and vomiting.

Nausea and vomiting has a very wide differential. Broadly speaking, what can cause nausea and vomiting?

The **vomiting centre** (mainly histamine and acetylcholine receptors) in the medulla oblongata can be activated by four main input systems shown in Fig. 13.1: the **vestibular system**, the **central nervous system**, the **chemoreceptor trigger zone** (in the fourth ventricle of the brain), and **cranial nerves IX and X**.

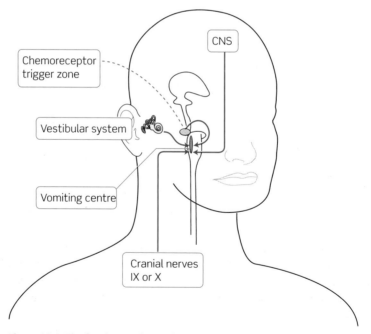

Figure 13.1 The four inputs that activate the vomiting centre: CNS, central nervous system.

With these four inputs in mind, it becomes easier to understand some of the pathologies that can activate the vomiting centre and cause nausea and vomiting, as is shown in Fig. 13.2.

13

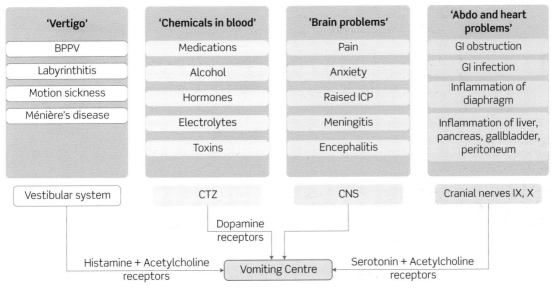

Figure 13.2 Causes of nausea and vomiting: BPPV, benign paroxysmal positional vertigo; CTZ, chemoreceptor trigger zone; ICP, intracranial pressure; CNS, central nervous system; GI, gastrointestinal.

What initial questions will help you narrow down your differential?

Details of the vomit:

- **Contents**
  - **Undigested:** oesophageal disorders, e.g. achalasia, pharyngeal pouch.
  - **Partially digested:** gastric outlet obstruction, gastroparesis (delayed stomach emptying, e.g. seen in diabetics).
  - **Bile (green):** small bowel obstruction (distal to the ampulla of Vater).
  - **Faeculent:** distal intestinal or colonic obstruction. Note the only time you will see faecal (i.e. true faeces), as opposed to faeculent (i.e. foul looking), vomiting is in patients with a gastrocolonic fistula ... or coprophagia.
  - **Blood/coffee-ground:** haematemesis (see Chapter 5)
  - **Large volume:** less likely to be functional.

- **Timing**
  - **Early morning:** classically in pregnancy and raised intracranial pressure:
  - **Duration:** this is useful in identifying the severity (patients with severe nausea and vomiting present early) and a longer time course makes conditions such as bowel obstruction less likely, as untreated this will either deteriorate or resolve.

- **Association with eating?**
  - Vomiting within an hour of eating suggests an obstruction high in the gastrointestinal (GI) tract proximal to the gastric outlet. If this is the case, you should ask about peptic ulcer disease as this can cause scarring and pyloric stenosis.
  - Vomiting after a longer post-prandial delay is consistent with an obstruction lower in the GI tract, usually in the small bowel.
  - Early satiety, post-prandial bloating, and abdominal discomfort together suggest gastroparesis or outlet obstruction.

13

Details of any pain:

- Use SOCRATES to characterize the pain (see Chapter 12).
- The site is indicative of certain pathologies (e.g. right upper quadrant suggests a hepatobiliary cause, epigastric suggests a pancreatic or gastroduodenal cause). However, localization of pain is far from accurate in abdominal pathology due to the neural wiring and embryology, and also anatomical variations.
- Relief after vomiting is consistent with obstruction.

Other symptoms?

- **Fever?** Any infectious or inflammatory cause: gastroenteritis, appendicitis, cholecystitis, cholangitis, pancreatitis, hepatitis, urinary tract infection (UTI), meningo-encephalitis.
- **Headache? Visual disturbance?** Meningitis, encephalitis, migraine, raised intracranial pressure.
- **Vertigo ('the room is spinning')?** Labyrinthitis, Ménière's, benign paroxysmal positional vertigo (BPPV).

Bowel movements?

You should always ask when a patient's bowels were last open. This includes passing both faeces and flatus.

- **Delay/absolute constipation:** a long delay could suggest bowel obstruction (either mechanical or functional, i.e. ileus). Constipation may simply be a feature of eating less and vomiting, but *absolute* constipation of faeces and flatus is a serious sign, suggesting bowel obstruction.
- **Diarrhoea?** Diarrhoea and vomiting suggests infectious gastroenteritis.

Exposure to infectious bowel pathogens?

- **Close contacts also suffering nausea and vomiting?** Suggests highly contagious aetiology such as rotavirus, Norwalk virus, etc. or sharing contaminated food (e.g. buffet food infected with *Staphylococcus aureus* endotoxin).
- **Living in close quarters?** Hospitals, army barracks, boarding schools, and cruise ships are all notorious for outbreaks of infectious GI pathogens.
- **Recent foreign travel?** Differing hygiene standards and local pathogens make travelling abroad a high risk for GI infections.
- **Unusual meals recently?** A recent barbeque, wedding buffet, late night kebab, restaurant meal, etc. may all suggest exposure to an infectious GI pathogen.
- **Antibiotic use?** Antibiotics can kill the healthy commensal flora of the GI tract, allowing pathogenic bacteria to take over (e.g. *Clostridium difficile*).

Exposure to potential drugs and toxins?

- **Medications?** Opiates, chemotherapy, anticonvulsants, antibiotics, etc. can all cause nausea and vomiting.
- **Industrial chemicals?** Arsenic and organophosphate fertilizers, for example, can cause vomiting.
- **Alcohol? Illicit drugs?**

History of previous abdominal surgery?

Previous surgery predisposes to adhesions between the peritoneum and the bowel, which can cause bowel obstruction.

The principal components of this approach are summarized in the flow chart in Fig. 13.3, along with some examples of the pathologies they could indicate.

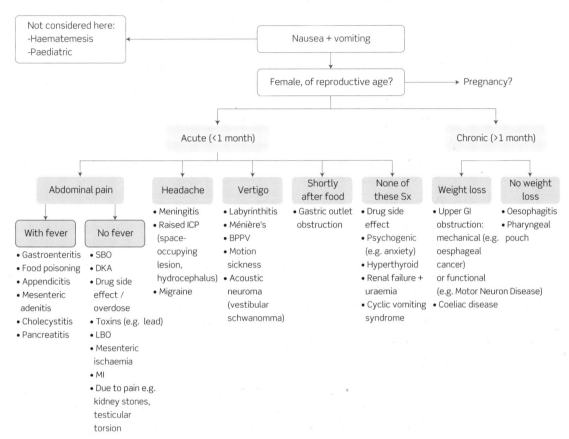

Figure 13.3 Flow chart for investigating nausea and vomiting: SBO, small bowel obstruction; DKA, diabetic ketoacidosis; LBO, large bowel obstruction; MI, myocardial infarction; ICP, intracranial pressure; BPPV, benign paroxysmal positional vertigo; Sx, symptoms; GI, gastrointestinal.

As mentioned above, the differential diagnosis for nausea and vomiting is very broad, including some potentially serious causes.

What signs and/or symptoms will help alert you to these?

First and foremost you will be concerned about any patient who requires resuscitation on a primary survey of their Airway, Breathing, and Circulation (ABC). In particular, persistent large-volume vomiting can result in dehydration, which may be severe enough to decrease the patient's consciousness.

13

Specific worrying symptoms and signs are shown in Table 13.1:

Table 13.1 Worrying signs and symptoms in nausea and vomiting

Features	Serious condition suggested
Motionless patient, rigid abdomen, absent bowel sounds	?Peritonitis (any cause)
Bilious or faeculent vomiting, distended abdomen, absolute constipation, abdominal pain	?Bowel obstruction
Very high fever (>38.5°C)	?Infection
Early morning vomiting, headache worse when lying down, nerve VI palsy	?Raised intracranial pressure
Central, crushing chest pain	?Myocardial infarction
Meningism (stiff neck, photophobia, headache)	?Meningitis
Reduced consciousness	?Diabetic ketoacidosis
Haematemesis	?Bleeding peptic ulcer ?Oesophageal varices

You should also be worried about a drug overdose; the signs and symptoms of overdose will depend on the drug taken.

Mr Price tells you that he started vomiting a couple of hours after eating dinner the night before last. The vomit was 'normal vomit', by which he means digested food, and is not obviously associated with meals although he has barely eaten during the past 36 hours. The pain has been 'cramping' and is vaguely umbilical but not well localized. He gets mild relief from vomiting, and says the pain is severe (8/10). He has felt generally unwell but has not taken his temperature. He has, however, had no night sweats. None of his close contacts have reported any vomiting. He last opened his bowels yesterday morning and he cannot recall passing any flatus today. About 20 years ago he had an appendicectomy, but has had no other surgery.

Mr Price tells you he takes sumatriptan for occasional migraines, when he needs to. He also uses some herbal remedies and aromatherapy. He takes no regular medications. He has no allergies and is a non-smoker who drinks about a bottle of wine a week at most. He denies taking any recreational drugs.

What signs would you specifically look for on examination?

You should of course conduct a full examination. However, specific signs you would look for in Mr Price's case include:

On inspection

- **Hydration status:** e.g. dry mucous membranes, sunken eyes
- **Abdominal distension:** suggestive of obstruction – but remember this can be caused by six Fs: faeces, flatus, fluid, foetus (not in Mr Price's case!), fat, filthy great tumour
- **Scars:** from previous abdominal surgery, which could be associated with adhesions
- **Hernias:** (particularly irreducible hernias) that could contain trapped bowel and cause the obstruction or which could appear due to obstruction and raised intra-abdominal pressure
- **Jaundice:** consistent with a hepatobiliary cause

On palpation

- **Tender abdomen:** suggesting inflammation somewhere in the peritoneal cavity
- **Masses:** could be causing an obstruction
- **Guarding:** could indicate peritonitis

On auscultation

- **Bowel sounds:** absent in ileus (e.g. due to peritonitis) and high-pitched or 'tinkling' in mechanical obstruction

13

> You examine Mr Price. He is lying in bed but in some discomfort from the 'stomach cramps'. He is not jaundiced but has an appendicectomy scar and mild distension of his abdomen. There are no other peripheral stigmata of disease. His abdomen is soft and non-tender, with no palpable masses or organomegaly. You hear high-pitched bowel sounds on auscultation.
>
> His observations are as follows: temperature of 36.5°C, heart rate 66 bpm, blood pressure 128/69 mmHg, respiratory rate 12/min, oxygen saturations 99% on room air.
>
> **In the light of the history and examination, which investigations would you request?**

You should request the follow investigations:

Bloods

- **Full blood count (FBC)** and **C-reactive protein (CRP):** raised inflammatory markers (white cell count (WCC), CRP) would indicate infection or inflammation.
- **Urea and electrolytes (U&Es):** in protracted or severe vomiting there may be some electrolyte imbalance; a baseline is also needed if the patient may go to surgery.
- **Liver enzymes:** hepatobiliary pathologies will lead to deranged liver enzymes, e.g. biliary disease causes alkaline phosphatase (ALP) to rise, hepatitis can cause alanine aminotransferase (ALT)/aspartate aminotransferase (AST) to rise (although prothrombin time is a better marker of liver function).

- **Amylase:** to help confirm or exclude pancreatitis.
- **Group and save:** Mr Price may need surgery on this admission, so it would be wise to 'group and save' his blood group, so that blood is available if he proceeds to theatre.

Imaging

- **Supine abdominal radiograph:** you must order this to look for signs of intestinal obstruction.
- **Erect chest radiograph:** this is used to look for air under the diaphragm, which may be seen if the bowel has perforated and is a serious sign.

Other potential investigations:

You would not initially order these for Mr Price but might consider them in patients with a different history and examination:

- **Pregnancy test:** you must consider (and test for) pregnancy in any woman of potentially child-bearing age. You should enquire if they are sexually active, and explain that you need to perform a pregnancy test if only to exclude pregnancy. It is worth noting that no contraceptive method is failsafe (e.g. the combined oral contraceptive pill, properly taken, still has a failure rate of 1 in every 100 women per year). It is interesting to note that β-human chorionic gonadotropin (β-HCG) is associated with the nausea and vomiting seen in pregnancy, and that the hyperemesis (exaggerated nausea and vomiting) seen with multiple pregnancies and molar pregnancies merely reflects the greater production of β-HCG in these states.
- **Toxicology screen:** if there is suspicion of accidental or deliberate overdose of medications.
- **Contrast studies:** e.g. small bowel follow-through, looking for obstruction if this was not evident on abdominal radiography.
- **Abdominal CT:** looking for intraperitoneal pathology.
- **Head MRI:** looking for intracranial disease such as dilated ventricles suggesting raised intracranial pressure.

Older textbooks may refer to the 'saline load test', which was used to distinguish gastric outlet obstruction from gastroparesis (delayed gastric emptying). The advent of endoscopy has made it redundant.

Stool gazing yields pitifully little information and is therefore (thankfully!) a dying art.

Mr Price's blood tests come back and show: white cell count 7.8 × 10^9 cells/L, CRP 22 mg/L, Na 138 mM, K 3.8 mM, AST 28 U/L, ALT 26 U/L, ALP 30 U/L, amylase 154 U/dL, urea 4.3 mM, creatinine 90 μM. His abdominal radiograph is shown in Fig. 13.4.

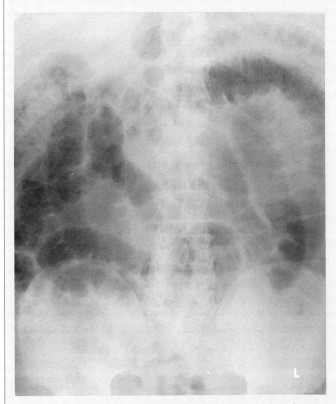

Figure 13.4 Mr Price's abdominal radiograph taken on admission.

What does the abdominal radiograph show? Based on all the information you have, what is the most likely diagnosis? What is a possible aetiology in Mr Price?

13

The abdominal radiograph shows centrally located loops of distended (>3 cm diameter) small bowel with valvulae conniventes.

The most likely diagnosis is **small bowel obstruction**. A possible aetiology is entanglement of a loop of bowel in **post-operative adhesions** from his previous appendicectomy. Post-surgical inflammatory response leads, over time, to the formation of fibrous 'adhesions' between the bowel and the parietal peritoneum. Obstruction may occur shortly after the operation or, as in the case of Mr Price, many years later if a loop of bowel gets twisted in a pre-existing adhesion.

Small bowel obstruction accounts for 20% of acute surgical admissions.

A surgical referral is made.

Whilst you await the surgeons, how should you manage Mr Price?

As always, you should have checked Mr Price's need for resuscitation (ABC) on admission (and on an ongoing basis as necessary).

You should also start the following:

- **Nil by mouth** (NBM), in case Mr Price needs to go to theatre (an empty stomach reduces the risk of aspiration on induction of anaesthesia) and to 'rest the bowel'.

- **Drip and suck,** i.e. IV fluids and aspiration of gastric contents via a nasogastric (NG) tube. He will need the fluids as he may be dehydrated from vomiting and is NBM, plus you may need to correct any electrolyte imbalance. Aspirating the gastric contents will relieve the gut and reduce the risk of aspiration following vomiting.

- **Analgesia.** You must not forget this – patients will be very grateful!

Mr Price goes to the surgical unit for review.

How are the surgeons likely to manage Mr Price?

A sensible approach would be:

1) **A trial of conservative management,** i.e. fluids and NG aspiration ('drip and suck'), to see if the obstruction resolves of its own accord. He should be reviewed regularly to ensure he does not deteriorate (e.g. bowel strangulation).

2) **Surgery,** if:
   - there are signs of strangulation or peritonism;
   - after ~48 hours the obstruction has not resolved; or
   - there is no history of abdominal surgery, making adhesions less likely and more sinister causes more likely.

In Mr Price's case, the surgeons attempted conservative management, but 48 hours later he was still in pain and had not been able to keep anything down. They then operated, dividing post-operative adhesions.

About a quarter of patients with small bowel obstruction will undergo surgery, to divide post-operative adhesions or repair hernias, with or without small bowel resection.

Short cases

Mrs O'Connor is a 35-year-old woman who is 32 weeks pregnant and presents with a 3-day history of nausea and vomiting. The vomit looks like digested food, and she has been unable to keep anything down other than a bit of water and some soup. She has had diarrhoea and abdominal pain, which she still complains of. In addition she believes that she has had a temperature, although she didn't actually measure it. She is multiparous, with four previous children and says she never had any morning sickness (or any other problems) during those pregnancies. Two of her children have also been unwell with vomiting and diarrhoea over the past week.

On examination, her pulse is 88 bpm, blood pressure 110/66 mmHg, temperature 37.7°C, respiratory rate 12/min, and oxygen saturations of 98% on room air. Her abdomen is soft and non-tender, and the fetal heart rate is present and normal.

Blood test results include: Na 136 mM, K 3.8 mM, urea 8.1 mM, creatinine 148 μM. Urinalysis is unremarkable.

What is the most likely diagnosis?

Mrs O'Connor has a 3-day history, probable affected contacts (her children), diarrhoea as well as vomiting, and is pyrexial but not peritonitic or tachycardic. The most likely diagnosis is **gastroenteritis** (i.e. infection of the bowel), particularly given the combination of diarrhoea and vomiting. It is unlikely to be 'morning sickness' as this is most common in the first trimester and she has no history of it in previous pregnancies; moreover this would not explain the diarrhoea. It is also unlikely to be 'food poisoning', i.e. due to a toxin in the food (which may be a bacterial or environmental toxin) rather than infection, as toxins do not usually persist for more than 24 hours, whereas infections often do.

Gastroenteritis is common – so much so that it is the highest cause of sick leave after the common cold. Mrs O'Connor is dehydrated (raised urea and creatinine at the upper end of normal). Given that she has tolerated water and soup, she should be encouraged to drink fluids in order to rehydrate. Infectious gastroenteritis hardly ever requires antibiotics as most cases resolve spontaneously within a few days. The most important management is adequate fluid intake to avoid dehydration.

13

Short case

A 16-year-old girl is brought into A&E after several episodes of vomiting. She is also becoming drowsy and difficult to rouse. She had a history of thirst and polyuria in the previous days, and had abdominal pain with her nausea and vomiting. Her parents say she has vomited her last meals but there has been no bile or blood in the vomitus.

On examination, her pulse is 103 bpm, blood pressure 111/63 mmHg, temperature 36.2°C, respiratory rate 25/min, and oxygen saturations of 100% on room air. She has dry mucous membranes but the rest of the physical examination was unremarkable.

The blood tests on admission record a haemoglobin of 11.7 mg/dL, red cell count of 4.1×10^{12} cells/L, white cell count 6.6×10^9 cells/L, Na 128 mM, K 4.9 mM, Cl 101 mM, glucose 19.4 mM, urea 10.1 mM, creatinine 168 µM. Urinalysis revealed ++ glucose and +++ ketones. An arterial blood gas (ABG) is performed and shows pH 7.25, arterial partial pressure of carbon dioxide (P_aCO_2) 2.1 kPa, arterial partial pressure of oxygen (P_aO_2) 17.1 kPa, HCO_3^- 7.2 mM (with a fraction of inspired oxygen (FiO_2) of 21%).

What is the most likely diagnosis? How would you interpret the ABG in the context of your diagnosis? What is the anion gap?

13

This girl has **diabetic ketoacidosis**, based on her symptoms, urinalysis, and the results of her blood tests (including ABG) which demonstrate *diabetes mellitus* (raised glucose), *ketosis*, and *acidaemia*. Diabetic ketoacidosis can present with vomiting, abdominal pain, polydipsia, polyuria, headache, and, in more extreme cases, decreased consciousness and Kussmaul breathing. The urinalysis shows ketone production, which is inhibited by even the smallest amount of insulin, and glucosuria, consistent with insufficient insulin. Her serum glucose is elevated (>11 mM). Her creatinine is also high, probably due to her dehydration (supported by the clinical finding of dry mucous membranes). Her sodium is low, probably artificially so ('pseudo-hyponatraemia') due to the high glucose in the serum that is distorting the readings made by the laboratory machine (blood gas machines are not prone to this artefact).

Her ABG shows an acidosis (pH <7.35). The low P_aCO_2 (<4.5 kPa) indicates that this is a metabolic acidosis, confirmed by the low bicarbonate (<22 mM). The P_aCO_2 is low as there has been some respiratory compensation. If the bicarbonate had been normal or raised that would suggest some renal compensation, but this takes longer. The anion gap is calculated as $[K^+] + [Na^+] - [Cl^-] - [HCO_3^-]$. In this case, it is raised (>16 mM) at 24.7 mM. Put simplistically, a raised anion gap suggests the presence of extra acid groups in the blood (e.g. ketone bodies, lactate, aspirin) rather than the loss of alkali (e.g. bicarbonate in diarrhoea).

The chronic management of type I diabetes mellitus is discussed in other textbooks. In the acute setting, diabetic ketoacidosis should be managed by giving IV fluids (normal saline) to rehydrate the patient and IV insulin infusion (not a bolus) to suppress ketosis, until the ketones have disappeared from repeat blood tests. In fact, such patients need extensive monitoring: of their fluid balance, capillary glucose, ketones, and serum potassium (in case of a drop in potassium while on IV insulin). Potassium therapy is often called for, but bicarbonate is rarely given to correct the acidosis. Patients should be transferred to subcutaneous insulin once capillary ketones and acidosis subside sufficiently (check local protocols for exact levels).

Miss Agar is a 15-year-old schoolgirl who presents to the hospital (she is worried her GP is overly friendly with her parents) with a history of several days early morning nausea and vomiting. The vomit consists of her last meal and sometimes 'some bile', which she describes as a slight yellowing (true bile, however, is green). She has had no abdominal pain, no fever, headache, visual disturbance, vertigo, or other symptoms except for feeling a bit tired. You ask her if she could be pregnant; she tells you she has had sex four times in the last month using the withdrawal method. Her last period was around 4 or 5 weeks ago, she cannot quite remember but says she is late.

Her pulse is 63 bpm, blood pressure 108/61 mmHg, temperature 36.1°C, respiratory rate 10/min, and she has oxygen saturations of 100% on room air. Her abdomen is soft and non-tender with no organomegaly, and the rest of her examination is unremarkable.

Blood test results include: haemoglobin (Hb) 10.9 mg/dL, red cell count (RCC) of 4.1×10^{12} cells/L, WCC 5.9×10^{9} cells/L, Na 138 mM, K 4.4 mM, urea 5.7 mM, creatinine 99 μM. No abnormalities are noted on urinalysis.

What is the most likely diagnosis and how would you confirm this? What medications could you use to treat Miss Agar?

The most likely diagnosis is **pregnancy**, and you must perform a pregnancy test. 70–85% of pregnant women suffer with nausea or vomiting and 50% have both, especially in the first trimester.

You need to be very careful about the drugs and doses you give in pregnancy. Antihistamines (e.g. meclizine or promethazine), electrolyte replacement, and thiamine supplementation are recommended for morning sickness. In severe cases (hyperemesis gravidarum) prochlorperazine, chlorpromazine, metoclopramide, or methylprednisolone can be used.

13

Mrs Bray is a 74-year-old lady brought in to her GP by her daughter who says she has been vomiting regularly over the last few days. This has happened mainly in the mornings, and she has also had a headache that is worst in the mornings. Mrs Bray has noticed no change in her vision but it is a little blurry in any case as she is developing cataracts. On questioning she tells you the vomit is small amounts of food, and is not accompanied with abdominal pain or fever. She can think of no recent head trauma and has no other symptoms. She is a diabetic for which she is on metformin, and also takes ramipril and simvastatin. She has been taking paracetamol for the headaches but it hasn't worked. She does not drink or smoke, but smoked 10 cigarettes a day until her husband died of a heart attack 25 years ago (a total of 30 years, or 15 pack years).

Her vital signs are pulse 86 bpm, blood pressure 138/63 mmHg, temperature 36.7°C, respiratory rate 12/min, and oxygen saturations of 99% on room air. On examination, her abdomen is soft and non-tender with no organomegaly. Her chest is clear, and her heart sounds are present with no added sounds. She has no focal neurological signs on examination of her limbs. Cranial nerve examination reveals double vision on extreme right gaze and failure of the right eye to abduct. The rest of her cranial nerve examination is normal.

What is the most likely cause of her vomiting? What bedside examination would help you confirm this?

You must suspect **raised intracranial pressure** as the cause of Mrs Bray's nausea and vomiting because she has two key features of this:

- Early morning nausea and vomiting
- Headaches that are worse on lying down

Mrs Bray has also has signs suggestive of a cranial nerve VI palsy. This is the commonest focal neurological deficit in raised intracranial pressure because of the long course of nerve VI, which increases the points at which it can be compressed. The most likely underlying cause is metastatic spread of a cancer to the brain, although it could also be a primary tumour or other space-occupying lesion.

At the bedside you should perform **fundoscopy**, to look for papilloedema. This is not always present but when it is, is a good sign of raised intracranial pressure. Mrs Bray will need an MRI of her head looking for a space-occupying lesion.

13

Mr Pitman is an electrical engineer in his mid-20s who comes into hospital suffering with severe abdominal pain and vomiting. He says it began 2 or 3 days ago but has been getting progressively worse. You ask about the pain and he tells you it was like a diffuse ache which he thought would pass, but is now much sharper and points to his right iliac fossa. It is uncomfortable whatever position he is in and has not been alleviated by eating, fasting, vomiting, or the large doses of paracetamol and ibuprofen he says he has tried. You ask about the journey to the hospital and he tells you it was very painful. He tells you he has vomited four times and brings up partially digested food, but there has been less of this in the past 24 hours as he has lost his appetite and not eaten. He adds that he has been feverish, although he did not actually take his temperature. He last opened his bowels the previous evening but has passed flatus since then. There is no history of affected contacts. He is usually fit and well, with no current diagnoses or surgical history. Other than the painkillers, he takes no medications.

His pulse is 94 bpm, blood pressure 113/65 mmHg, temperature 38.3°C, respiratory rate 14/min, and oxygen saturations of 99% on room air. He is lying very still when you examine him and his abdomen is rigid and tender to light palpation throughout, with rebound tenderness also present. Bowel sounds are decreased. The rest of your examination is unremarkable.

Blood test results include: Hb 14.7 mg/dL, RCC of 5.3×10^{12} cells/L, WCC 14.2×10^9 cells/L (69% neutrophils), Na 142 mM, K 3.9 mM, urea 8.6 mM, creatinine 81 μM.

What is the most likely diagnosis?

Mr Pitman gives a good history for **appendicitis**, reinforced by the clinical signs and investigations. Key symptoms include a pain that was poorly localized but now localizes to the site of the appendix, anorexia, fever, and vomiting. Clinically he is febrile and has signs of peritonism (he is motionless with a rigid, very tender abdomen), suggesting a perforated appendix.

Mr Pitman will require an urgent surgical referral and appendicectomy as well as antibiotics to treat his peritonitis and prevent abscess formation. In the meantime he will need analgesia, to be kept NBM (as preparation for surgery), IV fluids, and potentially an anti-emetic if the nausea and vomiting are severe.

13

Viva questions

If a dehydrated patient is able to tolerate oral fluids, what is the best fluid to use and why?

The best fluid is oral rehydration solution. This contains sodium, glucose, and water in the correct proportions to make optimal use of the sodium–glucose co-transporter in the gut wall that drives fluid absorption.

What is the basis of the pregnancy test available over the counter?

The pregnancy test measures β-HCG. This is produced by the placenta after implantation of the fertilized ovum and can be detected around 12 days after fertilization.

A patient with terminal lung cancer presents with nausea and vomiting. They have widespread metastatic disease and are receiving palliative chemotherapy. What mechanisms could be mediating their nausea and vomiting? (Hint: there are lots!)

There are a variety of mechanisms:

- Metabolic: hypercalcaemia (bone involvement), uraemia
- Intracranial: raised intracranial pressure due to metastatic brain lesions
- GI: gastric outflow obstruction, hepatomegaly (pressing on the stomach), constipation, bowel obstruction or ileus
- Psychogenic: anxiety
- Chemotherapy (particularly platinum-based) or opiate analgesia

Name the common surgical scars on the schematic diagram in Fig. 13.5, and give an example of the operations each approach might be used for.

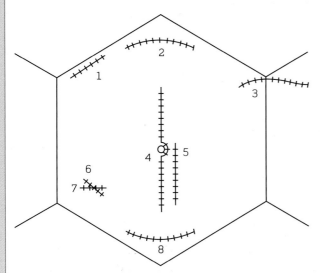

Figure 13.5 Common surgical scars. See text for key.

1) Kocher's (or subcostal) incision: cholecystectomy

2) Rooftop incision: Whipple's surgery, gastric surgery

3) Transverse abdominal incision for nephrectomy

4) Midline incision: laparotomy, e.g. exploratory, bowel obstruction, gynaecological

5) Paramedian incision: as for midline incision

6) Gridiron or McBurney's incision: appendicectomy

7) Lanz incision: appendicectomy

8) Pfannesteil incision: Caesarean section, gynaecological operation

Don't forget to look for porthole scars (including one in the umbilicus) for laparoscopic surgery.

What are the mechanisms of action of the following anti-emetics: cyclizine; metoclopramide; ondansetron; haloperidol? Based on this, give an example of a condition where each might be indicated.

- **Cyclizine** is an antihistamine and antimuscarinic that blocks acetylcholine receptors in vestibular and vomiting centres. It is useful in post-operative nausea, bowel obstruction nausea (as it is antikinetic), motion sickness and other labyrinthine aetiologies, and also in conditions causing raised intracranial pressure.

- **Metoclopramide** has agonist properties at 5-HT$_4$ (serotonin) receptors and antagonist properties at dopamine (D$_2$) receptors such as those found in the chemoreceptor trigger zone and myenteric plexus of the GI tract. It is prokinetic, particularly in the stomach, and therefore indicated in causes of delayed stomach emptying, e.g. as a side-effect of opiates, gastroparesis. Because it is a prokinetic, it is *contraindicated* in bowel obstruction.

- **Ondansetron** is a 5-HT$_3$ (serotonin) receptor antagonist that acts on receptors in the gut and the chemoreceptor trigger zone. It is useful for chemotherapy-induced and post-operative vomiting.
- **Haloperidol** is an antagonist of dopamine (D$_2$) receptors such as those found in the chemoreceptor trigger zone and myenteric plexus of the GI tract. At low doses (rather than the higher doses used in psychosis), it acts both centrally and on the GI tract to remove inhibition to normal motility. It is useful in treating drug-induced and metabolic causes of nausea and vomiting, and also vomiting due to raised intracranial pressure.

What are the potential complications of vomiting?

Vomiting can cause:

- Dehydration
- Electrolyte imbalance, particularly hypokalaemia and hypochloraemia
- Metabolic alkalosis
- Aspiration and aspiration pneumonia
- Mallory–Weiss tear in the mucosa of the upper oesophagus, leading to bleeding
- Boerhaave's syndrome – rupture of the oesophagus

Nausea and vomiting is common in post-operative patients. What factors might be contributing to this?

There are a number of reasons why post-operative patients might be expected to suffer from nausea and vomiting:

- Pre-operative factors
  - Patient factors, e.g. obesity, female, non-smokers
  - Prolonged pre-operative fasting
  - Anxiety
- Intraoperative factors
  - Pharyngeal irritation from intubation
  - Side-effect of opioid use or inhalation anaesthetic
- Post-operative factors
  - Pain
  - Post-operative opioid analgesia
  - Early post-operative intake of food
  - 'Dizziness'/light-headedness due to dehydration, hypotension
  - Ileus

For a range of Single Best Answer questions related to the topic of this chapter go to
www.oxfordtextbooks.co.uk/orc/ocms/

Jaundice

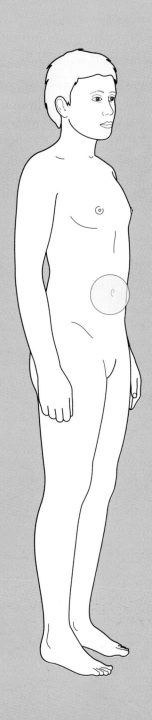

Core case

! *Read through the sections in red, covering up the sections in white that follow*
♦ *so that you don't see the answer. At the end of each red section, try to answer the*
   question before reading on.

Miss Watroba is a 28-year-old from Poland who has recently moved to the UK. She has attended her general practitioner (GP) because she has developed 'yellow eyes'. As soon as she walks into your office, you can see she is jaundiced. Jaundice is due to the excessive accumulation of bilirubin in tissues.

What is the normal metabolism of bilirubin?

The metabolism of bilirubin can be divided into three sequential steps:

1) **Production of unconjugated bilirubin.** Red blood cells are broken down by macrophages (mainly in the spleen), which degrade haemoglobin into iron and unconjugated (water insoluble) bilirubin. The iron is stored inside transferrin proteins. Unconjugated bilirubin travels to the liver bound to albumin.

2) **Conjugation of bilirubin.** Liver hepatocytes conjugate water insoluble bilirubin to glucuronate, thus making water soluble, conjugated bilirubin. Once conjugated, bilirubin is secreted into the bile canaliculi.

14

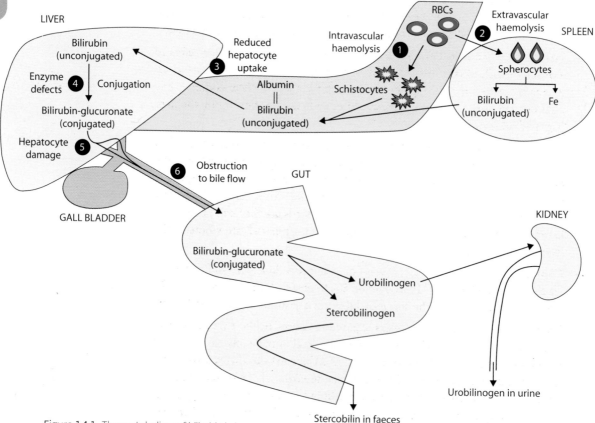

Figure 14.1 The metabolism of bilirubin in humans.

3) **Excretion of bilirubin.** Conjugated bilirubin flows with bile down the bile ducts and into the duodenum. Inside the bowel, conjugated bilirubin is metabolized by bacteria into colourless products (urobilinogen, stercobilinogen). Some of these can be reabsorbed by the gut and excreted via the kidneys, but the vast majority get oxidized in the gut into coloured pigments (urobilin, stercobilin) which give faeces their brown colour. Consequently, if there is *complete* obstruction of the bile ducts there will be no flow of conjugated bilirubin into the gut, no conversion into urobilinogen and therefore not even a trace of urobilinogen in the urine.

Clinicians often talk about jaundice being pre-hepatic, hepatic, or post-hepatic in origin; obstructive; cholestatic; and conjugated or unconjugated.

What does all this terminology mean?

The metabolism of bilirubin in humans is summarized in Fig. 14.1.

This is confusing terminology because different people mean different things. If you are going to use this terminology, make sure that you and your colleagues agree on the definitions. Nonetheless, this is what people usually mean:

- **Pre-hepatic jaundice:** this refers to jaundice caused by an excessive production of bilirubin. Remember that bilirubin is produced by the breakdown of haemoglobin in the spleen, hence the term pre-hepatic.

- **Hepatic jaundice:** for some people, this means any jaundice due to pathology in the liver (anatomically) and can thus include problems with hepatocytes (e.g. hepatitis) or with the bile canaliculi (e.g. primary sclerosing cholangitis, PSC). For other people, hepatic jaundice refers strictly to pathology affecting hepatocytes but not the bile canaliculi, which they consider part of the post-hepatic system.

- **Post-hepatic jaundice:** everyone agrees that post-hepatic jaundice refers to a problem with biliary flow. However, some people only talk of post-hepatic jaundice when the flow is obstructed outside the liver (e.g. common bile duct obstruction) whereas others would include obstruction inside the liver (e.g. PSC). Confusing!

- **Obstructive jaundice:** this refers to jaundice caused by the lack of bile flow into the gut, which manifests as pale faeces (lack of urobilin/stercobilin) and dark urine (conjugated bilirubin). Strictly, the obstruction can be anywhere in the biliary system and therefore can be in the liver (bile canaliculi) or after the liver (common bile duct). However, some authors use the term 'obstructive jaundice' to refer only to obstructions affecting the biliary system outside the liver. Again … confusing!

- **Cholestatic jaundice:** this refers to jaundice caused by bilirubin not flowing out via the common bile duct. This could be due to obstruction (e.g. a gallstone) or due to paralysis (ileus) of the common bile duct peristalsis (e.g. drug induced).

- **Unconjugated jaundice:** this refers to jaundice caused by the accumulation of unconjugated bilirubin (which is water insoluble, cannot dissolve in urine, and is thus sometimes called 'acholuric jaundice'). This can be due to excessive production of unconjugated bilirubin (increased breakdown of red blood cells) or due to decreased capacity to conjugate bilirubin (hepatocyte pathology). Thus, by definition, all pre-hepatic jaundice is unconjugated. Hepatic jaundice may be conjugated or unconjugated, depending on your definition of 'hepatic'.

14

- **Conjugated jaundice**: this refers to the accumulation of conjugated bilirubin. Thus, post-hepatic jaundice is always conjugated but hepatic jaundice can be conjugated or unconjugated depending, again, on your definition of 'hepatic'.

What is your differential diagnosis for jaundice?

It is helpful to divide your list into problems that affect either bilirubin production, bilirubin conjugation or bilirubin excretion.

The following list of differential diagnoses is not comprehensive but includes the most common causes of jaundice:

Increased production of bilirubin

Increased breakdown of red blood cells (haemolysis) can lead to excessive amounts of bilirubin in the circulation that the normal liver is unable to cope with. This can be due to:

- **Intravascular haemolysis**: if the increased haemolysis is taking place in the circulation, one might find *black urine* due to free haemoglobin being degraded via an alternative pathway into haemosiderin (which is very dark but water soluble), and *schistocytes* on a blood film (fragments of red blood cells).
  - **Congenital causes**: for example glucose-6-phosphate dehydrogenase (G6PDH) deficiency, pyruvate kinase (PK) deficiency, sickle cell disease, thalassaemia, etc.
  - **Acquired causes**: for example artificial heart valves, blood group mismatch, disseminated intravascular coagulopathy (DIC), malaria, medications, etc.
- **Extravascular haemolysis**: if the increased haemolysis is taking place in the spleen, one might find *splenomegaly* on examination and *spherocytes* on a blood film (due to the red blood cells being 'nibbled' at by splenic and liver macrophages):
  - **Congenital causes**: hereditary spherocytosis
  - **Acquired causes**: autoimmune haemolysis

Decreased conjugation of bilirubin

This is either because not enough unconjugated bilirubin is getting into the hepatocytes for conjugation (*reduced hepatocyte uptake*) or because the hepatocytes aren't conjugating bilirubin adequately (*enzymatic problems*). The excess bilirubin will be *unconjugated*. Decreased conjugation is rarely due to hepatocyte damage, because hepatocytes need to be *very damaged* before they stop conjugating bilirubin – so damaged that jaundice would be the least of one's problems.

- **Reduced hepatocyte uptake**: cholecystographic contrast agents, portosystemic shunts to bypass a cirrhotic liver
- **Congenital enzymatic problems**: Gilbert's syndrome (common), Crigler–Najjar syndrome (rare)

Decreased excretion of bilirubin

In this case, there are normal amounts of bilirubin being produced, and the liver can cope adequately with conjugating the bilirubin, but the conjugated bilirubin either cannot make it out of damaged hepatocytes (because the active exporter of bilirubin is very sensitive to damage) or cannot make it into the bowel (due to obstruction). The consequence is that faeces may become pale (due to lack of stercobilin), foul-smelling, and floating (steatorrhoea, due to lack of bile salts which normally solubilize fat in food) and the urine may become dark (due to conjugated bilirubin, which is water soluble, being excreted by the kidneys). The excess bilirubin is *conjugated*. There are many causes that can lead to reduced excretion of bilirubin from hepatocytes and into the duodenum. Congenital causes such as Dubin–Johnson syndrome are very rare. Acquired causes are much more common and different people have different ways of remembering them. Here, we offer a 'surgical sieve' using the acronym **INVITED MD** although as you can see, surgical sieves don't always work:

Infection: viral hepatitis, bacterial hepatitis (e.g. Weil's disease), ascending cholangitis, liver abscess, Echinococcus (tapeworm) infection

Neoplasia: metastatic liver cancer, hepatocellular carcinoma, pancreatic cancer, cholangiocarcinoma (cancer of the bile duct)

Vascular: Budd–Chiari syndrome (thrombosis in the hepatic vein)

Inflammation: primary biliary cirrhosis (PBC), PSC, autoimmune hepatitis, pancreatitis

Trauma: gallstones, stricture (e.g. after an endoscopic retrograde cholangiopancreatography (ERCP) or cholecystectomy)

Endocrine: there aren't really any endocrine causes

Degenerative: likewise, there aren't really any degenerative causes

Metabolic: Wilson's disease, haemochromatosis

Drugs: some drugs affect the ability of hepatocytes to excrete bilirubin (e.g. alcohol abuse, paracetamol overdose, valproate, rifampicin) whilst others can induce a paralysis (ileus) of the biliary system (e.g. co-amoxiclav, nitrofurantoin, oral contraceptive pill).

Having formulated a broad differential diagnosis for jaundice, you proceed to take a history from Miss Watroba. Your history will contain the usual elements of personal information, presenting complaint, past medical history, medications and allergies, family history, social history, and patient concerns.

Can you think of key clues in each of these sections that might suggest certain diagnoses?

Personal information

- **Ethnic background:** sickle cell disease affects mainly West African and Afro-Caribbean patients, whilst thalassaemias and G6PDH deficiency mainly affect Mediterranean, Far Eastern, and African patients.

Presenting complaint

- Is this an **acute** or **chronic** illness?

Ask about potential associated symptoms:

- **Right upper quadrant discomfort, nausea, vomiting,** and **pruritus** (itch) are all features of hepatitis of any cause (virus, autoimmune, drugs, alcohol).

- **Fever** or **diarrhoea** may additionally be present if the liver is infected (e.g. viral hepatitis, abscess).
- **Steatorrhoea** (pale, floating, foul-smelling faeces), **dark urine**, and **pruritus** are seen in obstruction to biliary flow.
- **Weight loss, fever,** and **night sweats** could indicate a malignancy of the liver, bile duct, or pancreas.
- **Bronzed skin** and **signs of diabetes mellitus** (polyuria, weight loss, infections) are suggestive of haemochromatosis. This condition is hereditary so check for family history.
- **Exposure to outdoor water/sewage** (that may be contaminated by rat urine and faeces) is a risk factor for Weil's disease.

Past medical history

- **Gallstones?** Consider obstructive jaundice due to gallstones or ascending cholangitis blocking the common bile duct.
- **Liver disease?** 'Fatty liver' (steatohepatitis due to chronic alcohol abuse or dyslipidaemia), hepatitis B and C, haemochromatosis, Wilson's disease, α_1-antitrypsin deficiency, PBC, and PSC are all causes of jaundice *per se* and also significant risk factors for liver cirrhosis.
- **Haemophilia?** Such patients may have received blood products contaminated with hepatitis C, a scenario which was tragically the case up until the 1980s.
- **Recent blood transfusion or surgery?** This may suggest a blood group incompatibility, although this is thankfully rare in hospitals today.
- **Ulcerative colitis?** This makes PSC more likely, as there is a strong association between these conditions.
- **Diabetes mellitus?** As mentioned above, this is seen in haemochromatosis.
- **Emphysema?** Suggests α_1-antitrypsin deficiency.
- **Psychosis?** May suggest Wilson's disease (rare!).

Medications

Medications can cause haemolysis by four mechanisms:

- **Intravascular haemolysis** (e.g. sulphonamides, aspirin in G6PDH-deficient patients).
- **Autoimmune, extravascular haemolysis** (e.g. methyldopa).
- **Hepatitis** (e.g. paracetamol overdose).
- **Cholestasis** (e.g. co-amoxiclav).

Family history

There are various familial conditions which can cause jaundice, such as: Gilbert's disease, haemochromatosis, Wilson's disease, sickle cell disease, thalassaemia, hereditary spherocytosis, G6PDH deficiency (although the latter is unlikely to affect Miss Watroba as it is X-linked).

Social history

- **Excessive alcohol consumption?** Quantify exactly how many units a week the patient consumes and remember that recommended levels are <14 units/

week for females and <21 units/week for males. Levels above 35 units/week for females or 50 units/week for males are very dangerous.

- **Intravenous drug use?**
- **Unprotected sex** or **multiple partners?**
- **Foreign travel?** You must consider the possibility of malaria, hepatitis A, and, if they have been to the Far East, hepatitis E.
- **Tattoos?** The unsterile conditions under which some tattoos are created, particularly those acquired abroad, increases the risk of blood-borne transmission (e.g. viral hepatitis).

Concerns

Firstly, patient concerns can provide important clues that can alter clinical management: a patient who is very worried that their jaundice is due to intravenous drug use or unprotected sex may need advising on the need to screen for a variety of pathogens such as hepatitis B, hepatitis C, HIV, *Chlamydia*, gonorrhoea, syphilis, etc.

Secondly, if you don't address a patient's concerns you are failing in your duty as a doctor. A patient whose jaundice is due to hepatitis A contracted abroad from contaminated food but who fears they have liver cancer needs reassurance.

Miss Watroba was born in Poznan, Poland. She has lived in Frankfurt for the past 4 years, and only moved to the UK 2 months ago. She has been well until 4 days ago when she began feeling nauseated and vomited a couple of times. She was initially worried that she might be pregnant, but then developed diarrhoea and mild discomfort in the right upper quadrant of her abdomen. She relaxed, assuming this meant she was suffering from an upset stomach. However, yesterday morning her flatmates noticed that her eyes were a bit yellow. The diarrhoea resolved, but by the evening, her eyes were more noticeably yellow and she decided to seek medical help. She has not lost any weight in the last few months, her faeces are brown, and she denies any urinary symptoms.

Her past medical history is remarkable only for chest infections as an infant. She has never had any surgery or transfusions of blood products. She takes paracetamol for occasional headaches but hasn't taken any in the past week. She is not allergic to any medications.

Her family are all from Poland. Her father and grandfather had heart problems and required coronary artery bypass surgery, and she has a younger brother with Down's syndrome. She does not recall anyone in her family ever being jaundiced or having hepatitis.

She shares a flat with three other Polish girls. She has smoked 10 cigarettes a day since she was 16 but says she never drinks more than 10 units of alcohol a week and she has never taken any recreational drugs. She does not have a boyfriend and appears reluctant to discuss her sexual history. You explain this information is important and that everything discussed is confidential. She hesitantly tells you that she has slept with three men in the last few months, and that some of the sexual encounters have involved unprotected intercourse. She does not undertake any regular exercise and has no history suggesting she is at risk of Weil's disease.

She is worried that she is pregnant or that she may have a sexually transmitted illness.

You examine Miss Watroba. Is there anything in particular that you will be looking out for?

14

Basic observations

- **Signs of dehydration:** tachycardia, a narrow pulse pressure, and hypotension (a late sign)
- **Fever**

On inspection

- Confirm the patient is **icteric** (yellow eyes) and **jaundiced** (yellow skin)
- Does the patient look **cachectic?** If so, consider malignancy
- Does the patient have **scratch marks,** suggesting pruritus (itch)?
- Does the patient have **needle marks,** suggesting intravenous drug use?
- Does the patient have **spider naevi, palmar erythema, clubbing,** or **bruising** that might suggest chronic liver disease?
- Does the patient have a **bronzed tan** to the skin, suggesting haemochromatosis?
- Does the patient have **Kayser–Fleischer** (green) **rings** in the iris, suggesting Wilson's disease?

On palpation

- Does the patient have any **hepatomegaly, splenomegaly,** or an **epigastric mass?** If so consider malignancy (liver or pancreatic respectively), extravascular haemolysis (splenomegaly) or acute hepatitis (hepatomegaly)
- Does the patient have **right upper quadrant tenderness?** Consider acute hepatitis or gallbladder disease (e.g. cholecystitis or cholangitis)
- Does the patient have **ascites?** Consider chronic liver disease
- Does the patient have **palpable lymphadenopathy?** Consider malignancy.

14

> On examination, Miss Watroba is jaundiced but has no other signs. Her basic observations show a regular heart rate of 75 bpm, a respiratory rate of 15/min, a blood pressure of 125/85 mmHg and a temperature of 36.8°C.
>
> **What investigations will you perform to help narrow your differential diagnosis?**

The history makes particular diagnoses unlikely (blood mismatch, alcoholic liver disease, drug-induced hepatitis, abnormal red blood cells, malaria, and G6PDH deficiency). The examination has been unhelpful in further narrowing your differential diagnoses, but the following investigations can help (key investigations for a jaundiced patient are summarized in Fig. 14.2):

Initial screen

Bloods:

- **Full blood count (FBC) and reticulocyte levels.** A low red blood cell (RBC) count with a high (>2%) reticulocyte count suggests increased RBC turnover consistent with haemolysis or a recent bleed. Remember that reticulocytes are precursors to RBCs and if the bone marrow is struggling to keep up with RBC destruction, it will end up throwing reticulocytes out into the circulation. A low RBC volume (microcytosis) would be consistent with thalassaemia (or iron-deficiency anaemia).
- **Serum bilirubin levels.** This will confirm that the jaundice is due to hyperbilirubinaemia. If the proportion of conjugated bilirubin is >20% of the total bilirubin, it suggests that the problem is obstruction to bile flow (as the liver

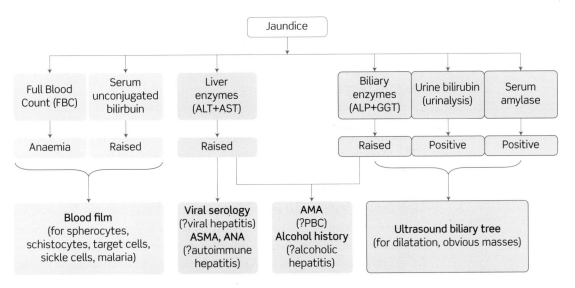

Figure 14.2 Key investigations for a jaundiced patient: ALT, alanine aminotransferase; AST, aspartate aminotransferase; ALP, alkaline phosphatase; GGT, gamma-glutamyl transferase; ASMA, antismooth muscle antibodies; ANA, antinuclear antibodies; AMA, antimitochondrial antibodies; PBC, primary biliary cirrhosis.

14

can cope with conjugating all the bilirubin that reaches it). In Gilbert's disease, total bilirubin levels will not be >100 μM.

- **Liver enzymes.** Alanine aminotransferase (ALT) and aspartate aminotransferase (AST) are raised if there is damage to hepatocytes, and are very high in acute viral hepatitis. In general, elevation of AST > ALT suggests excessive alcohol intake whereas elevation of ALT > AST suggests viral hepatitis.

- **Alkaline phosphatase (ALP) and gamma-glutamyl transferase (GGT).** ALP and GGT are useful enzymes if bile flow obstruction is suspected. ALP is released from damaged biliary epithelial cells, bones with high turnover, and/or a placenta (remember that she might be pregnant!). GGT is expressed almost exclusively by biliary epithelial cells. Consequently, a raised ALP and raised GGT suggest bile duct pathology (e.g. obstruction), whereas a raised ALP but normal GGT suggests increased bone turnover (e.g. malignant bone metastases, primary hyperparathyroidism) or pregnancy. Hepatitis is often associated with an element of intrahepatic obstruction and a rise in GGT and ALP. A raised GGT in isolation is seen after recent alcohol consumption.

- **Serum amylase or lipase.** Elevated levels of either of these pancreatic enzymes is highly suggestive (although not 100% specific) of pancreatic pathology (e.g. pancreatitis).

Urine:

- **Urinalysis.** Bilirubin in the urine (which may be visible to the naked eye as brown urine) is always pathological and indicates post-hepatic obstruction. Urobilinogen is sometimes found in the urine of healthy adults and is the result of bilirubin being metabolized by gut bacteria and then reabsorbed in the gut. Thus in post-hepatic obstruction, bilirubin cannot reach the gut and therefore no urobilinogen appears in the urine.

Second-line investigations

Bloods:

+ **Blood film.** If the initial screen suggests that the jaundice is due to haemolysis (anaemia, elevated unconjugated bilirubin), a blood film will allow you to directly assess whether there are schistocytes, sickle cells, target cells (thalassaemia), spherocytes, or malaria.

+ **Viral screen.** If the initial screen reveals elevated liver enzymes, it is worth checking serology for hepatitis A, hepatitis B, and hepatitis C in anyone with jaundice of unclear aetiology. Epstein–Barr virus (EBV, causing glandular fever) and cytomegalovirus (CMV) are also relatively common in the younger population and would be worth checking in a patient like Miss Watroba. Given the patient's confessed unprotected intercourse with multiple partners, you may wish to suggest that she has her HIV status checked too.

+ **Autoimmune screen.** Check antinuclear antibodies (ANA), antismooth muscle antibodies (ASMA), and antimitochondrial antibodies (AMA). These should be checked if the initial screen reveals elevated liver enzymes, i.e. hepatocyte damage. ASMA are positive in (type I) autoimmune hepatitis. AMA is elevated in 95% of patients with PBC and in some patients with autoimmune hepatitis.

+ **Congenital screen.** Check for haemochromatosis (high ferritin, high transferrin saturation), α_1-antitrypsin deficiency (low α_1-antitrypsin levels) and Wilson's disease (high Cu, low caeruloplasmin).

Imaging:

+ **Ultrasound of abdomen.** An ultrasound of the pancreas and biliary tree may be helpful, particularly if the history, examination, and blood results suggest problems with biliary outflow (pale faeces, dark urine, high ALP + GGT). If the common bile duct is dilated, it suggests mechanical obstruction. The cause may be obvious (e.g. gallstone) but if not, further imaging (e.g. magnetic resonance cholangiopancreatography (MRCP), endoscopic ultrasound, computed tomography (CT) scan of the abdomen) will be necessary. If the common bile duct is not dilated, but you think the problem is biliary outflow, you should think of other causes of cholestasis: drugs, PBC, PSC, cholangiocarcinoma, or a choledochal cyst.

Further investigations

+ **Pregnancy test.** This won't help with your diagnosis but you should address the patient's concern that she might be pregnant. You should also offer to refer her to a GUM clinic given her worries about sexually transmitted illnesses.

+ **Clotting studies.** The prothrombin time (PT) should be measured if liver pathology is suspected, as deranged PT is one of the earliest markers of compromised liver function.

+ **Albumin.** This is a reasonable marker of liver function (but takes about 20 days to fall). Decreased albumin suggests either reduced synthesis of albumin (e.g. liver damage, severe malnutrition) or increased albumin loss (e.g. nephrotic syndrome).

- **Liver ultrasound.** A useful, safe, non-invasive imaging modality that will show, for example, cirrhosis or liver carcinoma.
- **Liver biopsy.** This invasive procedure may be necessary to establish the diagnosis in liver disease.

Blood and urine samples are taken and sent off to labs. Initial results show:

Hb	12.6 g/dL
RBC	5.2×10^{12} cells/L
WCC	14×10^9 cells/L
Platelets	280×10^9 cells/L
MCV	92 fL
Total bilirubin	95 µM
Albumin	36g/L
ALT	1650 U/L
AST	1200 U/L
ALP	60 U/L
GGT	20 U/L
Serum amylase	36 U/L
PT	12 seconds
APTT	35 seconds

Urinalysis is positive for bilirubin. All other results are pending.

(Hb, haemoglobin; MCV, mean corpuscular volume; APTT, activated partial thromboplastin time)

How would you interpret these results? What is the likely diagnosis? What is your next step?

The presence of bilirubin in the urine is always pathological and suggests problems in conjugated bilirubin getting out of hepatocytes into bile and down to the duodenum. The high WCC suggests infection. The elevated ALT and AST suggest damage to hepatocytes. Thus, there appears to be an infection that is damaging hepatocytes and compromising the ability of conjugated bilirubin to reach the duodenum. Several infections could do this but the *very* high ALT and AST levels (>1000 U/L) are strongly suggestive of a **viral hepatitis**. If you haven't already, you should send for **viral serology** and a **liver autoimmune profile**.

Viral serology is requested and shows:

Anti-HepA IgM/IgG	Negative
HepC on PCR	Negative
HBsAg (HepB surface antigen)	Positive
HBeAg (HepB core antigen)	Positive
Anti-HBeAg IgM	Positive
Anti-HBsAg IgG	Negative
AMA	Undetectable
ASMA	Undetectable
ANA	Undetectable

What is the diagnosis and prognosis for this condition?

Miss Watroba is suffering **acute viral hepatitis B**. The prognosis for acute viral hepatitis B is:

- **'Full recovery'.** In the majority of cases, hepatitis B is a self-limiting condition with full *clinical* recovery, although evidence suggests that the virus is rarely cleared completely but kept in check by cytotoxic T-cells. Thus, immunosuppression at any stage in later life can lead to reactivation of the virus. However, if patients recover from acute hepatitis B and have undetectable levels of virus (HBeAg), the long-term sequelae are negligible.

- **Carrier status.** About 10% will become asymptomatic carriers (no symptoms but virus still detectable in the blood). In such patients, the long-term prognosis is good with most studies suggesting that the risk of long-term complications is <1%.

- **Chronic hepatitis B.** About 5–10% will develop chronic (symptomatic) hepatitis B. Rates are 90% if the infection was acquired at birth from the mother. Of the patients who develop chronic infection, about 20% will develop cirrhosis and 6% will develop hepatocellular carcinoma.

- **Fulminant hepatitis.** About 0.5% of patients with acute hepatitis B will develop fulminant hepatitis B, which has a mortality rate of 80%.

How should Miss Watroba be managed?

Miss Watroba needs referral to a specialist hepatologist. Management of the acute phase is supportive and largely involves:

- Practising 'safe sex' with barrier protection until her virus levels are undetectable (HBeAg negative)
- Minimizing alcohol consumption to <10 units/week during the acute phase
- Avoid sharing any toothbrushes or razors
- Contact tracing
- Vaccinate current sexual partners and children, who are at risk of exposure via cuts and scratches

Miss Watroba probably contracted hepatitis B during her unprotected sexual encounters. She should therefore be advised to attend a genitourinary medicine (GUM) clinic to screen for other sexually transmitted diseases and for advice on precautions during future sexual encounters.

14

Short cases

Jane is a 21-year-old female who attends her GP complaining of 'yellow eyes'. For the past few days she has been feeling unwell with a cough and fever, but she is most distressed about the unusual colour of her eyes. She has never received blood or coagulation factors, denies any intravenous drug use, and she denies any sexual intercourse in the last 6 months. Blood tests taken by the GP reveal:

Hb	13.7 g/dL
RBC	6.1×10^{12} cells/L
WCC	13×10^9 cells/L
Platelets	180×10^9 cells/L
Total bilirubin	60 μM
Conjugated bilirubin	2 μM

Markers for viral hepatitis are negative. Liver enzymes and reticulocyte count are within the normal range. A blood film is reported as unremarkable. A urine dipstick is normal.

What is the likely diagnosis? How should it be managed?

The most likely diagnosis is **Gilbert's syndrome**, a diagnosis of exclusion. Thus you need to demonstrate normal liver enzymes, normal haemoglobin levels, a serum bilirubin <100 μM and no bilirubin on a urine dipstick. This is an autosomal recessive condition affecting approximately 3–8% of Caucasians that results in the liver not being able to conjugate bilirubin at an adequate rate in times of physiological stress (e.g. acute infection, excessive alcohol, pregnancy, starvation). There is no need for management for Gilbert's syndrome as it is asymptomatic except for the occasional episode of icterus. Patients should be reassured there is nothing they can do beyond leading as healthy a life as possible.

14

Mrs Gupta is a 43-year-old marketing director who attends her local A&E complaining of yellow eyes, nausea, and pain in her abdomen. It all started a few days ago after dinner, when she developed a stabbing pain in the right upper quadrant. The pain 'comes and goes' several times a day, with each wave of pain lasting about 40 minutes. She has developed smelly, loose stools that are slightly pale and her urine is dark.

Her past medical history is unremarkable. She takes no medications and does not smoke or drink. On examination, she is afebrile but jaundiced. She is tachycardic and has tenderness on deep palpation of her right upper quadrant. The rest of her examination is normal.

Initial blood results show:

Hb	13.4 g/dL
RBC	6.1×10^{12} cells/L
WCC	11.8×10^9 cells/L
Platelets	320×10^9 cells/L
Bilirubin	134 µM
INR	1.2
ESR	21 mm/h
Albumin	32 g/L
ALT	98 U/L
AST	92 U/L
ALP	410 U/L
GGT	231 U/L

(INR, international normalized ratio; ESR, erythrocyte sedimentation rate)

An abdominal ultrasound reveals a common bile duct that is dilated proximal to an echogenic mass in the lumen of the duct, but no other pathology.

What is the diagnosis? What related surgical emergencies must you rule out?

Mrs Gupta has presented with jaundice, steatorrhoea, and dark urine. This suggests that the jaundice is due to reduced excretion of conjugated bilirubin via the normal route. The elevated ALP and GGT together suggest damage to biliary epithelia, and the raised ALT and AST suggest damage to hepatocytes. Put together, this suggests that the jaundice is due to obstruction in the biliary system (**obstructive jaundice**). Several aetiologies are possible, but the history of waves of right upper quadrant pain and nausea are suggestive of biliary colic due to a **gallstone**. The ultrasound confirms an echogenic mass in the common bile duct which is almost certainly a gallstone. If the ultrasound had been inconclusive, the next step would be to visualize the biliary tree and pancreas using MRCP. Most gallstones pass by themselves, but if they cause obstructive jaundice they need removing via **ERCP**.

In anyone presenting acutely with gallstone pathology you have to rule out two related conditions that are surgical emergencies:

- **Cholecystitis:** the patient will usually present with constant, unresolving (>6 hours) fever, a tender abdomen (Murphy's sign positive) that is often distended, nausea, and possibly vomiting. Cholecystitis is an emergency that requires prompt antibiotics, analgesia, nil by mouth, and intravenous (IV) fluids, plus a cholecystectomy (either urgently or electively). Mrs Gupta does not have cholecystitis (yet) as her symptoms are intermittent and she is afebrile.

- **Ascending cholangitis:** such patients often present with Charcot's triad of febrile rigors, jaundice, and right upper quadrant pain. This is also an emergency and requires blood cultures, careful monitoring, broad-spectrum antibiotics, and an ERCP to drain the common bile duct of pus. Mrs Gupta does not have ascending cholangitis: she is afebrile and far too well.

14

Short case

Mrs Gonzalez is a 48-year-old woman presenting with jaundice. She has become increasingly lethargic over the past month. For the past week she has had yellow, itchy skin and pale, offensive stools. Her past medical history is unremarkable and she takes no medications. She does not smoke and drinks less than 10 units of alcohol a week.

On inspection, she is jaundiced and looks unwell. Several spider naevi are evident on her chest and a number of bruises are noticeable on her limbs. Her liver is tender to palpation. The rest of her examination is unremarkable.

Her urine dipstick is positive for bilirubin, despite her urine not being dark to the naked eye. An abdominal ultrasound does not reveal any abdominal masses, gallstones, or dilated common bile duct. Her blood results are:

Hb	12.3 g/dL
RBC	5.2×10^{12} cells/L
WCC	11×10^9 cells/L
Platelets	220×10^9 cells/L
Bilirubin	120 μM
INR	1.7
ESR	62 mm/h
Albumin	41 g/L
Total cholesterol	4.1 mM
HDL cholesterol	2.8 mM
ALT	100 U/L
AST	85 U/L
ALP	320 U/L
GGT	210 U/L
AMA	60 IU/L
ASMA	Undetectable
ANA	Undetectable
Anti-HepA IgM/IgG	Undetectable
Anti-HBsAg	Positive
Anti-HBeAg	Negative
Anti-HepC PCR	Negative

What is the diagnosis? How should this patient be managed?

Mrs Gonzalez is jaundiced. The elevated ESR and a borderline high WCC suggest an inflammatory process. Her INR is elevated, suggesting poor liver synthetic function or decreased absorption of fat-soluble vitamin K. Her ALT and AST are elevated, suggesting active liver damage. Viral serology is negative (the positive anti-HBsAg but negative anti-HBeAg result indicates past vaccination), making viral hepatitis unlikely. ALP and GGT are elevated, suggesting damage to the biliary epithelial cells. She has bilirubin in her urine and steatorrhoea suggesting obstruction to the biliary tree.

There are multiple causes of post-hepatic (obstructive) jaundice but her positive AMA suggests this is a case of **PBC**. This is an autoimmune disorder characterized by T-cell-mediated destruction of the biliary ducts (the autoantibodies form as a secondary consequence of this damage). As the biliary ducts are destroyed (hence the high ALP and GGT), outflow of bile contents (including bilirubin) from the liver is obstructed. This explains the pale faeces (lack of urobilin and stercobilin), smelly faeces (undissolved fat due to lack of bile salts), itch (due to accumulation of bile salt in the skin), and jaundice.

Management of PBC involves:

- **Refer to hepatologist,** for ongoing care
- **Confirm diagnosis,** via MRCP and liver biopsy
- **Immunosuppression** (as this is an autoimmune condition), using agents such as corticosteroids, methotrexate, or ciclosporin
- **Bile salt replacement,** using agents such as ursodeoxycholic acid
- **Fat-soluble vitamin replacement:** supplement the fat-soluble vitamins A, D, E, and K
- **Pruritus (itch) management,** using agents such as cholestyramine (which sequesters bile salts in the gut lumen to prevent their reabsorption) and antihistamines
- **Liver transplant,** to be considered once the patient becomes cirrhotic.

14

Mr Al-Iqbal is a 38-year-old mathematics teacher with ulcerative colitis. He is attending his local hospital for his yearly colonoscopy, because patients with ulcerative colitis have a much higher risk of colonic cancer. The radiology registrar notices that Mr Al-Iqbal is icteric and offers to investigate this there and then. Mr Al-Iqbal denies feeling unwell, and had not even noticed his icterus. He has never received any blood transfusions or clotting factors and never drinks any alcohol. He has not noticed any change in his bowel motions or urine. The radiology registrar sends off bloods, which come back showing a normal full blood count, normal clotting screen, total bilirubin = 70 μM, ALT = 60 U/L, AST = 32 U/L, ALP = 200 U/L, GGT = 80 U/L, negative AMA, negative ASMA, negative ANA, and negative serology for viral hepatitis.

The mildly elevated ALT, ALP, and GGT suggest a post-hepatic (obstructive) cause to Mr Al-Iqbal's jaundice. Worried about potential gallstones, but concerned about an alternative diagnosis, the radiology registrar performs an MRCP study of Mr Al-Iqbal's liver, bile duct, and pancreas. The MRCP shows that the bile ducts are dilated in some areas but have strictures in others, all along their course from inside the liver down to midway along the cystic duct.

Why did the radiologist opt to perform an MRCP rather than an ultrasound? What is the likely diagnosis?

Mr Al-Iqbal appears to have jaundice caused by cholestasis due to pathology in the biliary system (hence his elevated ALP and GGT). The best way to determine the cause of the obstruction is to use some form of imaging. This usually involves ultrasound, which is good at showing masses (e.g. gallstones, tumours) but less good at showing the fine detail of the biliary tree. The radiologist knew that patients with ulcerative colitis are at increased risk of PSC, a disease which affects the biliary tree – hence this choice to do an MRCP, which will show any masses compressing the biliary tree but also any strictures within the bile ducts.

The MRCP did not show any masses, but instead multiple areas of biliary strictures that had led to dilatation upstream. This is highly suggestive of **PSC**. This is also a T-cell-mediated autoimmune destruction of biliary epithelial cells, leading to multifocal scarring of the biliary ducts. Approximately 90% of patients with PSC have underlying **ulcerative colitis** (although only 5% of patients with ulcerative colitis develop PSC). Patients with PSC also have elevated perinuclear antineutrophil cytoplasmic autoantibodies (pANCA) in 60–80% of cases.

Management of PSC is essentially the same as for PBC (see earlier).

Mr MacDonald is a 72-year-old gentleman referred to the surgical admissions unit by his GP. He is jaundiced and has noticed his trousers becoming looser over the past few months. He initially attributed his jaundice to excessive alcohol consumption, as he drinks 2 pints of Guinness every day before going to bed. He says that he is otherwise well, but on inspection you notice that he is severely cachectic, with the skin around his ribs and abdomen looking too big for him. Lymph nodes are palpable in his left supraclavicular fossa, and on deep palpation of his abdomen a mass is noted in his epigastrium.

What is the likely diagnosis? What initial investigations will you perform?

Few people successfully lose *significant* weight on purpose (despite many people dieting) and so weight loss should always alert you to the possibility of a catabolic (energy-consuming) process such as cancer. The combination of significant weight loss, an epigastric mass, Virchow's lymphadenopathy, and painless jaundice should make you suspicious of **pancreatic carcinoma**.

Initial investigations should include:

- **FBC:** cancer patients are often anaemic
- **Serum amylase:** this may be raised in any form of pancreatic disease
- **Liver enzymes:** to see if there is liver pathology secondary to the obstruction
- **Abdominal ultrasound:** to see if a cause for the obstruction is apparent

An abdominal ultrasound revealed a mass in the head of the pancreas compressing the common bile duct, which was later found to be a **pancreatic adenocarcinoma**. Pancreatic cancer has a very bad prognosis, despite heroic surgical attempts to remove it (known as a Whipple's procedure). Five-year mortality is around 97% without surgery and 80% (at best) with surgery.

14

Miss Hoeder is a 26-year-old journalist who presents to her GP complaining of increasing fatigue. She claims that she is usually a highly active individual who runs 10 km twice a week and is always 'up for a party'. Over the past month, she has become unusually tired. At first, she put this down to 'a flu or something' but her fatigue and lethargy have remained, and she is worried because she gets short of breath when she goes for even a gentle run. Her periods have not been unusual in any way but she has noticed that her eyes are yellow and she thinks her skin might be slightly yellow, too. Her family history is unremarkable.

On examination, Miss Hoeder is indeed icteric and jaundiced. Her spleen is palpable just below her left costal margin. The rest of the examination is unremarkable.

The GP sends off some blood for analysis. It reveals:

Hb	9.2 g/dL
RBC	3.6×10^{12} cells/L
MCV	95 fL
WCC	4.5×10^9 cells/L
Platelets	210×10^9 cells/L
Reticulocytes	6%
INR	1.05
Total bilirubin	72 μM
Conjugated bilirubin	7 μM
Blood film	Spherocytes and reticulocytes evident

What is the likely diagnosis? What is the next step?

Miss Hoeder has a normocytic anaemia with a reticulocytosis, spherocytosis, and jaundice. This suggests a **haemolytic anaemia**.

The next step is to diagnose the cause for her haemolytic anaemia by referring her to a haematologist. The combination of spherocytes and elevated bilirubin in Miss Hoeder suggests that she is suffering from extravascular haemolysis. This is either due to hereditary spherocytosis or due to an autoimmune haemolytic anaemia (including drug-induced). The lack of family history makes hereditary spherocytosis unlikely. Thus, autoimmune haemolytic anaemia is the most likely diagnosis, and hence tests to detect anti-erythrocyte antibodies (e.g. Coomb's test) should be performed.

Viva questions

A medical student is asked to take urgent bloods for cross-matching from an intravenous drug user and alcohol-dependent patient who has presented to A&E with bleeding oesophageal varices. Having successfully obtained the blood, the student cannot see a sharps disposal bin within easy access. Ignoring all previous health and safety advice, the student tries to resheath the used needle into its cap, and in doing so sustains a needlestick injury. What infections is the student most at risk of catching?

Most people worry about HIV transmission from needlestick injuries. This concern is understandable, because despite great advances in the management of HIV infection, there is still no cure. However, HIV is a rather fragile virus (it won't last more than a few hours at room temperature) and the risk of infection from a single needlestick injury is estimated to be 0.3%.

Hepatitis C has an infection risk following needlestick injury of 3%. Hepatitis B virus, by contrast, is a robust virus that will survive for up to a week at 44°C. Risk of infection after a needlestick injury is 30%. These statistics assume that the injury occurred from a patient who is a carrier for the virus, rather than the population as a whole.

If a patient is clinically jaundiced, how high will his bilirubin levels be at a minimum?

Jaundice is due to the accumulation of bilirubin above its normal range of 3–17 μM (of which at least 10% will be conjugated bilirubin). For jaundice to be visible to the naked eye, serum bilirubin levels must be >40 μM.

A medical student is asked to provide proof of his hepatitis B immunization status. As he has lost his relevant paperwork, Occupational Health take a blood sample for serological studies. These reveal that the student has

HBsAg	Positive
IgG anti-HBs	Positive
IgG anti-HBc	Positive
IgM anti-HBc	Negative

What do these results mean?

Like any virus, hepatitis B virus contains multiple proteins. The surface antigen (HBsAg or HBs) is present on the surface of the virus and is used, in isolation, for immunization. The core antigen (HBe or its precursor HBc) is buried deep inside the virus and is absent from the vaccine preparation.

He has positive IgG anti-HBs which could be due to vaccination or infection. However, he also has high levels of HBsAg suggesting either the presence of the virus or a *very recent* vaccination. Most importantly, he has positive IgG anti-HBc, suggesting infection with the hepatitis B virus (as HBc is *not* a part of the vaccine). The lack of IgM anti-HBc (remember that IgM is an acute antibody) suggests this is *chronic* hepatitis B. This has potential implications for his medical career, so he should seek advice from both a hepatologist and from occupational health, and practice safe sex at all times.

Which tumours could cause obstructive jaundice?

The most common tumours causing obstructive jaundice are carcinoma of the head of the pancreas and malignant lymph nodes at the porta hepatitis. Liver metastases or a carcinoma at the ampulla of Vater are less common, while cholangiocarcinoma (cancer of the biliary tree) is rare. For interest, a Klatskin tumour is a cholangiocarcinoma at the confluence of right and left hepatic ducts.

Why does obstruction of the common bile duct result in steatorrhoea?

Steatorrhoea is stool with a high fat content – it is typically foul-smelling, greasy, pale, and floats in water. Bile salts provide stool with its colour and normally emulsify (solubilize) fats in the intestine which facilitates absorption through the enterocyte brush border. If bile is not reaching the intestine then less fat will be absorbed and more will be excreted with the faeces. As a consequence, the patient will have steatorrhoea but may also develop deficiency of fat-soluble vitamins (A, D, E, K).

 For a range of Single Best Answer questions related to the topic of this chapter go to www.oxfordtextbooks.co.uk/orc/ocms/

14

Right upper quadrant (RUQ) pain

Core case

Core case

Mrs Cole is an overweight 38-year-old Caucasian woman who presents to accident and emergency (A&E) at 11 p.m. complaining of severe pain in the RUQ of her abdomen, nausea, and vomiting.

What is your differential diagnosis for this lady's current presentation? Think anatomically of which structures might give you pain in the RUQ of the abdomen. Try to arrange your list of possible diagnoses in order of likelihood given this patient's sex, age, and presentation.

We have arranged the differential diagnosis in order of likelihood in a woman of this age.

> ### Biliary colic
> ### Cholecystitis
> ### Duodenal ulcer
> Pancreatitis
> ### Basal pneumonia (irritating the right hemidiaphragm)
> Ascending cholangitis
> Gastric ulcer
> Small bowel obstruction
> Appendicitis
> Hepatitis (autoimmune, infective, or drug-induced)
> Pyelonephritis
> Ovarian pathology

15

Let us suppose that Mrs Cole was 68 years old, rather than 38 years old.

Would your differential diagnosis list change?

Yes, the likelihood of certain diseases would change considerably. In older patients, certain pathologies are relatively more common, such as pneumonia, cancer (e.g. cholangiocarcinoma), or vascular disease (aortic dissection, abdominal aortic aneurysm, inferior myocardial infarction). Of course, the differential would still include those diseases seen in a 38-year-old Mrs Cole.

What questions should you ask in a history to narrow your differential diagnoses?

Characterize the pain. One useful way is to follow the mnemonic SOCRATES:

Site of pain, and has it moved since it began?

Onset of pain – was it sudden or gradual, and did something trigger it?

Character of pain – stabbing, dull, deep, superficial, gripping, tearing, burning?

Radiation of pain – does the patient have pain elsewhere?

Attenuating factors – does anything make the pain better (position? medications?)

Timing of pain – how long has it gone on for, has it been constant or coming and going?

Exacerbating factors – does anything make the pain worse (moving? breathing?)

Severity – on a scale of 0–10, where 10 is the worst pain ever (e.g. childbirth).

Once you have characterized the pain, you should ask:

- **Has the patient had any symptoms other than pain?** (e.g. fever, weight loss). The reason is that certain other symptoms will help you refine your diagnosis. Thus, fever suggests an infective process and makes a myocardial infarction less likely. Significant weight loss over the preceding months may be due to a cancer, which is catabolic.

- **When did they last open their bowels or pass any flatus (wind)?** A patient who hasn't opened his or her bowels may be constipated, whilst a patient who isn't even managing to pass wind ('absolute constipation') may be obstructed – a surgical emergency.

- **Have they noticed any change in their stool recently?** (e.g. colour, floating, smelly). If the common bile duct is obstructed, bilirubin and fat-dissolving bile salts won't reach the bowel and thus stools will be pale, floating, and smelly (steatorrhoea). If blood is entering the bowel lumen via a bleeding ulcer, the iron (haemoglobin) in the blood will be oxidized, making stools appear very dark, black, tarry, and smelly (melaena).

- **If they are female, are they pregnant?** If the patient is a female of fertile age, you must exclude pregnancy, even if the patient insists they are not pregnant or sexually active. This is partly because radiography of a pregnant woman is legally irresponsible and partly because potentially fatal ectopic pregnancies are a major source of abdominal pain – even if pain in the RUQ would be an unusual presentation.

15

Mrs Cole's pain is in the RUQ of her abdomen. It came on gradually 16 hours ago when she went to bed. It is deep, sharp, constant, and 8/10 in severity. She also gets the occasional sharp stabbing sensation on her back and she points to her right scapula very specifically (this is known as Boas' sign). She has not found anything that makes it better or worse. She last opened her bowels before she went to bed but has been passing flatus this morning. She reports no significant weight change recently.

In the history, she also reveals that every couple of months, usually after a heavy, fatty meal, she develops a sharp, stabbing pain in the same area of her abdomen and which usually gets better after a few hours. Her past medical history includes heartburn (dyspepsia), which is well controlled with omeprazole (a proton-pump inhibitor, PPI). However, the pain this time 'feels different' and she feels 'very sick'.

Just from this history, particular diagnoses become very likely. The next steps will be to examine the patient and arrange first-line investigations with the aim of confirming your suspected diagnosis and ruling out those diseases that would require urgent management (those in red in our differential list above).

What key features on examination would you look out for?

- **Jaundice:** most easily seen in the whites of the eyes (sclera); it is typical of diseases that block the common bile duct such as choledocholithiasis, ascending cholangitis, acute pancreatitis, pancreatic cancer, or cholangiocarcinoma.
- **Bruising and discoloration around the umbilicus and flank** (Cullen's sign or Grey Turner's sign, respectively). Sometimes seen in severe pancreatitis.
- **A pulsatile and laterally expansile central mass.** This indicates an abdominal aortic aneurysm.
- **Murphy's sign:** palpate the abdomen just below the tip of the right ninth costal cartilage, apply pressure, and ask the patient to take a deep breath. This will cause the liver and hence gallbladder to descend and press against your fingers. If the gallbladder is tender it will cause the patient to arrest inspiration as the gallbladder strikes your fingers. This is strongly suggestive of an inflamed gallbladder (cholecystitis).
- **Peritonitis:** the patient will lie very still, have a rigid and exquisitely tender abdomen, and exhibit guarding when you try to palpate lightly. There may be no bowel sounds. In the case of Mrs Cole, this would suggest perforation of a peptic ulcer or the gallbladder.
- **Signs of small bowel obstruction:** a distended abdomen (which may be hard to appreciate in a patient with a high body mass index (BMI)) and absent or tinkling bowel sounds. If the bowel becomes strangulated, signs of peritonitis would predominate.

15

On examination, Mrs Cole is febrile (38.3°C) and tachycardic (108 bpm). Her cardiovascular and respiratory systems are otherwise unremarkable. She is not jaundiced, has no hernias, and no palpable abdominal masses. Her abdominal aorta is palpable but does not feel laterally expansile. Her RUQ is tender to light palpation with a positive Murphy's sign. A digital rectal examination in the presence of a female nurse reveals soft faeces in the rectum but no signs of blood.

Her history and physical examination are very typical of a particular diagnosis. The next step is to arrange first-line investigations that will confirm this diagnosis and help rule out other diagnoses that you should exclude because of their need for urgent management.

What investigations will you request?

Blood tests

- **Full blood count:** the patient may be anaemic from a chronically bleeding gastric or duodenal ulcer. Her white cell count will be elevated if she has any inflammatory condition (e.g. cholecystitis, ascending cholangitis, or basal pneumonia).

- **Serum amylase (or lipase) levels:** slight increases (200–600 U/L) in amylase levels are most commonly caused by pancreatitis, but also by various other pathologies such as bowel obstruction, mesenteric ischaemia, a posteriorly perforated duodenal ulcer, mumps, pancreatic carcinoma, or opiate medications. However, very high amylase levels (>1000 U/L) or elevated lipase levels (>300 U/L) are almost exclusively found in pancreatitis. (The exact cut offs will depend upon your local laboratory protocols).

- **Liver enzymes:** elevated levels of aspartate aminotransferase (AST) and alanine aminotransferase (ALT) suggest inflammation in the liver which could be due to viral hepatitis, autoimmune hepatitis, or obstruction of the common bile duct because of a gallstone, infection of the duct, tumour of the duct, inflammation of the pancreas or tumour of the pancreas. A raised alkaline phosphatase (ALP) level by itself can be due to increased bone breakdown (e.g. metastatic bone disease, Paget's disease). However, a raised ALP level that is more elevated than AST/ALT levels and/or accompanied by a raised gamma-glutamyl transferase (GGT) level suggests obstruction of the common bile duct.

- **Bilirubin:** elevated levels of *unconjugated* bilirubin suggest that the liver cannot conjugate it fast enough, either because there is too much breakdown of haemoglobin into bilirubin (e.g. haemolytic anaemia), because of a hereditary deficiency of conjugating enzyme (e.g. Gilbert's syndrome), intrahepatic (e.g. viral hepatitis) or extrahepatic (e.g. gallstones). Elevated levels of *conjugated* bilirubin suggest the liver is working (conjugating) but that there is obstruction of bile flow.

Imaging

- **Erect chest radiograph:** air under the diaphragm strongly suggests a perforated viscus such as a gastric or duodenal ulcer (but can also be a sign of recent abdominal surgery). Bear in mind that if this patient had suffered a perforated peptic ulcer we would have found signs of peritonism during the abdominal examination. A wide mediastinum and/or heart shadow can suggest aortic dissection. Don't forget to do a pregnancy test before any radiography on a woman of fertile age, no matter how much they insist they cannot be pregnant – this not only rules out certain gynaecological pathologies (e.g. ectopic pregnancies) but is important from a patient safety and medicolegal point of view.

- **Abdominal radiograph:** air on both sides of the bowel wall (Rigler's sign) strongly suggests a perforated gastric or duodenal ulcer. Small bowel loops with a diameter >3 cm suggests small bowel obstruction (possibly in conjunction with large bowel obstruction). Large bowel loops with a diameter >6 cm suggests large bowel obstruction. Not being able to see one of the two shadows caused by both psoas muscles may suggest retroperitoneal fluid (e.g. a ruptured abdominal aortic aneurysm or pancreatitis).

- **Ultrasound of pancreas, common bile duct, and gallbladder:** an ultrasound can reveal tumours in the pancreas or a dilated common bile duct due to obstruction (upper limit of normal is 6–7 mm diameter). An inflamed gallbladder (thick wall, fluid around it) may in some instances be apparent on ultrasound. Stones in the biliary tree should be visible if present.

15

Mrs Cole's blood tests, and chest and abdomen radiography are all normal. The abdominal ultrasound reveals a common bile duct of normal diameter, no masses in the pancreas but a gallbladder with a wall measuring an average of 4.5 mm (normal is ≤3 mm).

In light of the history, examination, and first-line investigations, what is the most likely diagnosis? How does this explain her symptoms?

This is a classical clinical picture for someone with **cholecystitis**: a middle-aged, Caucasian female with RUQ pain, positive Murphy's sign, fever, and a previous history of pains in this area after heavy, fatty meals. The normal serum amylase levels rule out pancreatitis. The lack of jaundice or raised serum bilirubin suggest that there is no obstruction of the common bile duct. There were no signs on examination suggestive of bowel obstruction or peritonism, and the abdominal and chest radiographs were normal, so small bowel obstruction or a perforated peptic ulcer are unlikely. The ultrasound did not reveal any pancreatic or common bile duct masses, suggesting that there is no pancreatic cancer nor cholangiocarcinoma. It did show a thick gallbladder wall suggesting it is inflamed.

Cholecystitis (*chole* = bile, *cyst* = bladder, *-itis* = inflammation) is inflammation of the gallbladder, caused in 95% of cases by a stone in the gallbladder. The gallbladder has a chemical inflammation and this may lead to subsequent infection affecting the surrounding tissue. The inflamed gallbladder irritates the parietal peritoneum, causing a *constant* pain. Irritation of the visceral peritoneum in the initial stages produces a poorly localized, dull, midline epigastric pain. As the irritation spreads outwards to the parietal peritoneum, the pain becomes sharply localized to the RUQ. The inflamed gallbladder can also irritate the liver capsule, which in turn can irritate the diaphragm above it. The diaphragm is supplied by nerve roots C3, C4, and C5 ('*3, 4, 5 keep the diaphragm alive*') which also supply sensation to the shoulder. The referred pain in the right scapula is believed to be because the central nervous system (probably the dorsal spinal cord, but perhaps the sensory cortex in the brain) confuses the incoming signals from the right shoulder and the right hemidiaphragm.

15

How will the team manage Mrs Cole's cholecystitis?

When asked about management in exams, remember that you must start from the beginning and not dive into drugs or surgery. Thus, having assessed her need for resuscitation (Airway, Breathing, and Circulation, ABC), taken a full history, examined the patient, carried out first-line investigations, and suggested a diagnosis of cholecystitis, Mrs Cole's therapeutic management can be divided into operative and non-operative:

- **Non-operative:**
  - **Nil by mouth.** Mrs Cole should avoid all food and have only sips of water. This is partly to avoid food in the duodenum triggering gallbladder contractions and partly to prepare her if there is a need for surgery.

- **Intravenous (IV) fluids.** To avoid dehydration, as she is nil by mouth (apart from sips).
- **Analgesia.** Opioids may be necessary in the initial stages, regular paracetamol will probably suffice later. Orally administered analgesics should be avoided if the patient is vomiting.
- **Antibiotics.** Broad-spectrum cover in accordance with local hospital guidelines. This will start to combat the infection if surgery is delayed and will reduce the risk of systemic or peritoneal infection as a consequence of the surgery.

- **Operative:** Mrs Cole should undergo a **laparoscopic cholecystectomy** to remove her inflamed gallbladder. Controversy exists over whether the best strategy is urgent laparoscopic cholecystectomy within the first 72 hours or treating the acute episode and then returning the patient for an elective cholecystectomy 6–12 weeks later. The arguments in favour of the latter are that conversion rates from laparoscopic to open surgery are reduced. However, waiting for an elective procedure may mean that patients have repeat admissions in the interim – and this entails increased morbidity, expense, and lost time (for the patient).

15

Short cases

Mrs Cole (from the above case) was admitted onto a surgical ward, and the admitting team opted not to perform an urgent laparoscopic cholecystectomy. During her stay in hospital for cholecystitis, Mrs Cole's RUQ abdominal pain becomes worse. She also becomes jaundiced, her temperature rises to 40.1°C, and she starts to shake uncontrollably with rigors.

What are the complications of cholecystitis, and what has happened to Mrs Cole? How must she be managed?

Complications of cholecystitis include empyema (a collection of pus in the gallbladder that will need draining), formation of a cholecystoduodenal fistula (a connecting fistula between the gallbladder and small bowel, which allows bowel air into the gallbladder – seen on radiography – but also allows gallstones to travel into the small bowel, eventually getting stuck in the terminal ileum and causing 'gallstone ileus'), or even gallbladder carcinoma. However, Mrs Cole has more likely developed **ascending cholangitis**, which is characterized by *Charcot's triad* of signs:

- RUQ pain
- Jaundice
- Fever with rigors

Ascending cholangitis (*chole* = *bile*, angio = vessel, -*itis* = inflammation) is inflammation of the common bile duct because of an infected stone in the common bile duct or due to spread from an infected gallbladder (cholecystitis). Inflammation in the common bile duct leads to it becoming obstructed, so that conjugated bilirubin can no longer drain through it, its build-up causing **jaundice**. Unlike cholecystitis, where the infection is confined to the gallbladder, in cholangitis the infection can easily spread up the common bile duct, into the liver, and thence into the systemic circulation – hence it being called *ascending* cholangitis. The presence of inflammatory markers in the systemic circulation leads to the swinging fever and rigors.

Management of ascending cholangitis: ascending cholangitis is a surgical emergency that carries a high mortality (~10–30%) if intervention is not started early, because of the high risk of the infection spreading upwards to the liver and ultimately entering the circulation (sepsis). Management should include:

- **Blood cultures** should be taken to try and establish the identity and antibiotic sensitivities of the infective bacteria.
- **Antibiotics.** The patient should then be started on broad-spectrum antibiotics (e.g. co-amoxiclav + metronidazole, but guided by local policy) until the exact antibiotic sensitivities of the bacteria are known.
- **Endoscopic retrograde cholangiopancreatography (ERCP) drainage.** The patient must have their blocked common bile duct physically drained via ERCP. An endoscope is passed via the oesophagus from the patient's mouth into the duodenum. From here, a fine catheter is passed via the sphincter of Oddi and into the common bile duct, where the pus is drained and sent for culturing to determine the identity and antibiotic sensitivities of the infective

bacteria. ERCP carries a risk of making matters worse if the pus is accidentally pushed upwards into the liver.

- **Monitoring.** Once the common bile duct has been drained, the patient is kept in hospital on antibiotics, nil by mouth, fluids (IV), and analgesia and the patient's vital signs are monitored carefully for any signs of systemic infection (sepsis).

Mrs Cole mentioned in her initial history that she often suffered from a sharp, stabbing pain in her RUQ, typically a few hours after a fatty meal. The pain came and went over a period of several hours but always self-resolved within half a day.

What pathological process was Mrs Cole most likely describing?

Mrs Cole was probably suffering from bouts of **biliary colic** due to **cholelithiasis** (*chole* = bile, *lithiasis* = stone formation). About 20% of the population have small stones in their gallbladder, but in 90% of cases these cause no problems at all. In some people, however, the stones can irritate Hartmann's pouch (where the gallbladder meets the cystic duct) or the common bile duct, causing a sharp, stabbing pain which, despite being called 'biliary colic', is rarely a true colic (i.e. waxing and waning pain), as the pain is usually fairly constant. In most patients the gallstone eventually passes into the small bowel but in some the gallstone requires removal via ERCP.

15

Mr Goldstone is a 52-year-old restaurant manager who presents to his hospital with severe RUQ pain. The pain started a few hours after lunch and has been present since. He says that for the last month he has been suffering from a burning pain in his upper abdomen, often after meals. This time, the pain is stabbing in nature and much worse in severity. He has not opened his bowels since the pain started, about 4 hours ago. He has a past medical history of osteoarthrosis of his right hip, for which he takes regular NSAIDs (diclofenac) whilst he awaits his hip replacement. Examination reveals only a mildly tender RUQ. His faecal occult blood test (FOBT) is positive but his chest and abdominal radiographs are normal, with no distended bowel loops or air under the diaphragm.

What diagnosis is likely in this gentleman? How would he be investigated?

Mr Goldstone gives a history of upper abdominal burning pain for the last month, which is highly suggestive of a peptic ulcer (you cannot tell if it is gastric or duodenal from associations with meals and times of the day, contrary to myth). His positive FOBT suggests that blood may have entered the bowel (or that he has consumed a lot of red meat), and this combined with his more severe, stabbing pain suggests that Mr Goldstone may have developed a **bleeding peptic ulcer**. However, Mr Goldstone's age means that other causes of blood in the gut lumen (haemorrhoids, angiodysplasia, large bowel cancer) must be considered too.

To investigate a positive FOBT, a **digital rectal examination** is essential, as this may reveal haemorrhoids, a rectal mass (rectal cancer?), melaena (dark tar-like stools, suggestive of an upper gastrointestinal (GI) bleed), or haematochezia (bright red stools, suggestive of a lower GI bleed). The next step would be to visualize the gut wall for sources of blood using **endoscopy.** An oesophagogastroduodenoscopy (OGD) will look at the oesophagus, stomach, and duodenum, whilst a colonoscopy will look at the entire colon. If both forms of endoscopy still don't reveal the source of bleeding, one can consider looking for a bleed in the jejunum and ileum using either an abdominal **computed tomography (CT) angiogram** (which will only pick up relatively large bleeds), **video capsule**, or a **red cell scan.**

Mr Goldstone was admitted to hospital and underwent an OGD. This showed a bleeding duodenal ulcer just distal to the pylorus which was injected with adrenaline to stop the bleeding. Biopsies of the ulcer were positive for *Helicobacter pylori* but showed no signs of malignancy. Mr Goldstone went on to receive triple eradication therapy for his ulcer: a PPI (e.g. omeprazole) and two antibiotics (e.g. amoxicillin and clarithromycin) for 1 week.

15

Viva questions

15

Explain the difference between biliary colic, cholecystitis, and ascending cholangitis.

Biliary colic occurs when the gallbladder attempts to contract against an obstruction – usually a gallstone at Hartmann's pouch. At this stage the gallbladder is not inflamed or infected. Pain only lasts until the stone falls back into the gallbladder or is passed along the cystic duct and then common bile duct – but this can be anything from minutes to hours.

Cholecystitis: a significant proportion of patients presenting with biliary colic go on to develop acute chole-cystitis – at which point the gallbladder is inflamed (*chole* = bile, *cyst* = bladder, -*itis* = inflammation). If a stone impacts in Hartmann's pouch or the cystic duct, the gallbladder may be full of bile that cannot escape. As water is absorbed by the gallbladder, the bile becomes very concentrated and irritates the gallbladder caus-ing a sterile, chemical cholecystitis. As the bile and gallstone cannot drain, they often become infected caus-ing an infective cholecystitis. Hence, both biliary colic and cholecystitis can be regarded as consequences of stones in the gallbladder (*cholelithiasis*; *chole* = bile, *lithiasis* = stone formation). Bowel rest (nil by mouth), antibiotics, and analgesia are sufficient in 90% of cases of cholecystitis, although many surgeons will opt for either urgent cholecystectomy or elective cholecystectomy at a later date to avoid repeated attacks.

Ascending cholangitis is usually a complication of *choledocholithiasis* (*chole* = bile, *docho* = duct, *lithiasis* = stone formation) – stone(s) in the common bile duct. These stones block the common bile duct causing jaundice, but they can also become infected by gut bacteria and the infection can spread via the liver into the circulation, causing high fever and rigors. This is the most serious presentation of gallstone disease and carries a mortality of about 15%. Ascending cholangitis may also occur if the common bile duct is blocked by a stricture (due to recent surgery) or a tumour, or if gut bacteria have been pushed up into the common bile duct by a doctor during an ERCP. Charcot's triad of fever, RUQ pain, and jaundice is present. The patient needs urgent drainage of the common bile duct, broad-spectrum antibiotics, and careful monitoring in hospital for signs of sepsis.

What is bile? How are bile salts conserved by the body?

Bile is made up of four main components:

- **Water:** although much of this is reabsorbed while bile is stored in the gallbladder
- **Fat:** mainly cholesterol and some phospholipids
- **Bile salts:** which serve to solubilize the fats in bile but also fats and fat-soluble vitamins (A, D, E, K) found in food
- **Conjugated bilirubin:** digested by gut bacteria into a brown pigment (stercobilin) which gives faeces its unique colour

Bile salts are absorbed from the terminal ileum and then travel back to the liver via the enterohepatic circula-tion. Bile salts may be recycled up to ten times each day.

Both liver disease or a blocked common bile duct (obstructive jaundice) can cause patients to have prolonged blood clotting times, but administering parenteral (not oral) vitamin K will only correct the problem in one of the cases: which one and why?

Remember that the extrinsic arm of the clotting cascade, as measured by the prothrombin time (PT), relies upon the liver making clotting factors II, VII, IX, and X. This process depends on vitamin K which is fat soluble and therefore absorbed thanks to bile salts. Liver disease may result in an increased PT due to impaired synthesis of these clotting factors within the liver. By contrast, if the patient is suffering from a blocked common bile duct (obstructive jaundice) then there will be little or no bile salts reaching the gut and emulsifying fats. Thus there will be severely impaired vitamin K absorption from the terminal ileum, and this in turn impairs clotting factor synthesis.

An increased PT due to liver disease will not be corrected by the parenteral administration of vitamin K as the problem is the liver, not the lack of vitamin K. Conversely, parenteral vitamin K will correct a prolonged PT that is due to obstructive jaundice (because clotting factor synthesis is only being impaired by a lack of raw material – vitamin K, rather than impaired synthetic ability).

What sorts of gallstones are there? Which groups of patients are prone to particular sorts of gallstones?

There are three main types of gallstones: approximately 5% are bile pigment stones, 20% are cholesterol, and 75% are mixed composition. Note that only about 10% of gallstones are radio-opaque and thus the vast majority will not show on plain abdominal radiographs. Contrast this with renal/ureteric stones, about 90% of which are radio-opaque.

Certain patients are predisposed to particular gallstones:

- **Bile pigment stones:** bile pigments are haemoglobin breakdown products and thus patients with haemolytic anaemias (such as hereditary spherocystosis, sickle cell disease, or G6PD deficiency) are predisposed to these sorts of stones. Long-term total parenteral nutrition (TPN) is also associated with pigment gallstone disease.

- **Cholesterol stones:** it is said that the classic cholesterol gallstone patient is a fair, fat, fertile female of forty (the five Fs). Some add 'flatulent' as a further alliterative compliment to the unfortunate patient. The use of oral contraceptive therapy further increases the risk of cholesterol stones. Patients with Crohn's disease may suffer higher rates of cholesterol stones because the terminal ileum pathology impairs reabsorption and enterohepatic circulation of bile salts, thus making bile-based stones less likely.

15

What are the potential consequences of gallstones?

Remember that gallstones usually cause no pathology – they may uneventfully pass down the biliary tree and then into the duodenum. Otherwise think anatomically. Stones may remain in the gallbladder and cause biliary colic, acute or chronic cholecystitis, a mucocoele (mucus-filled gallbladder), empyema (pus-filled gallbladder), or cholangiocarcinoma. Stones may pass into the common bile duct and block it (obstructive jaundice) or get infected (ascending cholangitis). If the stone travels down the common bile duct it may become lodged at the ampulla of Vater and thus cause acute pancreatitis. Lastly, the stone may cause gallstone ileus. This latter pathology causes some confusion and is worth elaborating on. When the gallbladder becomes inflamed, its neighbouring structures, namely duodenum, transverse colon, and omentum, may wrap around the gallblad-der to 'wall off' the inflammation. This raises the possibility of fistula formation. A stone that travels through a cholecystocolic fistula (to the large bowel) is unlikely to cause any problems, and will most likely be passed from the body with the next stool. However, if a stone passes through a cholecystoduodenal fistula (to the small bowel) it is liable to get stuck at the narrowest part of the intestinal tract – the terminal ileum. This represents a mechanical obstruction and the term 'gallstone ileus' is thus rather a misnomer as ileus usually refers to functional obstruction of the gut. Gallstone ileus can be diagnosed on a plain abdominal radiograph by looking for signs of small bowel obstruction, air in the biliary tree, and perhaps a stone at the terminal ileum (remembering that radio-opaque gallstones are rare).

Explain why the consumption of fatty foods can exacerbate the pain of biliary colic and chronic cholecystitis.

Cholecystokinin (CCK) is released from the duodenum in response to fatty foods. CCK stimulates the secre-tion of digestive enzymes from pancreatic acinar cells, and also stimulates contraction of the gallbladder and relaxation of the sphincter of Oddi. These last two actions would release bile into the duodenum to aid with fat digestion and absorption. However, CCK-induced gallbladder contraction can exacerbate the pain of biliary colic and chronic cholecystitis. It would also accentuate the pain of acute cholecystitis, but you are unlikely to be eating if you have this disease!

15

During cholecystectomy the surgeon will look for Calot's triangle – what is it?

Calot's triangle (see Fig. 15.1) is an anatomical zone used to define the usual path of the cystic artery, the cystic duct, and the common hepatic duct. It is essential to visualize and dissect this triangle during a chole-cystectomy so that one can be sure that one is ligating and cutting the cystic artery and cystic duct, and not the right hepatic artery, hepatic duct, or common bile duct. The superior border of the triangle is the liver, the inferior border is the cystic duct, and the medial border is the common hepatic duct. The cystic artery is a branch of the right hepatic artery, which usually passes behind the common hepatic duct. However, in about 25% of patients, the right hepatic artery passes in front of the common hepatic duct.

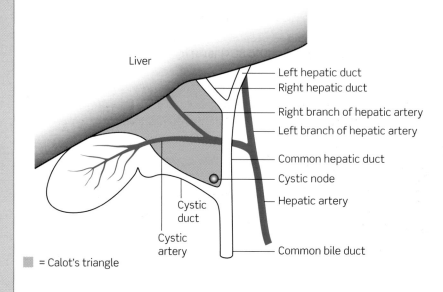

= Calot's triangle

Figure 15.1 Anatomy of Calot's triangle.

15

Where would a gallstone need to be in order to cause obstructive jaundice?

Typically the stone would need to be in the common bile duct or the ampulla of Vater. However, it is worth remembering that a stone in Hartmann's pouch (see Fig. 15.2) may also press extrinsically on the common bile duct (Mirizzi's syndrome).

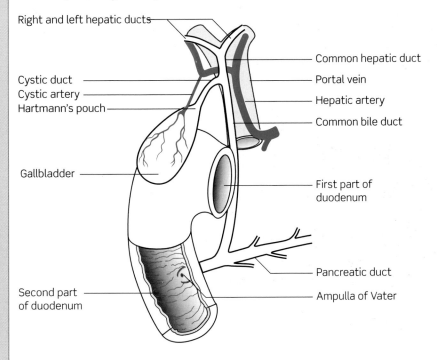

Right and left hepatic ducts

Cystic duct

Cystic artery

Hartmann's pouch

Gallbladder

Second part of duodenum

Common hepatic duct

Portal vein

Hepatic artery

Common bile duct

First part of duodenum

Pancreatic duct

Ampulla of Vater

Figure 15.2 Anatomy of the biliary tree.
From MacKinnon PCB, Morris JF (2005). *Oxford Textbook of Functional Anatomy, Vol. 2 Thorax and Abdomen*, 2nd edn, p. 162, Fig. 6.6.4.

15

What is Courvoisier's law?

This 'law' states that if the gallbladder is palpable in the presence of jaundice then the jaundice is unlikely to be due to stones. The rationale is as follows: if the obstruction is caused by a stone in the common bile duct then the gallbladder is likely to be thickened and fibrotic (as the gallbladder is the source of the stone) and thus not distended and palpable, but rather shrivelled up. By contrast, if the common bile duct is obstructed for some other reason, such as a tumour, then the gallbladder is likely to be normal and it will dilate due to back-pressure. Note the phrasing of Courvoisier's law – it does NOT state that if the gallbladder is not palpable then the jaundice is due to a stone. This is because it is perfectly possible for the gallbladder to be dilated (perhaps due to a distal tumour causing back-pressure of bile) but not palpable because it is obscured by the liver or layers of fat in the abdominal wall.

> **What is an ERCP? What is the advantage of ERCP over MRCP? What are the complications of ERCP?**
>
> **ERCP** is endoscopic retrograde cholangiopancreatography. A side-viewing endoscope is passed via the mouth, past the oesophagogastric junction and pylorus, and down to the second part of the duodenum. At this point a fine catheter emerges from the endoscope and is passed through the duodenal papilla and into the ampulla of Vater. It is possible to inject contrast medium directly into the biliary tree, which is then visualized radiographically.
>
> **MRCP** is magnetic resonance cholangiopancreatography. It enables detailed visualization of the biliary tree, but is purely a diagnostic procedure. ERCP has a therapeutic role as it is possible to both remove stones (using a Dormia basket) and perform endoscopic sphincterotomy (cutting the sphincter of Oddi with a fine diathermy wire in order to facilitate the passage of any stones within the common bile duct).
>
> Aside from being a rather unpleasant procedure to undergo, the **risks of ERCP** include bleeding, perforation of the biliary tree, cholangitis, and pancreatitis. There is about a 1–3% risk of pancreatitis and, for reasons that are not entirely clear, this pancreatitis carries a 20% mortality risk (which is higher than normal for pancreatitis).

For a range of Single Best Answer questions related to the topic of this chapter go to
www.oxfordtextbooks.co.uk/orc/ocms/

15

Right iliac fossa (RIF) pain

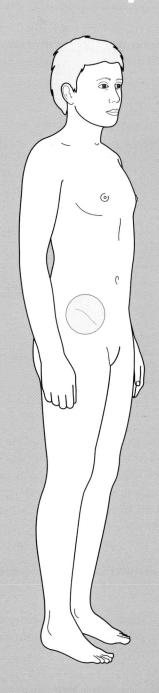

Core case

Core case

Mr Beck is a 28-year-old builder who presents at accident and emergency (A&E) on Sunday evening with a 3-hour history of right iliac fossa (RIF) pain. He is nauseated and has vomited once.

What is your differential diagnosis? Try to prioritize into those conditions that are most likely (or most common), those that you must exclude, and the remainder.

The diagnoses shown in red are all surgical emergencies that you must exclude as you clerk the patient. The most common are in large font at the top

Appendicitis
Gastroenteritis
Ureteric colic
Acute pancreatitis
Testicular torsion
Meckel's diverticulitis
Small bowel obstruction
Caecal volvulus
Perforated peptic ulcer
Pyelonephritis
Diabetic ketoacidosis
Acute onset ileitis (bacterial or Crohn's)
Constipation
Caecal diverticulitis
Mesenteric adenitis
Urinary tract infection
Cholecystitis
Shingles
Rectus sheath haematoma

Note that certain diagnoses are going to be more likely in different patient groups. Children and the elderly are more likely to have a longer differential as symptoms are often less pronounced and non-specific. Intussusception is almost exclusively seen in children, and the vast majority of cases of mesenteric adenitis are also seen in children. By contrast, caecal pathology (tumours, volvulus, or a solitary mesenteric diverticulum) is usually associated with advancing age.

What other diagnoses must you consider in a female patient?

You must of course consider gynaecological pathology, such as ectopic pregnancy, pelvic inflammatory disease/salpingitis, torsion/haemorrhage/rupture of an ovarian tumour or cyst, mittelschmerz (mid-cycle pain corresponding to a ruptured ovarian follicle), threatened abortion, fibroid degeneration, or uterine dehiscence.

In any woman of reproductive age you *must* perform a pregnancy test – this is not only to exclude particular diagnoses such as ectopic pregnancy, but is also essential if you wish to proceed to tests such as abdominal radiographs which would risk harm to the foetus.

On further questioning we establish that Mr Beck had a milder, poorly localized, central abdominal pain for about 12 hours prior to the onset of the RIF pain. The pain worsened about 3 hours ago, at which time he felt that it had shifted to the right. The pain has been constant ever since. He says that the pain doesn't radiate anywhere else, but struggles to give much more of a description when asked to characterize it – 'pain is pain'. He hasn't taken anything for the pain but states that he'd rate it as 8 out of 10. He is not aware of anything that makes the pain worse, but is reluctant to lie flat on the bed, and you notice that he keeps his right hip flexed. He had his customary Saturday night curry yesterday. He ordered the hottest dish on the menu, but says that he always does this and never suffers any ill-effects. None of his friends from the meal have had similar symptoms. He has completely lost his appetite today and has not opened his bowels either. He has felt otherwise well over the preceding week. Mr Beck's face appears flushed and, as already noted, he is reluctant to lie flat.

With this history in mind, you need to examine Mr Beck to try and narrow your differential. In particular, you need to establish the site and extent of abdominal tenderness. How will you do this?

Note that tenderness is a sign whereas pain is a symptom.

It is very useful to have an idea of the degree of abdominal tenderness before you even lay a hand on the patient. Remember that you will win no prizes if you actually cause a patient pain. So, start by asking the patient to suck their tummy in as far as possible and then puff it out again (this is particularly useful in children). A patient with board-like abdominal rigidity secondary to generalized peritonism will only make very minor movements. Now ask the patient to cough – patients with inflammation of the parietal peritoneum will find this rather painful and may well place their hands over the area of tenderness.

Whether you palpate the abdomen in quadrants or nine zones, be sure to start in the opposite area to that which the patient states is most painful. Start by palpating gently and keep looking at the patient's face for a reaction. Patients are likely to demonstrate guarding (involuntary muscular rigidity in tender areas of the abdomen). Percussion tenderness, when percussion over an area causes the patient pain, is a sensitive means of demonstrating parietal peritoneum irritation and is far kinder to the patient than assessing rebound tenderness.

What else will you be looking for on examination?

- **Is he ill?** As a first line you should establish whether Mr Beck is febrile and/or tachycardic, hypotensive, or tachypnoeic. Also quickly note any fetor oris (bad breath), which can indicate abdominal sepsis (such as appendicitis).

- **Scars:** scars in particular anatomical sites can be particularly informative – for example, has this patient still got an appendix? Remember that any previous

16

abdominal surgery will also make small bowel obstruction more likely as post-surgical adhesions predispose to obstruction.

- **Abdominal distension or visible peristalsis:** in a thin patient you may be able to observe these signs of small bowel obstruction.
- **Cervical lymphadenopathy:** particularly important for trying to rule out mesenteric adenitis, which is inflammation and enlargement of the mesenteric lymph nodes. It often follows an upper respiratory tract viral infection (hence cervical lymphadenopathy may be present) and is one of the most difficult conditions to differentiate from appendicitis in young patients.
- **Masses:** the greater omentum can wrap around inflamed organs, hence creating a localized mass (such as an appendix mass). Other palpable masses may be due to a tumour or a rectus sheath haematoma. The history in Mr Beck's case is rather short, but in someone with a longer history of constipation you may be able to palpate faecal loading in the sigmoid and colon.
- **Bowel sounds:** these will be absent if there is functional bowel obstruction (ileus) or perhaps 'tinkling' if there is small bowel obstruction.
- **Hernias:** a particularly important cause of small bowel obstruction.
- **Rectal exam:** provides three key pieces of information:
  - Is the rectum full of faeces, thus suggesting constipation?
  - Is there any blood? If so, think of pathologies such as a bleeding Meckel's diverticulum or caecal diverticulum.
  - Is there any local tenderness? Remember that the appendix can lie in a number of positions relative to the caecum. An inflamed pelvic appendix may not result in any abdominal tenderness to palpation, and the only sign may be right-sided rectal tenderness. However, the lack of rectal tenderness does not rule out appendicitis.
- **External genitalia:** you *must* examine the testicles for signs of torsion – particularly in young men. Torsion can present with referred pain to the abdomen via T10 sympathetic innervation. The window of opportunity for surgical rescue of torted testes is slim.

16

Mr Beck is febrile (37.8°C), tachycardic (102 bpm), and normotensive (134/78 mmHg) with a respiratory rate of 20/min. He has fetor oris. He's asked to cough and finds this incredibly painful – clutching his hands over his right side. There is guarding in the RIF. In addition, palpation in the left iliac fossa results in greater pain in the RIF than the left (Rovsing's sign positive). There are no palpable cervical lymph nodes and no abdominal masses. Owing to the tenderness of Mr Beck's abdomen, it is difficult to palpate for the liver, spleen, and kidneys. Nevertheless, this is attempted and no organomegaly is detected. His abdominal aorta is pulsatile but not expansile. Percussion tenderness is maximal over a point approximately two-thirds of the distance from the umbilicus laterally towards the anterior superior iliac spine (McBurney's point). Bowel sounds are normal. Examination of the external genitalia and hernial orifices is unremarkable. Once it is explained why a digital rectal examination would aid diagnosis, Mr Beck consents to the procedure. The rectum is empty, there is no blood, and no focal tenderness.

Although Mr Beck's history and examination are highly suggestive of a particular diagnosis, there are still a number of other contenders to rule out. What investigations would you like to request to refine your differential diagnosis?

Blood tests

- **Full blood count (FBC):** the white cell count may be elevated in response to any inflammatory condition (e.g. appendicitis, cholecystitis, or basal pneumonia).

- **C-reactive protein (CRP)/erythrocyte sedimentation rate (ESR):** elevated inflammatory markers point towards an inflammatory picture although, as with the white cell count, they are non-specific regarding the cause.

- **Urea and electrolytes (U&Es):** useful for establishing the baseline electrolyte status of the patient (remembering that a number of the diagnoses on our differential will require intravenous (IV) fluids and/or surgery). Urea is also used as a prognostic indicator for pancreatitis as part of the modified Glasgow criteria.

- **Serum amylase (or lipase) levels:** high amylase (or lipase) levels are strongly suggestive of pancreatitis, although they are non-specific and thus must be viewed in the context of the clinical picture. Slight increases (200–600 U/L) in amylase levels are most commonly caused by pancreatitis, but also by various other pathologies such as bowel obstruction, mesenteric ischaemia, a posteriorly perforated duodenal ulcer, mumps, pancreatic carcinoma, or opiate medications. However, very high amylase levels (>1000 U/L) or elevated lipase levels (>300 U/L) are almost exclusively found in pancreatitis. (The exact cut-offs will depend upon your local laboratory protocols.) If you have any clinical suspicion of pancreatitis you should also request markers used in the modified Glasgow score for pancreatitis severity (FBC, calcium, urea, liver enzymes, lactate dehydrogenase (LDH), albumin, glucose, arterial blood gas).

- **Glucose:** remember that diabetic ketoacidosis can present with an acute abdomen and that infection is likely to cause disturbed glycaemic control in diabetic patients. Glucose levels are also part of the Glasgow pancreatitis criteria.

- **Liver enzymes:** within the context of a raised amylase, these provide useful prognostic information for pancreatitis (which can result in elevated aspartate aminotransferase (AST) and low albumin). Liver enzymes are also essential if there is any clinical suspicion of biliary pathology.

Urine

- **Urinalysis:** in the context of the acute abdomen, haematuria may result from infection, renal/ureteric calculi, or rarely an inflamed pelvic appendix that is irritating the bladder or retrocaecal appendix irritating the ureter. Glucose and ketones are indicative of diabetic ketoacidosis. A combination of leucocyte esterase and nitrites suggests a urinary tract infection. Both urinary tract infection and appendiceal irritation of the bladder can result in proteinuria but these could be distinguished by performing urine microscopy looking for bacteria, which would confirm the urinary tract infection.

Imaging

- **Abdominal radiograph:** look for signs of a perforation (resulting in air in the peritoneal cavity), small bowel obstruction, or volvulus. Dilatation of a few 'sentinel' loops reflects a response to inflammation of other local structures such as the pancreas or appendix. Approximately 80% of renal/ureteric calculi are radio-opaque and thus visible on a plain abdominal radiograph. It may also be possible to see an appendiceal faecolith that is causing appendicitis.

16

- **Abdominal ultrasound:** this can be a very useful test if there is an atypical history such that renal or biliary pathology are likely differentials. Appendicitis *can* be suggested by ultrasound scanning. Ultrasound is also a useful test for detecting free fluid in the abdomen. Ultra sound may be particularly useful in female patients, where the differential diagnosis is broadened by gynaecological pathology.

Other investigations to consider are:

- **Erect chest radiograph:** request if there is any clinical suspicion of a perforated viscus. Air under the diaphragm could result from a perforated peptic ulcer, Meckel's diverticulum, caecal diverticulum, or appendix. Lung consolidation from a basal pneumonia would also be visible.

- **Abdominal CT:** CT scans involve a considerable dose of radiation, and the delay in requesting a scan may be unacceptable for some diagnoses such as acute appendicitis. However, CT is useful for pre-operative incision planning, aiding discussion of stomas, diagnosis of metastatic tumour deposits, etc.

- **ECG:** although this would be a very atypical presentation of myocardial infarction, one must be wary (particularly in elderly patients).

> Blood tests are taken. The white cell count is 13.2×10^9 cells/L (neutrophils 10.5×10^9 cells/L), CRP 32 mg/L, and amylase 200 U/L. All other blood tests are unremarkable. Urine dipstick is negative for protein, blood, leucocyte esterase, nitrites, glucose, and ketones. A plain abdominal radiograph shows a single dilated loop of small bowel in the RIF, but nothing else of note. There are no signs of pneumoperitoneum.
>
> **In light of the history, examination and first-line investigations, what is the most likely diagnosis?**

This is a classical clinical picture for **acute appendicitis**: low-grade central abdominal pain that gradually migrates to the RIF over 12–24 hours and becomes more intense. Anorexia is a reliable feature. The patient is flushed, febrile, tachycardic, has foetor oris, and is lying still. Examination reveals guarding and percussion tenderness in the RIF – perhaps over McBurney's point. Digital rectal examination may also show right-sided tenderness. Rovsing's sign may be positive but is an unreliable sign. Bear in mind that this classical presentation is only seen in about 50% of patients. The appendix can lie in various positions relative to the caecum and thus produces various different examination findings when inflamed. Furthermore, there is no single test that is diagnostic for appendicitis.

> **What features of the history, clinical examination, and investigations help you rule out other diagnoses?**

We can go through the differential diagnosis given initially and try to rule out alternatives to appendicitis:

- **Mesenteric adenitis?** Typically follows an upper respiratory tract infection or sore throat, thus cervical lymphadenopathy may be present. It is most common in children less than 15 years old. In truth, it is very difficult to distinguish between appendicitis and mesenteric adenitis, with the final diagnosis being made intraoperatively in many cases. The pain with mesenteric adenitis is often more diffuse than that of appendicitis, and signs of peritonitis are often

16

absent. Mesenteric adenitis doesn't result in rectal tenderness, but appendicitis doesn't always result in this sign either. Fever is said to be slightly higher in mesenteric adenitis (>38.5°C), but this too is unreliable. Mesenteric adenitis often settles quickly.

- **Meckel's diverticulitis?** As with mesenteric adenitis, it is almost impossible to definitively exclude an inflamed/ruptured Meckel's diverticulum pre-operatively. Signs and symptoms are classically indistinguishable from appendicitis.

- **Constipation?** This would not cause a migration of pain to the RIF. We would also expect to feel faeces in the rectum and see faecal loading of the colon on plain abdominal radiographs. Constipation virtually never results in fever or tachycardia.

- **Acute onset Crohn's disease?** Although the acute signs and symptoms would mimic appendicitis, there is often a history of diarrhoea and weight loss for weeks/months leading up to the acute presentation.

- **Gastroenteritis?** Vomiting and diarrhoea would usually predominate. The shifting nature of pain, and localized abdominal tenderness are not typical. In addition, you may expect to see similar symptoms in other family members or close contacts.

- **Renal/ureteric colic?** The patient would typically be writhing in pain (rather than lying still). Pain would not migrate from the central abdomen. Urine dipstick would likely show haematuria, and plain abdominal radiograph would show a stone or stones in about 80% of cases.

- **Pancreatitis?** The migration of the pain to the RIF would be atypical for pancreatitis. Furthermore, if there is RIF pain we'd also expect there to be epigastric pain. Although the serum amylase is very slightly raised, it is not high enough to raise suspicions of pancreatitis (typically >1000 U/L, but levels may be normal even in severe pancreatitis). It is worth remembering that other intestinal pathology such as appendicitis, intestinal infarction, and perforated duodenal ulcer can also cause raised amylase levels, as can head injury, diabetic ketoacidosis, and drugs such as opioids. If Mr Beck did have pancreatitis it would be a very mild version as his Glasgow score is zero (see Chapter 12).

- **Testicular torsion:** there are no signs of testicular tenderness (see Chapter 25).

How will the surgical team manage Mr Beck?

The first step is to assess the need for resuscitation (**Airway, Breathing, and Circulation, ABC**). IV fluids would be given if required. He would then be given adequate **analgesia**. The first-line treatment for appendicitis is **appendicectomy**, either open or laparoscopic. Patients should be **nil by mouth** for 6–8 hours prior to surgery, although most appendicitis patients have usually lost their appetite anyway. Intraoperative mortality in the UK is <0.2%, but rises to about 5% in the very young or elderly as the difficulty of diagnosis in these patient groups means that they are more likely to present with perforation. Peri-operative **broad-spectrum antibiotics** should be used in all appendicectomies as they reduce wound infection and abscess formation. The patient should also be prescribed some form of **deep vein thrombosis (DVT) prophylaxis**.

16

Short cases

Mr Briggs is a 46-year-old solicitor admitted to the surgical unit at the same time as Mr Beck. He describes a similar history of central abdominal pain that migrated to the RIF. However, he has waited 3 days before seeking help. He has been taking paracetamol 1 g q.d.s. (four times a day) at home, but this has not controlled his pain. He has not eaten a proper meal for 3 days, and has only passed minimal amounts of stool. On examination, he is flushed, tachycardic, and febrile. There is marked halitosis. There is muscular rigidity in the RIF, and a tender mass is palpable in the RIF. The rest of the abdomen is soft and non-tender. Per rectum, genital, and hernial orifice examinations are all unremarkable.

What has happened to Mr Briggs?

It is likely that Mr Briggs has also had acute appendicitis but that he has suffered a complication and has now developed an **appendix mass**. The greater omentum, caecum, and/or adherent loops of small bowel wrap themselves around the inflamed or perforated appendix to form a localized mass. CT or ultrasound scan may clinch the diagnosis. The fact that Mr Briggs has waited 3 days before presenting to hospital does not necessarily mean that he is any more stoical or able to tolerate more pain than our previous patient. Rather patients who develop an appendix mass are usually those who have had a less intense pain resulting from 'milder' inflammation of the appendix.

Initial conservative therapy is usually indicated for an appendix mass. This involves keeping patients nil by mouth, ensuring adequate IV fluids, antibiotic cover, analgesia, and DVT prophylaxis, and then marking out the size of the mass on the abdominal wall. Surgery is indicated if the mass increases in size, if the patient becomes more septic, or if the patient develops small bowel obstruction due to the adhesions.

If early surgery is not indicated and the mass resolves with conservative treatment, it is usual to perform an elective appendicectomy 6–8 weeks after resolution of the mass, although elective removal of the appendix following resolution of the mass remains controversial.

It is worth emphasizing the difference between an appendix mass and appendix abscess. The former is a phlegmon (an inflammatory mass) whereas an abscess contains pus. Hence a conservative approach can be adopted for an appendix mass but an abscess must be drained – either as an open procedure or percutaneously.

16

Mr Fuhr is a 16-year-old student who presents to the surgical emergency unit with a 3-hour history of RIF pain. He has vomited once. He was specifically asked whether he had any central abdominal pain prior to the RIF pain but he is unsure. He was playing rugby earlier in the day and, as he doesn't like to play with a full stomach, says that it is usual for him to have some rumbling stomach pains prior to a big match. He has otherwise been fit and well. On examination, his temperature is 37.4°C and pulse is 134 bpm, regular. His is in obvious discomfort. However, abdominal examination is unremarkable – there are no local areas of tenderness; no palpable masses; bowel sounds are present. Urine dipstick is negative. Bloods are sent for analysis.

Which critical examination has not yet been performed? Which diagnosis must we consider?

Mr Fuhr is exactly the right sort of age to present with **testicular torsion**. It is absolutely critical that all boys/young men have their testes examined when presenting with an acute abdomen. A thorough gastrointestinal examination of patients of any age should feature inspection of external genitalia and hernial orifices, and a digital rectal examination if appropriate.

Signs of testicular torsion include an exquisitely tender testicle and scrotal erythema. The abdominal pain is referred via the T10 sympathetic supply and reflects the embryological origin of the testes. Nausea and vomiting are commonplace. The affected testis will lie higher in the scrotum than a normal testis. A testis that lies horizontally is more likely to tort, so examine the other testis as well. Prehn's sign is said to help distinguish between epididymitis and testicular torsion: elevating the affected scrotum relieves the pain of epididymitis (positive Prehn's), but will not relieve the pain of torsion. However, although you may hear Prehn's sign being mentioned on the wards, it is not a reliable sign. More information would be gleaned by attempting to elicit the cremasteric reflex (downwards stroking of the superomedial aspect of the thigh should result in elevation of the ipsilateral scrotum/testicle). Although the absence of the cremasteric reflex does not diagnose torsion (as it is very frequently absent), it has a negative predictive value of 96% – in other words, its *presence* is strongly suggestive of another pathology.

Although the majority of testicular torsions appear to happen spontaneously (often at night), they may follow minor trauma. Doppler ultrasound of the testes may aid diagnosis, but if there is any suspicion of torsion it is safest to send the patient to theatre as time really does matter (90% chance of rescuing testis at 6 hours, 5% at 24 hours). If there is a delay in reaching theatre it may be appropriate to attempt manual de-rotation of the testis. It is important to warn patients and parents prior to theatre that both testicles will need fixing to avoid future torsions, and that the affected testicle may need to be removed if it appears necrotic.

16

Miss Bakewell is a 12-year-old girl who presents to her GP with RIF pain. It is difficult to establish much of a pain history, but it seems as though she has had this pain for about a day. The GP notes that one of his colleagues saw Miss Bakewell last week and diagnosed a suspected viral pharyngitis. Upon examination today there is moderate peri-umbilical and RIF tenderness to light palpation, but no guarding or rebound. The GP decides that it would not be appropriate to perform a digital rectal examination. He does, however, ask her for a urine sample. With her consent he then performs a pregnancy test and this is negative. In addition there are no signs of urinary tract infection on urine dipstick testing. Miss Bakewell has a fever of 38.6°C and pulse 121 bpm, regular. The rest of the examination is unremarkable, except for a palpable right-sided submandibular lymph node. The GP decides to refer Miss Bakewell to the local hospital. He rings the admissions unit to warn of her arrival.

What is he likely to mention as the differential diagnoses?

Given that we can rule out ectopic pregnancy or threatened miscarriage, our most likely diagnoses would be **appendicitis** or **mesenteric adenitis**. The slightly higher fever, lack of guarding, and history of upper respiratory tract infection perhaps swing the pendulum in favour of mesenteric adenitis, but Miss Bakewell will need admitting for observation in case this is appendicitis. Miss Bakewell may proceed to surgery (laparoscopy) if her condition worsens enough to warrant it (so that appendicitis can be ruled out). It is, however, rare to need surgery in cases of mesenteric adenitis.

16

Mrs Riley is a 36-year-old housewife who presents with a 7-hour history of RIF pain that she rates as 7 out of 10. She also describes a 5-month history of painless loose stools that she has self-diagnosed as irritable bowel syndrome and is treating with probiotic yoghurts and peppermint tea (with minor benefit). She is nauseated and has vomited twice since the onset of the pain. She is not aware of any radiation of the current pain. There are no particular alleviating or aggravating factors.

On examination she is febrile (37.8°C) and tachycardic (103 bpm regular). There are no peripheral stigmata of gastrointestinal disease. Abdominal examination reveals guarding and percussion tenderness in the RIF, but no palpable masses. The abdominal aorta is pulsatile but not expansile. Rectal examination is performed and is unremarkable. There are no hernias.

Blood samples show a white cell count of 12.3×10^9 cells/L and CRP of 45 mg/L. Potassium is 3.3 mM and sodium is 129 mM. Other blood results are within normal ranges. Urine analysis shows nothing abnormal. A pregnancy test is arranged and is negative. Stool samples are sent for culture. A plain abdominal radiograph is requested but is inconclusive. The surgical team decide to perform laparoscopy. The appendix appears normal, but the terminal ileum is inflamed. The pattern of inflammation is discontinuous, and there are also isolated patches of inflammation in the proximal colon.

In light of the laparoscopy findings and clinical history, what is the most likely diagnosis?

It is most likely that Mrs Riley is suffering from an acute presentation of **Crohn's disease**. While only about 5% of Crohn's patients present in this way, it is important to consider the diagnosis when you have patients with a chronic history of disturbed bowel habit. Further tests such as barium meal and follow through, and ileo-colonoscopy with biopsy would be required to confirm the diagnosis. Mrs Riley's low sodium and potassium are most likely due to her diarrhoea.

16

Short case

Miss Jackson is a 23-year-old company secretary who calls her GP, requesting a home visit because she has abdominal pain. On further questioning, she describes how the pain started quite suddenly, and has now been present for about 2 hours. The pain is focused in her RIF, and has not radiated. It is not influenced by her body position. When asked to rate the pain out of ten, she gives it a four. She says that she feels slightly embarrassed calling the GP for a pain that is only 4/10, but explains that she has had similar pain a couple of times over the last few months and that she wanted the doctor to see her during one of these painful episodes in order to make sure that nothing sinister was going on. The last time that she had similar pain was about a month ago – it was also in her RIF, lasted about 4 hours, and was relieved by ibuprofen that she bought from the chemist. Prior to that, she remembers a similar unprovoked episode of abdominal pain about 2 months ago, but mentions that this pain was on the left side of her abdomen.

When specifically asked whether she could be pregnant, Miss Jackson says that this is impossible as she has not been sexually active since her last period. She has regular 28-day menstrual cycles and had her last period 2 weeks ago.

The GP explains that he feels that Miss Jackson is probably well enough to visit the surgery, rather than requiring a home visit, but that he will gladly see her if she is able to come in. While waiting for her to arrive, he looks through her medical record and establishes that she has no significant medical history and takes no regular medications. When Miss Jackson arrives at the surgery she looks well. She is, however, still complaining of abdominal pain and the GP therefore examines her. An abdominal examination is performed and nothing abnormal is noted.

What is the most likely diagnosis given the history and examination findings?

16

The most likely diagnosis is that Miss Jackson is suffering from **mittelschmerz**. This is a relatively common condition, affecting as many as one in five menstruating women. The key points in the history are that the pain is relatively mild, short-lived, and cyclical in nature – she has regular periods and reports how the pain appears around the time of ovulation (day 14 in a 28-day cycle). The fact that previous painful episodes have been on both the right and left sides is entirely consistent with mittelschmerz. Although some women experience a generalized lower abdominal pain mid-cycle, other women are able to perceive which of their ovaries has provided the egg in any given month. Whether the right or left ovary provides the egg each month is relatively random. The absence of any findings on abdominal examination is also consistent with mittelschmerz.

Viva questions

What are the main causes of appendicitis?

The main cause is thought to be obstruction by a faecolith or foreign body in the lumen of the appendix. Other important causes are lymphoid hyperplasia of Peyer's patches, or fibrous strictures at the base of the appendix following previous inflammation. A rare cause is a carcinoid tumour: such tumours are rare, but when they do occur, it is most often in the appendix.

What is the neuroanatomical basis of the shifting location of the pain in appendicitis?

The key to understanding the shift in location is to think about the distinction between visceral and somatic pain. There are two pain sensation systems in the abdomen – the splanchnic system, which only senses stretch and spasm, and the cerebrospinal pathway that can sense the same array of painful stimuli as skin. The embryonic gut arises as a midline organ and its splanchnic innervation is bilateral, thus visceral pain is felt in the midline. The splanchnic nerves carrying this information synapse on neurons which also receive inputs from the anterior abdominal wall – the brain misinterprets this visceral signal as arising from the anterior abdomen. The appendix, being an embryological midgut organ, is innervated by the lesser splanchnic nerve (T10–T11) and thus initial pain is felt around the umbilicus. There is no somatic innervation of the visceral peritoneum, but as the appendix progressively distends and the inflammatory process extends to involve the parietal peritoneum the pain signals are carried in somatic nerves and inflammation can be localized to the actual site of the appendix – usually in the RIF. This shift in pain location usually occurs in less than 24 hours.

Are you aware of any reliable scoring system to help decide which appendicitis patients require appendicectomy?

Alvarado published a scoring system for appendicitis in 1986 that was intended to minimize the number of people subjected to an unnecessary operation while also minimizing the number of people who progressed to appendiceal perforation due to delayed appendicectomy (see Table 16.1). Those with a score of 7 or more require an operation according to Alvarado's criteria. Those scoring 5 or 6 should be observed, whilst a diagnosis of appendicitis is unlikely in those scoring 4 or less. However, whilst this scoring system no doubt has heuristic value in that it forces us to collect a full complement of data, its actual value for selecting those in need of surgery is in doubt.

Table 16.1 The Alvarado scoring system for appendicitis

Feature	Score
Migration of pain	1
Nausea/vomiting	1
Anorexia	1
RIF tenderness	2
Rebound pain	1
Temperature >37.3°C	1
White cell count >10 ×10^9 cells/L	2
Neutrophil count ≥75%	1

Which two incisions are commonly used for appendicectomy?

The classic approach was the gridiron incision, which is made perpendicular to the imaginary line between the umbilicus and anterior superior iliac spine (ASIS), and centred over McBurney's point. This is rarely performed now. More commonly you will see a Lanz incision – this is placed slightly lower in the RIF, starting about 2 cm medial to the ASIS, and follows a more horizontal course than the gridiron. The Lanz produces better cosmesis as it sits in a natural skin crease. The laparoscopic approach is becoming more commonplace.

At the time of the operation, in the presence of a normal appendix, the surgeon also inspects the distal 2 feet of the terminal ileum – why?

Remember that one of the differential diagnoses of appendicitis is an inflamed/ruptured Meckel's diverticulum. This remnant of the vitelline duct is often said to follow the 'rule of 2s' – it occurs in 2% of the population, may contain two types of ectopic cells (pancreatic and gastric), is typically situated within 2 feet of the ileocaecal valve, is about 2 inches long, and is usually symptomatic by 2 years. Cynics would also add that the rule is only true 2% of the time! Surgeons are only likely to look for an inflamed Meckel's if the appendix is not inflamed at the time of operation (a non-inflamed appendix is said to look 'lily white').

If the appendix does not look inflamed at the time of open operation why would the surgeon remove it anyway?

It is possible for an appendix that is inflamed due to a faecolith to spontaneously resolve without surgical intervention. However, even a non-inflamed appendix is usually removed if the patient proceeds to theatre. This is to help future surgeons as it would be all too easy to assume that a patient no longer had an appendix if a gridiron or Lanz scar is visible.

What is an interval appendicectomy?

Some surgeons advocate electively removing the appendix at some time after the successful conservative treatment of an appendix mass or abscess. The rationale is that this prevents recurrence, but the approach is controversial as only 10–35% of patients suffer further attacks.

Are you aware of any relationship between appendicectomy and inflammatory bowel disease?

Epidemiological studies indicate that appendicectomy appears to protect against the development of ulcerative colitis.[1–4] Patients who do develop ulcerative colitis post-appendicectomy are less likely to develop recurrent symptoms and less likely to require colectomy.[5]

The risk of Crohn's disease appears to be increased during the first few years after appendicectomy,[6] although this is probably because many patients with Crohn's disease initially present with a clinical picture that strongly resembles appendicitis but is in fact their first presentation of Crohn's disease.[7]

[1] Andersson RE, Olaison G, Tysk C, Ekbom A (2001). Appendectomy and protection against ulcerative colitis. *New Engl J Med*, **344**: 808–814.

[2] Baron S, Turck D, Leplat C *et al.* (2005). Environmental risk factors in paediatric inflammatory bowel diseases: a population based case control study. *Gut*, **54**: 357–363.

[3] Hallas J, Gaist D, Sorensen HT (2004). Does appendectomy reduce the risk of ulcerative colitis? *Epidemiology*, **15**: 173–178.

[4] Russel MG, Dorant E, Brummer RJ *et al.* (1997). Appendectomy and the risk of developing ulcerative colitis or Crohn's disease: results of a large case-control study. South Limburg Inflammatory Bowel Disease Study Group. *Gastroenterology*, **113**: 377–382.

[5] Radford-Smith GL, Edwards JE, Purdie DM *et al.* (2002). Protective role of appendicectomy on onset and severity of ulcerative colitis and Crohn's disease. *Gut*, **51**: 808–813.

[6] Kaplan GG, Jackson T, Sands BE, Frisch M, Andersson RE, Korzenik J (2008). The risk of developing Crohn's disease after an appendectomy: a meta-analysis. *Am J Gastroenterol*, **103**: 2925–2931.

[7] Kaplan GG, Pedersen BV, Andersson RE, Sands BE, Korzenik J, Frisch M (2007). The risk of developing Crohn's disease after an appendectomy: a population-based cohort study in Sweden and Denmark. *Gut*, **56**: 1387–1392.

16

For a range of Single Best Answer questions related to the topic of this chapter, and hyperlinks to a selection of key papers go to **www.oxfordtextbooks.coc.uk/orc/ocms/**

Left iliac fossa (LIF) pain

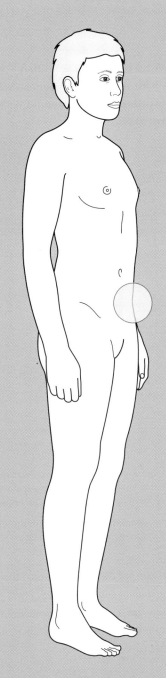

Core case

Mrs Hamilton is a 76-year-old lady who presents at her local accident and emergency (A&E) with left iliac fossa (LIF) pain.

What is your differential diagnosis for LIF pain? As we have done for previous presentations, try to think anatomically of what structures might give you pain in the LIF. Try to prioritize into those conditions that are most likely (or most common), those that you must exclude, and the remainder.

We have arranged the differential diagnosis in order of likelihood in a lady of this age, with more likely diagnoses in larger font and less likely diagnoses in smaller font. Pathologies that should be excluded at the earliest possible opportunity are shown in red.

Acute diverticulitis†
Constipation
Inflammatory bowel disease (IBD)
Ischaemic colitis
Pseudomembranous colitis‡
Leaking abdominal aortic aneurysm (AAA)
Locally perforated sigmoid carcinoma
Urinary tract infection
Ureteric colic
Pyelonephritis
Irritable bowel syndrome (IBS)
Shingles
Rectus sheath haematoma
Diabetic ketoacidosis

† A quick note on nomenclature. *Diverticulosis* refers to the presence of diverticula in the bowel (which may be asymptomatic). *Diverticular disease* is symptomatic diverticulosis, which can manifest as painless bleeding, altered bowel habit, or painful inflammation (*acute diverticulitis*).

‡ Pseudomembranous colitis is an acute inflammatory condition of the bowel that is usually, but not always, caused by *Clostridium difficile*.

If Mrs Hamilton had been pre-menopausal would there have been any other diagnoses to consider?

There are a number of gynaecological pathologies that can cause acute LIF pain. Some, such as ectopic pregnancy, mittelschmerz (mid-cycle pain), or haemorrhage into a functional ovarian cyst, can only occur in menstruating women. Others, such as pelvic inflammatory disease or torsion/rupture of an ovarian cyst, are far more likely to be seen in women younger than Mrs Hamilton, but can be kept in mind as rare differentials for someone of her age.

Is there any pathology peculiar to males that may cause LIF pain?

Testicular torsion can cause referred pain to either the left or right iliac fossa and tends to occur in boys and young men. Thus, don't forget to examine the testes.

What questions would you like to ask Mrs Hamilton about the pain in order to help narrow your differential diagnosis?

You should ask the standard array of questions about the pain – remember the mnemonic **SOCRATES**:

Site: Where is the pain, and has it always been there? Pain that is initially poorly localized, midline, and colicky but which then migrates to the LIF and becomes constant is highly suggestive of acute diverticulitis (akin to left-sided appendicitis). Pain that migrates down the left flank and iliac fossa is more consistent with the migration of a ureteric stone.

Onset: Gradual or sudden? Sudden onset of pain is suggestive of perforation of a viscus, or of acute haemorrhage (into an ovarian cyst) or torsion (of an ovary or testis).

Character: Is the pain colicky or constant? Is it sharp or dull? Acute diverticulitis is often preceded by colicky midline pain. Ureteric calculi may result in colicky pain. Established diverticulitis, and the other differential diagnoses from our list would all produce constant abdominal pain. Sharp pain is most suggestive of haemorrhage, perforation, or torsion.

Radiation: Does the pain radiate to the groin (typical of ureteric pain)?

Alleviating factors: Does anything make the pain better? Discomfort due to IBS may be relieved by defecation. Peritonitic patients will be most comfortable when lying still.

Timing: How long has the pain been present? Have there been any previous similar episodes? Patients with IBS may have suffered from abdominal discomfort for many months or years. Patients with acute diverticulitis often give a history of 2–3 days of LIF pain, and may have had a previous episode.

Exacerbating factors: Does anything make the pain worse? Patients with peritonitis (e.g. due to colonic perforation) are very sensitive to motion and may mention that the car journey to the hospital was painful (i.e. every time they hit a bump).

Severity: How severe is the pain (e.g. on a scale of 1–10)? Ureteric colic is excruciatingly painful, as is colonic perforation secondary to diverticulitis or a sigmoid carcinoma.

17

> Mrs Hamilton's pain started about 24 hours ago. She woke in the morning with 'vague stomach cramps'. By mid-morning she was suffering from constant pain in her LIF. She took some paracetamol at home, but this did not relieve the pain, which she reports as dull but 7/10 intensity. The pain does not radiate.
>
> **Having characterized the pain, what other symptoms should you enquire about?**

- **Nausea and vomiting?** Nausea and, to a lesser extent, vomiting, are seen with acute diverticulitis. They may also accompany pelvic inflammatory disease.
- **Fever?** Indicating an underlying infective or inflammatory disease such as acute diverticulitis.
- **Change of bowel habit?** A relatively non-specific symptom of most of the colonic diseases in our differential. IBS, diverticular disease, IBD, and colorectal carcinoma may all result in prolonged changes in bowel habit.
- **Rectal bleeding?** Overt rectal bleeding may be seen with acute diverticulitis, but is more likely to be seen in the context of bloody diarrhoea with ulcerative colitis, pseudomembranous colitis, ischaemic colitis, or colorectal carcinoma.
- **Bloating?** This is a characteristic feature of IBS.
- **Weight loss?** Although acute pain is an atypical presentation of colorectal carcinoma, a history of unintentional weight loss may raise your suspicions.
- **Gynaecological symptoms?** New vaginal discharge and/or pain during sex (dyspareunia) are consistent with pelvic inflammatory disease. In women who are menstruating, ask about the timing of the last menstrual period, regularity of periods, painful periods, and whether there is any possibility that the woman could be pregnant.

17

> **Are there any particular medicines to look out for in the drug history?**

The most important class of drugs to be aware of are **steroids** as these can dampen the inflammatory response, thus masking signs and symptoms. Bear in mind that patients taking steroids may be more ill than they appear by clinical examination.

Recent use of **antibiotics** (or **proton-pump inhibitors**) may raise your suspicions of pseudomembranous colitis (*Clostridium difficile* colitis) in patients presenting with LIF pain and diarrhoea.

> On further questioning, Mrs Hamilton explains that she has felt nauseated since this morning, but has not actually vomited. She feels feverish. She has not had any diarrhoea or felt constipated, and has not passed any blood per rectum. There are no gynaecological symptoms to note. She says that she is otherwise fit and well, and that her weight has not changed recently. She takes no medications, does not smoke, and enjoys an occasional glass of wine.
>
> Mrs Hamilton reports that she suffered from a similar pain last year, and that her GP had then advised her to drink lots of clear fluids and had prescribed her antibiotics and painkillers. However, Mrs Hamilton feels worse on this occasion, and thought that she should go to hospital instead of her GP.
>
> **What in particular will you look for when examining Mrs Hamilton?**

General examination

- **How unwell** is Mrs Hamilton? Check her basic observations: HR, BP, T, RR and Sats.
- Does she appear to have **generalized peritonitis**? Is she lying very still, taking shallow breaths, and looking pale?
- Is the patient **writhing in pain**, unable to keep still? This is typical for ureteric colic.

Abdominal examination

- You should examine the abdomen for any **focal tenderness**. Typically, uncomplicated acute diverticulitis presents with local tenderness and/or guarding.
- Does the patient have **generalized peritonitis** (tender, rigid abdomen with absent bowel sounds)? If so, you should suspect perforation of a colonic diverticulum, sigmoid carcinoma, or AAA.
- Are there any **masses**? A mass may be palpable in the LIF in patients with acute diverticulitis, even in the absence of a local abscess. A sigmoid carcinoma may also be palpable. A central, laterally pulsatile mass is an AAA until proven otherwise.

Rectal examination

- It may be possible to detect a pelvic abscess in patients with acute diverticulitis, and may also be possible to palpate a rectal malignancy.

Vaginal examination

- This is not indicated in Mrs Hamilton, but would be required in women presenting with LIF pain and new vaginal discharge, as cervical motion tenderness would lend weight to a diagnosis of pelvic inflammatory disease.

17

> Mrs Hamilton is febrile (38.2°C) and tachycardic (113 bpm regular), and looks flushed. Her blood pressure is 135/72 and her reopiratory rate is 21/min. She does not appear to have generalized peritonitis. Her LIF is tender to palpation, but the rest of the abdomen is soft and non-tender. There is no guarding or percussion tenderness. No masses are palpable, there is no organomegaly, and no palpable AAA. Bowel sounds are present. A digital rectal examination is unremarkable.
>
> **Which blood tests would you like to request?**

There are very few blood tests that are actually informative or necessary given this history:

- **Full blood count (FBC)**: the white cell count may be elevated in response to any inflammatory condition (e.g. acute diverticulitis, pseudomembranous colitis).
- **Urea and electrolytes (U&Es)**: useful for establishing the baseline electrolyte status of the patient (remembering that a number of the diagnoses on our differential will require intravenous (IV) fluids and/or surgery).

Blood tests are performed. The white cell count (WCC) is 14.1 × 10^9 cells/L (neutrophils 11.2 × 10^9 cells/L), and U&Es are unremarkable.

In light of the history, examination, and first-line investigations, what is the most likely diagnosis?

It is most likely that Mrs Hamilton has **acute diverticulitis**. She is an elderly patient with constant LIF pain, preceded by vague midline colicky pain, which is associated with nausea and fever. Examination confirms the LIF tenderness and shows no evidence of peritonism or an abscess. The leucocytosis confirms the underlying inflammatory response. Furthermore, there is a suggestion from the history that Mrs Hamilton has suffered from a previous episode of acute diverticulitis that was treated in the community.

Which imaging studies may be requested in the acute phase?

Mrs Hamilton appears clinically to have relatively mild diverticulitis, and there are some surgeons who would start empirical medical therapy without requesting any further imaging in the acute phase. However, a radiologically confirmed diagnosis is useful for determining whether surgery is indicated (see later in this case), and is also invaluable in more severely unwell patients, in those refractory to treatment, or those with a different history:

- **Abdominal computed tomography (CT) with contrast**: this is the imaging modality of choice for diagnosing acute diverticulitis and planning future elective surgery. If there is a suspicion of an abscess complicating acute diverticulitis, or if the patient is seriously ill, clinically deteriorates, or the diagnosis is unclear, then abdominal CT is also invaluable.
- **Erect chest radiograph**: request this if there is any clinical suspicion of a perforated viscus, looking for air under the diaphragm.
- **Abdominal radiograph**: useful for ruling out bowel obstruction if this is clinically suspected.

If Mrs Hamilton had been pre-menopausal are there any other imaging modalities that you would request to investigate her LIF pain?

Transabdominal ± transvaginal ultrasound are particularly useful investigations in young female patients, where the differential diagnosis is broadened by gynaecological pathology.

Could Mrs Hamilton have had a colonoscopy or double-contrast barium enema to confirm the diagnosis in the acute phase of her illness?

Mrs Hamilton **should not** have had either investigation in the acute phase. Colonoscopy and double contrast barium enema are contraindicated in the acute setting as there is a risk of perforating the acutely inflamed colon.

17

How should Mrs Hamilton be managed in the acute phase?

Mrs Hamilton should be treated as follows:

- **Analgesia**
- **Bowel rest**: by clear fluids only
- **IV fluids**: if Mrs Hamilton is unable to maintain a sufficient oral intake
- **Antibiotics**: to cover Gram-negative bacteria and anaerobes (e.g. co-amoxiclav plus metronidazole, but consult local guidelines)
- **Monitor**: if symptoms do not improve within 48–72 hours, further investigation is required to establish whether an abscess is present, or whether the initial diagnosis was flawed.

How will Mrs Hamilton be followed up? Is there any advice that she should be given?

Given that the diagnosis of acute diverticulitis has been made on clinical grounds, Mrs Hamilton will be offered a **colonoscopy or double-contrast barium enema 2–6 weeks after resolution of this episode**. This is to assess the extent of diverticulosis and the degree of stricturing secondary to inflammation, and can exclude other potential diagnoses such as colitis or carcinoma. CT colonography is being investigated as a potential alternative to conventional colonoscopy.

Mrs Hamilton should be advised to maintain a high intake of dietary fibre as this may reduce the chance of future episodes of diverticular disease.

Should Mrs Hamilton be offered an elective colonic resection?

17

Following the successful conservative treatment of an episode of acute diverticulitis, about a third of patients will remain asymptomatic, a third will develop occasional abdominal cramps, and a third will suffer a further attack of acute diverticulitis. Further attacks of acute diverticulitis are less likely to respond to conservative treatment than the first episode. Various authorities have therefore recommended that patients with two *proven* episodes of acute diverticulitis should be offered elective resection of the affected portion of bowel (if no emergency surgery has already been performed). Elective resection may be offered to patients <40 years of age following a single confirmed episode. Mrs Hamilton did not have *proven* diverticulitis last year, and thus is not yet a candidate for elective surgery. Mrs Hamilton was admitted to hospital and received IV fluids, analgesia, and antibiotics. She made an uneventful recovery and was discharged from hospital after 4 days. An outpatient colonoscopy 5 weeks later confirmed extensive diverticulosis of the sigmoid colon.

Short cases

Mr Arnold is a 67-year-old retired lecturer who presents to A&E with severe LIF pain. He reports that he has been in pain for the last 2 days, but that the pain suddenly increased in severity 1 hour ago. The pain is now sharp, does not radiate, and appears to be worsened by any degree of movement. Mr Arnold rates it as the worst pain he has ever experienced. For the past couple of days he has felt nauseated and feverish, but has not vomited. He has had slight diarrhoea, but has not noticed any blood in his stool. He reports no recent weight loss.

His past medical history is remarkable for two previous episodes of LIF pain. The first episode was 5 years ago and the second was 1 year ago. Mr Arnold reports that on both occasions the pain was very similar to that which he has had for the preceding 2 days – but was nowhere near as severe as the pain that he has experienced for the last hour. The episode 5 years ago was managed by his GP 'with anti-biotics and paracetamol' and the second episode resulted in a 3-day hospital admission but no surgery.

Mr Arnold has no other significant medical history and takes no regular medications. He is a smoker with a 15-pack-year history, and is teetotal. He has no allergies.

On examination, Mr Arnold looks pale and clammy. He lies still on the examination couch and is taking shallow breaths. He is reluctant to cough as this causes him considerable pain. His basic observations are: heart rate 107 bpm regular, blood pressure 92/53 mmHg, temperature 38.3°C, respiratory rate 19/min, and oxygen saturation 96% on room air. Examination reveals widespread guarding and absent bowel sounds.

What is the most likely diagnosis? How should Mr Arnold be managed?

Mr Arnold is **peritonitic** – he is shocked, lying still, displaying generalized guard-ing, and has absent bowel sounds. The sudden increase in pain and worsening of his symptoms suggests that Mr Arnold has probably perforated a viscus. More pre-cisely, the combination of his past medical history and pain over the previous 2 days suggests that he has probably developed **perforated diverticulitis**.

Appropriate management differs considerably from the uncomplicated acute diverticulitis of the previous case. Mr Arnold will need to be treated as follows:

* **Fluid resuscitation**
* **Blood tests**: request FBC, U&E, clotting, and cross-match
* **Analgesia**
* **Antibiotics**
* **CT**: provided that imaging is readily available and doesn't delay transfer to theatre
* **Emergency laparotomy**

The advantage of pre-operative scanning is that a more precise diagnosis may be reached, hence the surgeon is better informed and the patient may be fully consent-ed (for example, for a stoma). Pre-operative knowledge aids the surgeon in planning incisions, choosing stoma sites etc.

There are two most common surgical options for the emergency treatment of per-forated diverticulitis. Most patients have a Hartmann's procedure (see Chapter 21). In some patients it is safe to perform a primary anastomosis. To protect the primary anastomosis, the surgeon can also form a proximal loop ('defunctioning') ileostomy, which drains bowel contents before they pass via the primary anastomosis.

17

Miss Sellers is a 31-year-old sales assistant who presents to her GP with LIF pain. She has suffered from the pain intermittently for several months, and rates it as of moderate intensity. In addition, she often also has vague cramping abdominal pains. The pain does not radiate anywhere. The pain often follows meals, and may be relieved by defecation. She also reports feeling bloated. She has not felt nauseated or feverish. Her bowel habits are rather irregular – sometimes she has diarrhoea while at other times she tends towards constipation. She has not noticed any rectal bleeding. Her weight has been stable. She reports no unusual vaginal discharge or itch, no intermenstrual bleeding, and no post-coital bleeding or pain. Her last menstrual period was 2 weeks ago.

She suffers from asthma, for which she uses fluticasone and salbutamol inhalers. She is otherwise well. She also takes the combined oral contraceptive pill and has no allergies. She does not drink alcohol or smoke.

Examination is unremarkable. Miss Sellers is afebrile, normotensive, and has a pulse of 71 bpm regular. Her abdomen is soft and non-tender. Bowel sounds are audible. The GP does not perform a rectal or gynaecological examination as he does not feel that they are indicated in this instance.

Given the history and examination findings, which diagnosis do you feel is most likely? What investigations would you like to request to confirm the diagnosis?

Miss Sellers has a history of chronic abdominal pain, with cramping, bloating, and altered bowel habit. She is otherwise well and has no signs on examination. It is most likely that Miss Sellers is suffering from **IBS**, but **IBD** should also be considered (in an older patient diverticular disease could lead to a similar presentation). The LIF pain is not a universal feature of IBS, but is consistent with the diagnosis. The fact that Miss Sellers is otherwise well, has lost no weight, and has passed no blood per rectum, favours IBS over IBD.

Before diagnosing Miss Sellers with IBS it is necessary to exclude other causes of chronic abdominal pain and altered bowel habit. Thus, as a first line, it would be appropriate to request the following investigations in a patient of Miss Sellers' age, explaining to her that you expect all the blood tests to be entirely normal:

- **Bloods**:
  - **FBC**: any signs of infection, inflammation, or anaemia of chronic disease?
  - **Liver function tests (LFTs)**: albumin is used as a marker of malabsorption.
  - **Erythrocyte sedimentation rate (ESR)**: any underlying chronic inflammation?
  - **Anti-endomysial antibodies** or **tissue transglutaminase (TTG)**: a positive result has a sensitivity and specificity of over 90% for coeliac disease. (Antigliadin antibodies have been used to test for coeliac disease but are less sensitive and specific.) You must always check **IgA levels** too, because IgA deficiency can cause a false negative result.
- **Stool culture**: does she have a chronic infection such as *Giardia*, which may account for her abdominal pain and altered bowel habit?
- **Flexible sigmoidoscopy**: any structural disease of the sigmoid, such as IBD?

17

Short case

Mrs Martinez is a 27-year-old housewife who presents to A&E with acute LIF pain. She woke at 5 a.m. that morning with moderate dull pain in the LIF. The pain did not radiate, and was not relieved by simple analgesia. The pain has been constant for the past 4 hours. Mrs Martinez has not felt nauseated, and has not experienced any change in bowel habit. She last opened her bowels last night. She does not feel feverish.

Her last menstrual period was 35 days ago, and her usual menstrual cycle is 3–4/28 (bleeding for 3–4 days of a 28-day cycle). On direct questioning, she mentions that she has passed blood per vagina this morning, but that this is lighter than her usual period. She does not use any form of contraception with her husband. She reports no other gynaecological symptoms.

She had a laparoscopic appendicectomy 2 years ago, but has no other significant past medical history. She takes no regular medications, and has no allergies. She does not smoke, and drinks about 10 units of wine each week.

Mrs Martinez's observations are unremarkable, and she appears able to move with minimal discomfort. Her abdomen is tender to palpation in the LIF, but is otherwise soft and non-tender. There is no percussion tenderness or guarding, and bowel sounds are present. A rectal examination is not performed.

What single investigation must you request? How would you proceed with the results of this test?

Mrs Martinez is a sexually active young woman who presents with lower abdominal pain, vaginal bleeding, and amenorrhoea (her period is late). While it is possible that this morning's vaginal bleed represents the start of her period, the fact that she has pain should ring alarm bells that this is an **ectopic pregnancy**. Thus you must request an urgent **urine pregnancy test** to exclude this diagnosis. The fact that Mrs Martinez shows no signs of shock and has stable observations is reassuring as there is no current evidence that she has developed a perforated ectopic (a surgical emergency).

Mrs Martinez's pregnancy test was positive and thus she should be referred to the gynaecologists to confirm whether the pregnancy is intrauterine or ectopic.

17

Miss Efran is a 29-year-old salsa instructor who presents to her GP with LIF pain. She has had the pain for 3 days, and says that she decided to seek help as the pain has gradually become more uncomfortable for her. The pain is a dull ache that does not radiate. She can think of nothing that alleviates or exacerbates the pain. She has not taken any analgesia at home.

Miss Efran has vomited three times today. She says that she feels feverish, and that she has also been shaking/shivering. On direct questioning, she mentions that she has had some yellow vaginal discharge for the past 2 days, but has not passed any blood. She is sure that she cannot be pregnant because she is using the combined oral contraceptive pill with her new boyfriend. She reports no urinary symptoms and no change of bowel habit.

Miss Efran is otherwise fit and well. She has no significant past medical history, takes no regular medications other than the contraceptive pill, and has no allergies. She smokes about 10 cigarettes each day and drinks about 20 units of alcohol each week.

On examination, Miss Efran appears flushed, and is febrile (38.5°C). Her heart rate is 103 bpm regular and her blood pressure is 123/71 mmHg. Her respiratory rate is 15/min. Her abdomen is soft, but tender to palpation in the LIF. There is no percussion tenderness. No organomegaly is detected. A digital rectal examination is not performed, but Miss Efran is consented for a bimanual pelvic examination that reveals marked adnexal tenderness.

A urinary pregnancy test is negative, and urinalysis reveals nil leucocytes, nitrites, protein, or blood.

In light of history and examination, what is the most likely diagnosis? How would you manage this?

It is most likely that Miss Efran has **acute pelvic inflammatory disease** – she is a sexually active woman (with a new partner), who has acute lower abdominal pain, new vaginal discharge, vomiting, and fever, combined with adnexal tenderness on vaginal examination. Her pregnancy test is negative.

The most likely causes of acute pelvic inflammatory disease are sexually transmitted bacterial infections such as *Chlamydia* or gonorrhoea. Appropriate further management of Miss Efran may involve the following steps:

- **Vaginal, urethral, and endocervical swabs**: to identify the pathogen
- **Empirical antibiotics**: to cover likely pathogens until culprit identified
- **Referral to a genitourinary medicine (GUM) clinic**
- **Avoid sexual intercourse while being treated**
- **Partner notification**: sexual partners from the preceding 6 months should be traced and offered testing in a GUM clinic; if they test positive they too should avoid sexual intercourse until they have completed their treatment
- **Consider alternative contraception:** condoms offer protection against sexually transmitted infections

17

Viva questions

How common is diverticulosis? Are there any known risk factors?

It is difficult to assess the true prevalence of diverticulosis as most patients are asymptomatic, but some data are available from autopsy series. Many patients are diagnosed incidentally. The prevalence is age dependent, such that about 5% of 40-year-olds, about 30% of 60-year-olds, and about 65% of 85-year-olds have colonic diverticula (mostly asymptomatic). There is a huge difference in prevalence between 'developed' and 'developing' countries, such that diverticulosis appears to be rare in 'developing' countries. Much of this difference in prevalence is said to be due to variation in fibre intake – diets in the 'developed' world are relatively fibre-depleted and this leads to high intraluminal colonic pressures that favour the development of pulsion diverticula.

What is the natural history of diverticulosis?

There are a number of possible outcomes for patients with diverticulosis:

- 70% remain asymptomatic
- 15–25% develop acute diverticulitis, 75% of which is 'uncomplicated' (as in Mrs Hamilton's initial presentation) and 25% of which is 'complicated' (as in Mr Arnold's initial presentation)
- 5–10% develop rectal bleeding (see Chapter 21)

What are the main complications of diverticulitis?

The main complications of diverticulitis are as follows:

- Perforation
  - May be localized/contained/walled-off as an abscess
  - May lead to generalized peritonitis
- Abscess formation
- Fistulation into adjacent structures (e.g. bladder)
- Chronic inflammatory strictures resulting in bowel obstruction
- Haemorrhage

Colovesical fistulas are the most common type of fistula caused by diverticulitis. Are they more common in men or women? Why?

A fistula can form between adjacent areas of inflammation. Colovesical fistulas are more common in men. This is thought to be because the uterus sits between the sigmoid and the bladder, forming a barrier to colovesical fistula formation.

Acute diverticulitis is sometimes nicknamed 'left-sided appendicitis'. Both are typically preceded by colicky midline abdominal pain. Would you expect this initial pain to be peri-umbilical for both presentations?

This question relates to the embryological anatomy of the gut. Remember that the initial midline colicky pain caused by inflammation of the gut is mediated by autonomic innervation. This pain is approximately referred to the epigastrium, umbilicus, or hypogastrium according to whether the inflamed structure is within the embryological foregut, midgut, or hindgut. As the appendix is a midgut structure you would expect the initial colicky pain to be peri-umbilical, whereas acute diverticulitis would cause referred colicky pain in the suprapubic area. In practice, it may be difficult to differentiate these sites from the patient's account of the history of the pain. In addition, diverticulitis may yield right-sided pain if the sigmoid loop is long and extends to the right iliac fossa.

What are the risk factors for ectopic pregnancy?

The main risk factors include:

- Previous ectopic pregnancy
- Pelvic inflammatory disease
- Tubular procedures, e.g. sterilization (some women may still become pregnant)
- Endometriosis
- Pelvic surgery
- In vitro fertilization (IVF)
- Intrauterine contraceptive device

The underlying mechanism for several of these risk factors is an alteration to the normal anatomy of the Fallopian tubes. Inflammation or surgical manipulation of the tubes can lead to strictures or kinks that disrupt the normal passage of the egg.

17

What is Hinchey's classification?

This classification represents an assessment of peritoneal contamination at the time of surgery in the context of acute diverticulitis. As such, it may be used as a guide to the suitability for primary anastomosis following resection. Four classes are recognized:

   I   Pericolic or mesenteric abscess
   II Walled-off pelvic abscess
   III Generalized purulent peritonitis (~5% mortality)
   IV Generalized faecal peritonitis (~35% mortality)

 For a range of Single Best Answer questions related to the topic of this chapter go to
www.oxfordtextbooks.co.uk/orc/ocms/

Flank pain

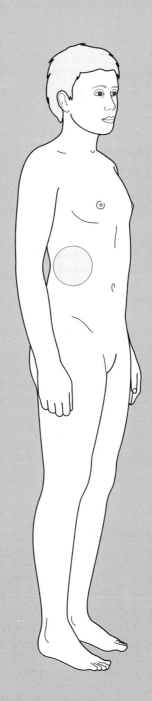

Core case

!

Read through the sections in red, covering up the sections in white that follow so that you don't see the answer. At the end of each red section, try to answer the question before reading on.

Core case

Mr Kirk is a 61-year-old pilot who comes to accident and emergency (A&E) complaining of severe flank pain just below his ribs.

What is your differential diagnosis for acute flank pain? Are any of your diagnoses life threatening?

The diagnoses shown in red are all surgical emergencies that you must exclude as you clerk the patient.

> Muscular sprain
> Nephrolithiasis/ureteric colic
> Leaking/ruptured abdominal aortic aneurysm (AAA)
> Spinal pathology (fractures, metastases, disc prolapse)
> Testicular torsion (very unusual in an elderly person)
> Pyelonephritis (unusual in a man)
> Perforated peptic ulcer
> Renal cancer
> Abscess (perinephric, renal)
> Basal pneumonia

In women, you should consider gynaecological causes, e.g. ectopic pregnancy, ovarian torsion. Also, bear in mind that other abdominal pathology can occasionally present as flank pain (e.g. pancreatitis, diverticulitis, appendicitis).

What questions will you ask about the presenting complaint (i.e. flank pain) to help you narrow your diagnosis?

You should ask the standard array of questions about the pain – remember the mnemonic **SOCRATES**:

Site: Where is the pain, and has it always been there? Is it unilateral or bilateral? Kidney stones are almost always unilateral, but the location of the pain may radiate from loin to groin. Often they start with a vague discomfort that is ignored until it becomes a severe pain. Appendicitis classically starts as a poorly localized midline pain due to irritation of the visceral (inner

18

layer) peritoneum but sharply localizes once the parietal (outer) peritoneum becomes irritated.

Onset: Any trauma or other trigger, or spontaneous? Gradual or sudden? Trauma may lead to musculoskeletal pain or internal bleeding.

Character: Is the pain colicky or constant? Is it sharp or dull? Ureteric stones give a colicky (waxing and waning) pain because of periodic spasms of the ureteric smooth muscle walls trying to dislodge the blockage. A constant pain is more consistent with a stone lodged in the kidney, which does not periodically contract like the ureters, or an inflammatory cause. Musculoskeletal pain is more typically an ache, while nerve impingement causes shooting pains.

Radiation: Does the pain radiate to the groin (typical of ureteric pain)? Does it radiate down the leg (typical of lumbar nerve root pain)?

Alleviating factors: Does anything make the pain better, e.g. a given posture, eating/drinking, any medications etc?

Timing: How long has the pain been present? Musculoskeletal back pain can last many weeks, whereas a leaking AAA is unlikely to persist for more than a day without resolution, one way or another.

Exacerbating factors: Does anything make the pain worse? Patients with peritonitis (e.g. due to appendicitis or a perforated peptic ulcer) are very sensitive to motion and may mention that the car journey to the hospital was painful (i.e. every time they hit a bump).

Severity: How severe is the pain (e.g. on a scale of 1–10)? Kidney stones are said to be excruciatingly painful, comparable to childbirth.

Mr Kirk's pain is unilateral. It is localized to his right flank, and has not moved. He says it came on spontaneously whilst he was watching television. At first it was just a dull constant ache, but a couple of hours ago it became colicky and started radiating from his flank into his groin. There is nothing he can do to make it better or worse.

Having characterized his pain, what further questions should you ask in the history?

18

History of presenting complaint

- **Fever, rigors, night sweats?** A markedly raised fever indicates an inflammatory process, potentially pyelonephritis or sepsis. The fever of malignancies (e.g. renal cell carcinoma) is typically intermittent, unlike in infection.

- **Dehydration?** Persistent dehydration predisposes to concentrated urine and therefore to kidney stones.

- **Nausea and vomiting?** This is more typical of visceral organ pathology (e.g. ureteric stones, biliary colic, appendicitis) but rare in other causes of pain (e.g. musculoskeletal pain, nerve root compression, shingles).

- **Haematuria?** Whilst 70–90% of patients with kidney/ureteric stones are reported to have haematuria, this is usually microscopic (i.e. not visible to the naked eye). Nonetheless, it is worth asking whether they have had any macroscopic haematuria, as this can occur.

- **Lower urinary tract symptoms?** Urinary frequency, urgency, and dysuria are common in urinary tract infection. Hesitancy, reduced flow, dribbling, and incomplete voiding are more typical of ureteric obstruction (e.g. due to stones or tumours).
- **Cloudy or offensive-smelling urine?** Another sign of infection.
- **Leg weakness?** This could suggest spinal pathology.

Past medical history

- **Previous kidney stones?** A strong risk factor for future episodes of nephrolithiasis.
- **Recurrent cystitis?** Recurrent episodes of urinary tract infection predispose to stones of the struvite type.
- **Atherosclerotic disease (e.g. angina, myocardial infarction, stroke, claudication)?** A strong risk factor for AAA.
- **Long-standing back pain?** This is usually due to pathology affecting the muscles, ligaments, and bones.
- **Kidney disease?** Polycystic kidney disease predisposes to pyelonephritis. If the patient only has one kidney, you need to know as obstruction of the only functional ureter is a medical emergency.

Drug history

- Indinavir, aciclovir, and acetazolamide can lead to kidney stone formation.

Family history

- **Family history of kidney stones?** This may indicate a (rare) inherited condition such as cystinuria.

Mr Kirk says he has been feeling sick, although he has not actually vomited. He adds that he has never had anything like this before. He has type 2 diabetes mellitus which is well controlled by diet and daily metformin. His family history is unremarkable. He concedes that he probably doesn't drink enough fluids, but doesn't feel especially dehydrated.

You proceed to examine Mr Kirk.

What signs are you looking for on examination?

- **Position?** Whether your patient is restless or still can be very informative. Those with ureteric colic are unable to sit still and thus tend to writhe in pain. Those with peritonitis (e.g. from appendicitis or a perforated peptic ulcer) are rigid and motionless, as any movement causes pain.
- **Tenderness?** Individuals with renal or ureteric stones may have flank or loin tenderness (particularly in the costovertebral angles), but tend not to have any other abdominal signs. Abdominal tenderness suggests a peritoneal cavity problem (e.g. appendicitis, pancreatitis). Any testicular tenderness should be mild if it is due to referred pain from renal tract stones; otherwise suspect a testicular cause, e.g. torsion.

- **Masses?** You should look specifically for a central, laterally expansile mass which could be a leaking AAA. This must be suspected in anyone >55 years of age. It is possible for the pain from an AAA to be misdiagnosed as ureteric colic. Note that physical examination does *not* exclude a ruptured aneurysm; if it is suspected, the patient should undergo imaging.

- **Spine?** You must also exclude spinal pathology by testing range of movement (e.g. straight leg raise) and feeling for tenderness along the vertebrae.

- **Lower limbs?** Conduct a neurological exam on the lower limbs, in case of spinal pathology causing the flank pain (e.g. a prolapsed intervertebral disc). Also conduct a vascular examination of the lower limbs, as an AAA can compromise blood supply to the lower limbs. If you can easily feel the popliteal pulse, you should suspect a popliteal aneurysm and remember that about 50% of patients with popliteal aneurysms also have AAAs.

- **Temperature?** Indicates whether an inflammatory process, potentially pyelonephritis, is ongoing.

Mr Kirk is restless, consistent with the description of his pain. His right flank is tender to palpation but his abdomen is otherwise soft and non-tender with no masses. Bowel sounds are present and normal. He is apyrexial. Examination of his lower limbs is unremarkable. Judging from the way Mr Kirk is writhing on the bed, he has a full range of motion in his back, and although you are not able to assess his spine formally, you establish there is no tenderness to palpation over bony landmarks.

What diagnosis do the history and examination suggest so far? What investigations will you arrange?

Mr Kirk has presented with a history of spontaneous, sudden-onset, 'loin to groin', colicky, severe pain that is highly suggestive of **ureteric colic**. The lack of fever, and abdominal tenderness, and lack of an expansile abdominal mass and lower limb signs makes other diagnoses far less likely. Therefore, the following investigations would be appropriate in this patient:

Urine

- **Urinalysis:** you should note the presence of haematuria, white blood cells (pyuria), leucocyte esterase, and nitrites. You may also want to note the urine pH, as patients with urate stones usually have acidic urine; an alkali pH suggests the presence of urease-producing bacteria (e.g. *Proteus, Pseudomonas, Klebsiella*) that can predispose to stone formation.

- **Urine microscopy, culture, and sensitivity (MC&S):** look for blood, evidence of infection (white cells, bacteria), and crystals. Identifying the type of crystal helps particularly in understanding the aetiology and secondary prevention of future stones. The presence of red cell casts or white cell casts indicates that the red or white cells are coming from the kidney, rather than the ureters or bladder. Thus red cell casts indicate glomerular damage and white cell casts suggest pyelonephritis (although these are rarely found).

18

Bloods

- **Full blood count (FBC) and C-reactive protein (CRP):** look for a raised white cell count (WCC) and CRP, indicating infection or sepsis.

- **Urea, creatinine, and electrolytes:** assess renal function, as obstruction by a renal stone can precipitate renal damage. Renal failure is a medical emergency!

- **Serum calcium, phosphate, and urate:** these provide valuable clues as to the aetiology of kidney stones.

Imaging

- **CT-KUB (kidneys, ureters, and bladder):** this will show any stones in the kidney or ureter, but also any rare causes of ureter obstruction causing renal colic (e.g. a retroperitoneal tumour). It will also detect any AAAs. CT has a greater sensitivity and specificity than plain KUB radiographs for kidney stones, but KUB radiographs are still useful for following the progression of known stones in a way that involves less exposure to ionizing radiation. A magnetic resonance urogram (MRU) can be used if the patient is pregnant and therefore unsuitable for any form of ionizing radiation. Although intra-venous urography/pyelography (IVU or IVP) used to be the gold standard for detecting kidney stones, it has now been superseded by CT-KUB.

*Remember! If pancreatitis is suspected, you should order a **serum amylase** level. If a perforated peptic ulcer is a concern, you should order an **erect chest radiograph** to look for air under the diaphragm.*

You take Mr Kirk's basic observations. His heart rate is 68 bpm and regular, his blood pressure is 126/84 mmHg and his respiratory rate is 12/min with oxygen saturation of 99% on room air. He is afebrile.

Urinalysis shows microscopic haematuria, a urine pH of 6.0, and is weakly positive for white cells (+). His while cell count is normal. Reassuringly, his urea and electrolytes (U&Es) are all within the normal ranges.

A CT-KUB scan is performed and a single slice is shown in Fig. 18.1.

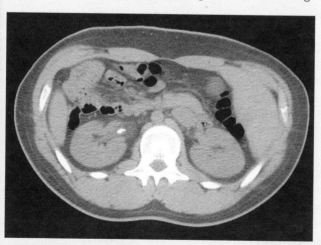

Figure 18.1 A computed tomography scan of kidneys, ureters, and bladder (CT-KUB) (single slice) for Mr Kirk.

What is the diagnosis?

18

Mr Kirk has ureteric colic caused by a **kidney stone** (aka *nephrolithiasis* or *ureteric calculus*), lodged at the right pelvi-ureteric junction (PUJ).

How should Mr Kirk be managed during the acute episode? Does he require admission?

Having assessed his need for resuscitation (Airway, Breathing, Circulation, ABC), you should decide whether or not to admit him. He should be admitted if:

* there is evidence of upper urinary tract infection (cloudy urine ± white cell casts, high WCC in blood, high CRP, fever) ... infection proximal to an obstruction is a surgical emergency, requiring drainage;
* there is evidence of renal failure (high creatinine, high urea, high K⁺);
* there is refractory pain (despite analgesia);
* there are bilateral obstructing stones (or a single obstructing stone if only one kidney present);
* the patient is elderly, a child, or otherwise unwell (e.g. unable to tolerate oral fluids), for closer monitoring.

Mr Kirk **does not need admitting**.

Your next step should be to provide **analgesia** (e.g. paracetamol + non-steroidal anti-inflammatory drugs (NSAIDs)) – remember this is as painful as childbirth! NSAIDs and paracetamol are preferred to opiates as studies show they provide equally adequate analgesia in the context of kidney stones (see viva question), may have some additional effect of decreasing ureteric smooth muscle tone, and lack some of the adverse effects of opiates, notably respiratory and central nervous system (CNS) depression, vomiting, and disorientation. Despite frequent patient concerns, long-term dependence of opiates is not an issue when they are used in the acute setting.

You should also **encourage fluid intake**. If they cannot tolerate oral fluids, you should admit them and prescribe intravenous (IV) fluids.

18

Mr Kirk is given NSAIDs and paracetamol and his pain subsides over the next hour. He now rates it as 3/10 in severity and is happy to 'put up' with this.

What should be the next step in his management?

Having achieved adequate pain relief and excluded emergencies requiring admission, a **management plan for dealing with the stone**(s) can be put in place. The two major prognostic factors are stone size and location:

1) Stones <0.5 cm diameter
   - Start with a **trial of conservative management** (analgesia and encourage oral fluid intake). Ninety per cent of stones <0.5 cm pass spontaneously, although only 10% of larger stones do. Patients should be asked to strain their urine to recover the stone for analysis.
   - You may consider adding medication to relax the smooth muscle of the ureter, either an **α-blocker** (e.g. tamsulosin) or a **calcium-channel blocker** (e.g. nifedipine).

– **Follow up** patients after 2–3 weeks and request a plain KUB radiograph to minimize the radiation exposure of repeat CT-KUB.

2) Stones >0.5 cm diameter (or if smaller but not passed after 4–6 weeks and continuing discomfort)

– **Lithotripsy**, otherwise known as extracorporeal shock wave lithotripsy (ESWL) if small enough (renal stones <2 cm, ureteric stones <1 cm).

– **Ureterorenoscopic removal** (using a fine telescope inserted via the urethra) with a dormia basket, holmium laser, mechanical lithotripsy etc., if too large for ESWL. Note that this commonly requires a post-operative ureteric stent as it can cause ureteric stricture.

– **Percutaneous nephrolithotomy** (PCNL) is rarely used nowadays as it is invasive and thus there are risks of bleeding and damage to the collecting system and neighbouring structures.

– **Stenting** (using a JJ stent) or percutaneous nephrostomy may be performed in order to prevent hydronephrosis, if the obstruction cannot be resolved surgically.

– **Antibiotic cover** if an invasive procedure is employed.

Of interest, certain occupations, notably pilots, do not permit people to work even with an asymptomatic stone for fear of the unpredictable onset of incapacitating pain while they are involved in a crucial task. Thus, patients such our 'Captain Kirk' (a pilot) will require early definitive therapy rather than a more conservative approach.

18

The stone in Mr Kirk's right ureter was 0.7 cm so the urologists decided to remove it the following morning using a ureteroscope and dormia basket.

How should Mr Kirk be managed in the longer term? Are any further investigations or measures for secondary prevention appropriate?

All patients should be advised to increase their fluid intake.

In addition, it is appropriate to try to identify the underlying cause in those patients at greatest risk of recurrence, as there are some treatments available. Appropriate criteria for further testing could include:

• strong family history

• multiple stones at first diagnosis

• recurrent stone formation/passage

Mr Kirk has none of the above and so can be discharged without further investigation.

Short cases

> Mr Kirk was discharged home after successful removal of his ureteric stone by the urologists. One month later he returns to hospital. He has a 2-day history of a dull ache in his right flank and is worried he has developed another kidney stone. However, this time he additionally has urinary frequency, dysuria, and a fever. He says he has vomited repeatedly. His heart rate is 104 bpm, blood pressure is 88/60 mmHg, respiratory rate of 18/min and his temperature is 40.2°C. His urine dipstick reveals microscopic haematuria, pyuria (white cells +++), and nitrites (+++).
>
> **What is the most likely diagnosis? How should he be managed?**

Mr Kirk has presented with a dull flank pain, high fever, and urinalysis suggestive of a urinary tract infection. He has most likely developed **acute pyelonephritis** secondary to obstruction from his previous kidney stone(s). The most common causal organism by far is *Escherichia coli*. Pyelonephritis requires rapid diagnosis and treatment as progression to septicaemia can be swift.

Management as always should begin with an assessment of Mr Kirk's need for resuscitation. This patient is hypotensive and needs to be given fluids. Given that he is hypotensive, has an active infection, and has vomiting that precludes oral therapy, he will need admission.

You should then take a full history, conduct a thorough examination, request investigations, and instigate treatment:

- **IV fluids** to restore his blood pressure, then orally if tolerated.
- Pyelonephritis should be treated with **antibiotics** for 2 weeks, initially on an empirical basis until the urine cultures return. Consult your local hospital guidelines for the appropriate antibiotic regimen.
- Don't forget the **analgesia!** (see viva questions)
- **Monitor** his renal function and urine output to assess his renal function. If his ureter is obstructed, he will need a percutaneous nephrostomy tube to give the urine an outlet and relieve pressure on the kidney.
- During his admission, you should maintain a high index of suspicion for intrarenal or perinephric abscess. Watch out for a persistently high fever, bacteraemia (positive blood cultures), very high initial WCC, severe tenderness on examination, or failure to improve after appropriate therapy. If an abscess develops, it will require surgical drainage.

18

> Mr McCoy is a 50-year-old truck driver with a high body mass index (BMI) who attends his GP complaining of right flank pain. The pain has been present for over a week, although he cannot remember a specific trigger. He describes it as an ache, worse in the morning or after a long day's drive. He has tried ibuprofen and this helps a little but he is unhappy as he sees it as only a temporary fix. Otherwise nothing relieves the pain.
>
> He has no associated symptoms. In particular, he has not had any urinary or bowel symptoms, and has not noticed any weakness or changes in sensation in either leg. Examination is unremarkable except for limited flexion of the spine.
>
> **What is the most likely diagnosis? How should this gentleman be managed?**

This gentleman is most likely suffering with **musculoskeletal back pain**. This will affect up to 80% of the population at some point. The majority will recover within 6 weeks, but 60% will have relapses in the future. Management should involve:

- **Maintaining activity and exercise.** It is better to avoid bed rest in patients with musculoskeletal lower back pain. Inactivity will make the problem worse. The key is to find mild, gentle exercise that they can tolerate on a regular basis. If the back pain becomes chronic there is also a proven role for cognitive behavioural therapy (CBT) to correct unhelpful negative beliefs regarding the back pain.

- **Regular analgesia.** Most over-the-counter analgesics (NSAIDs and paracetamol) work well for lower back pain but only if they are taken *regularly*. Back pain can take up to 6 weeks to recover, so opiates should be avoided if possible to avoid tolerance and dependence.

- **Build up core muscles.** 'Core stability' muscle groups such as transversus abdominis, the internal and external obliques, and multifidus are crucial in maintaining the lower spine in a stable 'neutral position'. Weakness in these muscles predisposes to musculoskeletal back injury. Encourage patients to lose weight and strengthen their core muscles at a gym or via a physiotherapy directed programme such as an integrated back stability programme.

- **General back care.** Most idiopathic back pain is the result of a combination of repeated bending (lumbar flexion) actions leading to accumulated strain on lumbar soft tissues. Recommend that a patient practices good back care – limit bending (bend the knees instead), and sit upright in a chair (don't slouch). When lifting or carrying, an object should be held close to the body to reduce leverage effects.

- **Avoid surgery.** For the overwhelming majority of patients, surgery is no better than conservative management involving exercise regimes, even when the lower back ache is due to clearly defined anatomical abnormalities such as herniated intervertebral discs or spondylolysis ± spondylolisthesis.

Mrs Chekov is a 76-year-old lady who presents to A&E with acute flank pain that came on suddenly and woke her at night. She has had back pain for many years, but this feels very different – it is sharper and more severe. Her initial observations are a heart rate of 116 bpm regular, blood pressure of 116/88 mmHg on lying, oxygen saturations of 98% on air and temperature of 36.4°C.

She has been feeling fine recently, although she has a past medical history of lower back pain, angina, hypertension, and 'indigestion', for which she takes aspirin, simvastatin, propanolol, diclofenac, co-codamol, and omeprazole. On examination, she is obese and has pitting oedema affecting both legs up to her knees. The oedema makes it impossible to palpate any pulses in her legs. Her body habitus makes it impossible to determine any masses on palpation of her abdomen, but she does have mild epigastric tenderness. Her back is free of tenderness on palpation. Her spine has a very limited range of motion, but this is apparently longstanding. An urgent CT abdomen is done and is shown in Fig. 18.2.

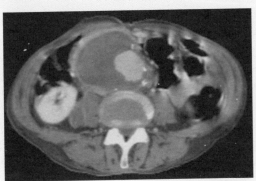

Figure 18.2 Abdominal computed tomography (CT) scan for Mrs Chekov.
O'Connor and Urdang Handbook for Surgical Cross-Cover, 2008, P139, Figure 4.2. By permission of Oxford University Press.

What is the diagnosis? How will you proceed?

18

Mrs Chekov is an elderly lady with a past medical history of ischaemic heart disease and hypertension who now presents with a sudden-onset, sharp flank pain. Her history and examination do not point to any clear diagnosis, but her age and risk factors do suggest the possibility of either a **perforated duodenal ulcer** (indigestion, epigastric tenderness, use of NSAIDs) or a **leaking AAA** (age, atherosclerotic disease, hypertension). The fact that she is an elderly and female patient who is presenting with acute flank pain should raise alarm bells that this may be a leaking aneurysm and hence an urgent CT abdomen was done. This shows an enlarged abdominal aorta and blood that has leaked into the peritoneal cavity. Mrs Chekov thus has a **leaking AAA** which is a surgical emergency that carries a mortality rate of 50%.

The next step is to obtain two large-bore IV access cannulae and **cross-match** 10 units of blood (= 5 L of blood or enough to replace the entire circulating volume), insert a **urinary catheter** (to monitor renal function), and to **immediately notify** the vascular surgeon and anaesthetist on call.

Viva questions

18

What different types of kidney stones are there? How might you treat them?

In decreasing order of occurrence:

- **Calcium** (75–85%), which may be calcium oxalate, calcium phosphate, or mixed. These may be treated in different ways depending on the presence of an underlying metabolic imbalance. Patients with hypercalciuria should be investigated to exclude hyperparathyroidism. They then can be treated with thiazides (which decrease renal excretion of Ca^{2+}) and a low-calcium diet. Those with hyperuricosuria can be given allopurinol (which inhibits the production of uric acid during the breakdown of nucleic acids). Those with hypocitraturia can be given potassium citrate (citrate alkalinizes the urine and inhibits the formation of crystals).

- **Struvite** (10–20%), which is ammonium magnesium phosphate. These are most common in women and are secondary to infection with a urease-producing bacteria (e.g. *Proteus*, *Pseudomonas*, *Klebsiella*) which can break down urea into ammonium. Treatment of the underlying infection is indicated.

- **Urate** (5–10%). Urate crystals form in the presence of acid urine, so potassium citrate may be given to alkalinize the urine. Allopurinol can be used to lower urate production and subsequent excretion.

- **Cystine** (1%). These stones form secondary to cystinuria, a rare autosomal recessive disorder with increased cystine excretion. Patients should be advised to increase fluid intake as a means to diluting the urinary cystine concentration. As with urate stones, the solubility of cystine is pH dependent and so potassium citrate can also be given. Cystine-binding drugs may be given if all else fails, e.g. tiopronin.

A number of medical conditions can predispose to stone formation – can you name them?

- Metabolic:
  - Hypercalciuria
  - Hyperuricosuria
  - Hypocitraturia
  - Hyperoxaluria
  - Gout and other hyperuricaemic states e.g. malignancy, glucose-6-phosphate dehydrogenase (G6PDH) deficiency (urate stones)
  - Cystinuria
- Primary hyperparathyroidism
- Crohn's disease (often oxalate stones, although the exact mechanism for this remains unclear)
- Chronic UTI due to urease-producing bacteria (struvite stones)
- Medullary sponge or polycystic kidneys (resulting in static collections in which stones form)
- Renal tubular acidosis (stones result from hypercalciuria, alkalinization of the urine causing precipitation of calcium phosphate, and low urinary citrate)
- Sarcoidosis (causes a hypercalcaemia that can lead to stone formation)

What radiographical findings would you look for in a patient with suspected kidney stones? What are the 'soft-tissue rim' and 'tail' signs?

- The stones themselves
- Hydronephrosis and/or hydroureter (dilated ureters) due to obstruction
- Perinephric fluid

In the '**soft-tissue rim**' sign stones may be surrounded by a rim of soft tissue, which can help differentiate stones in the ureter from a calcified pelvic vein (phlebolith).

The '**tail' sign** is where a soft tissue opacity extends away from the stone like a tail. This is consistent with a pelvic phlebolith (calcification of a previous thrombus in a vein) and is not a ureteric stone.

What are the complications of kidney stones? How are they managed?

- **Ureteric stricture** from the passage of the stone (or ureteroscopic removal of a stone). If necessary a stent can be inserted.
- **Acute or chronic pyelonephritis**, potentially leading to sepsis. Managed as per the first short case.
- **Renal failure**, due to obstruction and back-pressure causing hydronephrosis and kidney damage. This requires stone removal and close medical management including monitoring of renal function and ensuring good renal perfusion.
- **Intrarenal or perinephric abscess**. Abscesses may occur as a complication of pyelonephritis, particularly if there are large 'staghorn' stones present blocking the ureters. As suggested by the name, a perinephric abscess forms when the pus discharges through the renal capsule into the perinephric fat. Patients present with systemic features and pyuria. Diagnosis is by finding a renal mass with a fluid level on ultrasound or radiology. Patients require drainage of the abscess.
- **Xanthogranulomatous pyelonephritis**. This is a type of chronic bacterial pyelonephritis characterized by the destruction of renal parenchyma and the presence of granulomas and abscesses. Patients are chronically ill with systemic symptoms. Nephrectomy is the standard treatment.
- **Urine extravasation** into the pelvic cavity. Although uncommon, this has severe consequences, as the combination of urine and the subsequent infection produces severe oedema, high fever, and dehydration. The extravasated urine must be drained and the urine flow diverted so that it does not continue to extravasate. The patient will also need fluids and antibiotics.

18

NSAIDs are now the first-line analgesic treatment for renal colic pain. What are the cautions and contraindications to NSAID use?

NSAIDs are contraindicated in:

- Asthma
- History of anaphylaxis with any NSAID
- Previous or active peptic ulcers
- Severe heart failure

- COX-2 selective inhibitors (a subtype of NSAID) should not be used in ischaemic heart disease, cerebrovascular disease, or peripheral arterial disease as they are associated with an increased risk of thrombotic events

NSAIDs should be used with caution in:

- Coagulation defects: may be exacerbated due to antiplatelet effects.
- Renal, cardiac, or hepatic impairment: NSAIDs may impair renal function and cause fluid retention, leading to pulmonary oedema in patients with cardiac failure. This is more likely to occur if the patient has poor liver function (hepatic impairment) or pre-existing kidney disease (renal impairment).
- During pregnancy and breast-feeding: closure of the ductus arteriosus can occur in response to NSAIDs and this is a problem if it occurs *in utero*. There may also be delayed onset and increased duration of labour. NSAIDs are sometimes found in breast milk but there is little information on the risks presented. Nonetheless most manufacturers advise avoiding them if breast-feeding.
- The elderly: as the risk of bleeding is more common and is more likely to have a serious outcome.

Where along the renal tract are stones most likely to cause obstruction?

Stones are most likely to obstruct in the narrowest parts of the collecting system. These are:

- the PUJ
- the pelvic brim
- the vesico-ureteric junction (VUJ).

At what diameter is surgical intervention advisable for an unruptured AAA? What is the evidence for this?

Elective surgical repair of an AAA is a major operation that carries a 5% mortality rate. Left alone, AAAs with a diameter <5.5 cm have an annual risk of rupture <1%. However, AAAs with a diameter >6 cm have an annual risk of rupture of 25%(!). Thus the indications for surgery are:

- AAA diameter >5.5 cm
- AAA diameter growing >1 cm per year
- Symptomatic AAA

The evidence for this comes from the **UK Small Aneurysm Trial**[1] and the **US Aneurysm Detection and Management Study**[2]. Both showed that aneurysms <5.5 cm are best managed non-operatively, finding no mortality benefit from surgery.

[1] UKSAT Investigators (1998). Mortality results for randomised controlled trial of early elective surgery or ultrasonographic surveillance for small abdominal aortic aneurysms. The UK Small Aneurysm Trial Participants. *Lancet*, **352**: 1649–1655.

[2] Lederle FA, Wilson SE, Johnson GR, Reinke DB, Littooy FN, Acher CW et al. (2002). Immediate repair compared with surveillance of small abdominal aortic aneurysms. *New Engl J Med*, **346**: 1437–1444.

18

What is the 'psoas sign' on abdominal radiographs?

You may occasionally hear reference to the 'psoas sign'. This is where one of the two psoas shadows on an abdominal radiograph is not visible. This can represent an AAA, as in the example in Fig. 18.3. However, the 'psoas sign' is also present in patients with other abdominal pathology (e.g. acute pancreatitis) and quite a few healthy individuals, too. It is thus an *unreliable* sign for AAA. Instead, AAAs are best assessed using either abdominal ultrasound (for simple detection and screening), plain abdominal CT (to visualize the AAA in detail pre-operatively) or contrast abdominal CT (if a leaking AAA is suspected).

a)
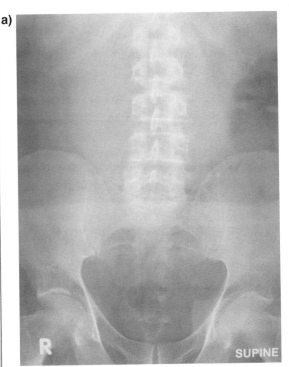

b)
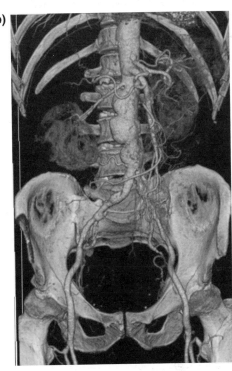

Figure 18.3 (a) Plain abdominal radiograph of a patient with an abdominal aortic aneurysm (AAA). (b) Three-dimensional reconstruction of a pre-operative abdominal computed tomography (CT) scan of a patient with an AAA.

Part (a) from Callaghan, Bradley, and Watson 2008. *Emergencies in Clinical Surgery*, p. 329, Fig 18.1. Oxford University Press.

Part (b) from Gardiner MD, Borley NR (eds) (2009). *Training in Surgery*, p. 161, Fig. 7.8. Oxford University Press.

18

A patient visits his GP complaining of ongoing lower back pain that is worse on the right side. What are the 'red flags' of back pain that warrant referral for further investigation?

Table 18.1 Back pain: the 'red flags'

Red flags	Referral time
Sphincter problems	Immediate
Patient unable to self-care or walk	
Weight loss	Within 1 week
Fever	
Back tenderness to palpation	
Thoracic spinal pain	
Violent trauma (e.g. car accident)	
Age <20 years or >50 years	As soon as possible
Severe morning stiffness	
Structural deformity (e.g. scoliosis)	
Nerve root pain not resolving >6 weeks	

What medications would you prescribe for any patient in pain?

When prescribing analgesia, you should keep in mind the WHO pain management ladder (Fig. 18.4):

Paracetamol ± NSAID + strong opioid (e.g. morphine)	Severe pain
Paracetamol ± NSAID + weak opioid (e.g. codeine)	Moderate pain
Paracetamol ± NSAID	Mild pain

Figure 18.4 The WHO pain ladder.

The WHO pain management ladder suggests you should start at the bottom of the ladder and work your way up until pain is controlled. The pain from ureteric colic is very severe, but studies[3] have shown that NSAIDs are just as effective as opioids for the vast majority of patients with ureteric colic. So there is rarely the need to go up a further step on the ladder. Secondly, because patients with opioid dependence have often presented to casualty pretending to have ureteric colic in an attempt to obtain opioids, it is best to start with paracetamol + NSAIDs and try to confirm the ureteric stone before prescribing opioids. Obviously, opioids should be added if the pain is not controlled by paracetamol + NSAIDs alone. Also, there are circumstances in which NSAIDs will be contraindicated (see Viva question above) and when an opioid will be better.

[3] Holdgate A, Pollock T (2004). Systematic review of the relative efficacy of non-steroidal anti-inflammatory drugs and opioids in the treatment of acute renal colic. *BMJ*, **328**: 1401.

For a range of Single Best Answer questions related to the topic of this chapter, and hyperlinks to a selection of key papers go to **www.oxfordtextbooks.co.uk/orc/ocms/**

Constipation

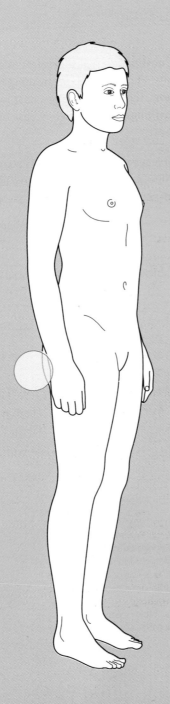

Core case

! *Read through the sections in red, covering up the sections in white that follow so that you don't see the answer. At the end of each red section, try to answer the question before reading on.*

Mrs Crabbe is a 62-year-old retired secretary who has been referred by her general practitioner (GP) to the gastroenterology department of her district general hospital, where you are one of the junior doctors. Her main complaint is constipation.

What does 'constipation' mean?

Constipation typically refers to stool that is passed infrequently and/or with difficulty. The most important thing to elucidate is what the patient means by 'constipation'. Therefore, writing 'constipation' in the notes is inadequate – you must say something about frequency, ease of passage, and volume.

Normal defecation requires that a person has adequate bowel peristalsis, relatively soft faeces, no obstruction to outflow, and the will and ability to push. With this in mind, it is possible to think of various mechanisms that might cause someone to be constipated.

What is your initial differential diagnosis for constipation in any patient?

Table 19.1 shows the differential diagnosis for constipation.

Table 19.1 Differential diagnosis for constipation

Abnormal bowel peristalsis	Hard faeces	Bowel obstruction	Patient not pushing
• Irritable bowel syndrome • Medications (e.g. opiates, iron supplements, calcium-channel blockers) • Hypothyroidism • Hypercalcaemia • Hypokalaemia • Spinal cord compression • Multiple sclerosis • Parkinson's disease • Diabetic neuropathy • Idiopathic megacolon • Idiopathic slow transit	• Lack of dietary fibre • Dehydration	• Colorectal adenocarcinoma • Sigmoid volvulus • Other pelvic masses (e.g. uterine fibroids, ovarian tumour) • Colonic strictures (e.g. radiotherapy, Crohn's disease, diverticular disease)	• Haemorrhoids • Anal fissure • Pelvic floor dysfunction (e.g. after hysterectomy)

19

Bear in mind that, in a hospital setting, some of the most common causes of constipation will not be due to any pathology *per se* but rather the embarrassment or discomfort of having to open one's bowels on a bed pan within earshot of others.

Equally, patients who are immobile for any reason (e.g. spinal pathology, elderly) are prone to constipation, although the mechanism for this is unclear.

> Constipation is a very common symptom. It usually has a benign aetiology (lack of fibre, dehydration) and is successfully managed in primary care.
>
> **What 'red flags' would cause the GP to refer a patient with constipation for further investigation?**

There are a number of features from the history that should alert you to potentially sinister causes of constipation (especially colorectal cancer) and which warrant further investigation:

- Severe, persistent constipation that is unresponsive to treatment
- Rectal bleeding, tenesmus, or intermittent mucoid diarrhoea
- Significant weight loss, iron-deficiency anaemia, and/or night sweats
- Past medical history of ulcerative colitis or colonic polyps
- Strong family history of colon cancer or colonic polyps, particularly if affected family members were <60 years old.

> The GP has referred Mrs Crabbe because of persistent constipation that has been refractory to primary care management with increased dietary fibre and lactulose. You take a fresh history from Mrs Crabbe about her constipation.
>
> **What key clues will you look for in the history?**

About the constipation

- **Characterize what the patient means by 'constipation'.** Passing hard, lumpy stools suggests lack of fibre or dehydration, but not obstruction. No longer passing any faeces nor flatus ('absolute constipation') suggests complete bowel obstruction.
- **When did this start?** Recent change in bowel habit suggests pathology, whereas chronic constipation is usually benign.

Associated symptoms

- **Weight loss, night sweats, fevers?** May suggest malignancy.
- **Diarrhoea?** Intermittent diarrhoea and constipation can suggest irritable bowel syndrome (in younger patients), colorectal cancer (in patients >45 years, especially if the diarrhoea is mucoid), or diverticular disease (in patients >60 years, especially if they have had episodes of left iliac fossa pain).
- **Tenesmus?** Suggests a persistent mass in the rectum (e.g. tumour).
- **Blood on faeces, per rectum, or when wiping?** May suggest haemorrhoids, anal fissure, diverticular disease, or colorectal cancer (see Chapter 21).

19

- **Bloating?** A feature of irritable bowel syndrome.
- **Feeling cold, reduced appetite, gaining weight?** May suggest hypothyroidism.
- **Bone pains?** Could suggest bone metastases, which would lead to hypercalcaemia that can cause constipation.
- **Polyuria, thirst?** May suggest hypercalcaemia.

You should note any **abdominal pain** but it is unhelpful in narrowing the diagnosis as constipation itself can be a source of pain.

Risk factors for constipation

- **History of bowel disease, neurological disorders, back problems, or endocrine disease?**
- **Family history of bowel disorders?** In particular, look for a family history of bowel disorders that increase the risk of colorectal cancer such as colorectal cancer *per se*, familial adenomatous polyposis (FAP), hereditary non-polyposis colorectal cancer (HNPCC), or Peutz–Jegher's disease.
- **What medications are they on?** Check the British National Formulary (BNF) to see if the patient's medications can cause constipation as a side-effect. Opiates, anticholinergics, tricyclic antidepressants, calcium-channel blockers, and iron supplements are notorious for causing constipation.
- **Diet?** Do they eat a healthy, varied, fibre-rich diet? Do they keep adequately hydrated? Ask what colour their urine is (persistently yellow urine can suggest a degree of dehydration).

19

Mrs Crabbe tells you that she has always found it relatively hard to pass faeces, having had to strain and take her time on the toilet for most of her adult life. Despite this, she has always managed to pass faeces three or four times a week. However, for the past 2 months she has found it very difficult to pass any faeces at all, saying that she has only opened her bowels perhaps once a week. When she finally opens her bowels it is painless but only small amounts of 'surprisingly soft' faeces come out. She last opened her bowels 3 days ago but is still passing wind every day. Her faeces are not mucoid and she has not noticed any blood on her faeces or when she wipes.

Mrs Crabbe has not noticed any weight loss, fevers, or night sweats. She has not been unusually thirsty nor has she had any aches or pains. Her appetite has been reduced but she has not felt cold or lethargic. Her urine passes without difficulty and she thinks it is pale yellow in colour.

Mrs Crabbe has type 2 diabetes mellitus and hypertension. She had a kidney stone a few years ago but 'it passed' and no cause was ever found. She has two daughters, both of whom were delivered vaginally and weighed about 8 lb (3.6 kg), albeit requiring an episiotomy for the first. She takes metformin for her diabetes, bendroflumethiazide for her hypertension, and low-dose aspirin and simvastatin because of her cardiovascular risk factors. She has never had any surgery.

Mrs Crabbe lost her husband 6 months ago quite suddenly and unexpectedly. She has since been living with her eldest daughter and her family. She describes her mood as having been low since her husband passed away, although the recent arrival of a granddaughter to the family has improved things. There is nil of note in her family history.

Mrs Crabbe smoked two packs of cigarettes a day from her teenage years until her father's death 20 years ago. She drinks a glass of sherry every evening and says her diet is 'very healthy' now that she is living with her daughter, who makes sure she eats plenty of 'greens'. She walks a couple of miles every day with her daughter and their dog.

Mrs Crabbe's main concern is that she will become completely constipated and need some sort of surgery.

Can you narrow your initial differential diagnosis based on the information so far?

Based on her history, sex, and age, Mrs Crabbe's differential diagnosis can be narrowed down to:

Dehydration
Colorectal cancer
Pelvic mass
Diabetic neuropathy
Hypothyroidism
Hypercalcaemia
Hypokalaemia

You move on to examination.

What clues should you look for on examination of someone with constipation?

General inspection
- **Cachexia?** Suggests malignancy.
- **Signs of hypothyroidism:** loss of hair (especially the outer third of eyebrows), brittle hair, dry skin, puffy eyes, malar flush?

Abdominal examination
- **Virchow's node** (left supraclavicular fossa)? Enlargement can suggest gastrointestinal (GI) malignancy.
- **Abdominal mass?** In the context of constipation, this could be impacted faeces, a colonic tumour, a Crohn's mass, or an ovarian mass.
- **Anal fissures or haemorrhoids?** This may explain the constipation – it can be too painful to push.
- **Mass on digital rectal examination?** This may suggest a rectal carcinoma or impacted faeces.
- **Lax or asymmetric anal tone?** This suggests neurological pathology, such as diabetic neuropathy, multiple sclerosis, or cauda equina compression.

Neurological examination
- If the history is suggestive of diabetic neuropathy, multiple sclerosis, cord compression, or Parkinsonism.

19

There is nothing unusual on inspection of Mrs Crabbe. Her abdominal examination is remarkable only for what feels like a colon loaded with faeces down the left side of her abdomen on deep palpation. No other masses or organomegaly are present. There is no ascites, clubbing, or lymphadenopathy.

You explain to Mrs Crabbe that it would be wise for you to perform a rectal examination (as you have felt a mass which you think is just faeces – but you want to make sure it isn't anything sinister). She consents but it reveals no anal fissures or fistulae and an empty rectum.

What investigations will you arrange for Mrs Crabbe, and why?

Ideally, no investigations will be necessary for the vast majority of patients with constipation, as the common diagnoses can be made clinically (diet, drugs, etc.). However, given that no obvious diagnosis can be made for Mrs Crabbe, a number of investigations may be useful:

- **Blood tests:**
  - **Full blood count:** a colonic mass can bleed and cause anaemia
  - **Electrolytes and calcium:** hypokalaemia and hypercalcaemia can cause constipation
  - **Thyroid function tests:** the history and examination do not suggest hypothyroidism as a cause of constipation, but it is easily excluded biochemically
  - **Glucose and HbA1c:** not routine examinations for constipation, but as Mrs Crabbe is a diabetic you should investigate her diabetic control at present (glucose) and over the last few months (HbA1c).

The following investigations are not routinely requested when first investigating constipation but may be requested if the history and examination warrant them:

- **Faecal occult blood test (FOBT):** although this test is increasingly being used to screen for asymptomatic colon cancer, it should be remembered that faecal blood can also be due to colonic angiodysplasia, colonic polyps, haemorrhoids, aspirin, or warfarin. The test has a low specificity and sensitivity for colon cancer, but a positive test warrants further investigation.
- **Carcinoembryonic antigen (CEA)/CA19-9/CA125:** these are all markers of colon cancer. However, they lack specificity (e.g. CA125 is more commonly elevated in ovarian malignancy) and sensitivity and therefore are *not* used in diagnosis. They are, however, used to monitor response, relapse, and recurrence in patients with confirmed GI cancer.

The blood results and FOBT results for Mrs Crabbe are shown below:

Hb	10.4g/dL
MCV	72 fL
Ferritin	3 µg/L
RBC	4.3×10^{12} cells/L
WCC	12.1×10^9 cells/L

Platelets	190×10^9 cells/L
Na	137 mM
K	3.7 mM
Cl	98 mM
Ca (corrected)	2.2 mM
ALT	25 U/L
AST	22 U/L
ALP	98 U/L
GGT	18 U/L
TSH	2.1 mU/L
Free T_4	10 pmol/L
Glc	6.2 mM
HbA1c	5.9%
FOBT	Positive

(Hb, haemoglobin; MCV, mean corpuscular volume; RBC, red blood cell [count]; WCC, white cell count; ALT, alanine aminotransferase; AST, aspartate aminotransferase; ALP, alkaline phosphatase; GGT, gamma-glutamyl transferase; TSH, thyroid-stimulating hormone)

What is your next step?

Mrs Crabbe has iron-deficiency anaemia in the context of a positive FOBT and constipation, although the positive FOBT could be due to her low-dose aspirin. Given these factors and her age, your next step should be to request **imaging** of her upper and lower GI tract such as:

- **Proctoscopy.** A transparent dilator is used to visualize the anus. Can be done in the clinic or on the wards.

- **Rigid sigmoidoscopy.** Visualizes as far as the sigmoid colon. Can also be done in the clinic or on the wards.

- **Colonoscopy.** This involves a flexible colonoscope, often with sedation (but not general anaesthetic) and bowel preparation, and can visualize as far as the ileo-caecal valve. Can be done as an outpatient.

- **Computed tomography (CT) colonography.** Also known as 'virtual colonoscopy' or 'CT pneumocolon'; this involves an abdominal CT scan after bowel preparation and insufflation (filling the colon with air). It shows the bowel lumen and surrounding structures (e.g. liver, ovaries).

- **Double-contrast barium enema (DCBE).** As the name suggests, a barium enema is given to the patient and plain radiographs are taken at various times. Thus the lumen of the bowel can be visualized.

- **Oesophagogastroduodenoscopy (OGD).** An endoscope is inserted via the mouth and used to visualize as far as the duodenum. An OGD should always be performed in the context of iron-deficiency anaemia to exclude an upper GI bleed.

19

You arrange for Mrs Crabbe to have a colonoscopy. The report is below:

Anal canal:	Internal, grade 1 haemorrhoids
Rectum:	Normal
Sigmoid colon:	Normal
Descending colon:	Large suspicious polypoid mass [see Fig. 19.1]. Biopsy taken
Spenic flexure:	Normal
Transverse colon:	Normal
Hepatic flexure:	Normal
Ascending colon:	Normal
Caecum:	Normal

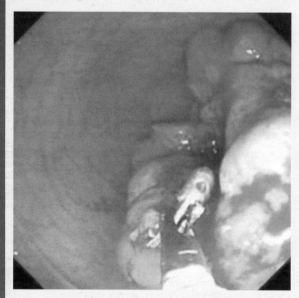

Figure 19.1 Photograph of colon mass at colonoscopy.
From Gardiner MD, Borley NR (eds) (2009). ***Training in Surgery***, p. 105, Fig. 15.3. Oxford University Press.

Pathology report:
Focalized adenocarcinoma, grade 2. The biopsy shows involvement of the mucosal lamina propria by neoplastic glands. The muscularis propria was clear of invasion in the biopsy specimen.

What will you tell Mrs Crabbe? What is the next step?

Mrs Crabbe must be told that she has **colon cancer** but this must be done with care. Telling patients they have a serious condition (particularly cancer) can be devastating, so make sure you provide:

- **The right people.** Get an experienced and senior doctor (e.g. your Consultant) to deliver the news. Involve the senior nurse, who will have more contact with the patient than doctors and can thus provide more support. Ideally, offer for family or friends to be present at the time so that they can offer support.

- **The right place.** Telling someone they have cancer on a rushed 'business' ward round and then leaving them to ponder the news is not good practice. Take patients into a quiet room.

- **The right time.** Make time to deliver bad news so that you don't have to rush off during the process (e.g. once your jobs are done, and don't be afraid to hand your bleep over to a colleague). Choose the right time for the patient, too: make sure the patient is able to understand, and await the arrival of family or friends.

- **The right message.** Make sure that Mrs Crabbe understands what she is being told as many patients complain that doctors are euphemistic when talking about serious diseases such as cancer, which only confuses them. Find out how much she knows already. Explain to Mrs Crabbe that the colonoscopy found a mass in her bowel, on the left-hand side. The laboratories have confirmed it is a colon cancer. Explain that the spread of the cancer needs assessing, various treatment options are available, and the outcomes are nowadays very good if colon cancer is caught before it spreads. You can explain that, if caught early and before it spreads, colon cancer has a good prognosis (75–90% survive more than 5 years) as the affected segment of bowel can be surgically removed. Unfortunately, you cannot say how far the cancer has spread from the pathology report, as the report reflects only a small biopsy. The next step is therefore to assess how far the cancer has spread.

Staging the cancer is important because it influences subsequent management and prognosis (see below). Staging needs to look at the main areas where the cancer might spread. In the case of colon cancer this is the liver and lungs, the ovaries in women, and the lymphatics that drain the colon. Previously, staging was done by a combination of exploratory laparatomy (very invasive), liver ultrasound, and chest radiography. Nowadays this has been substituted by combined chest and abdomen CT scans, which offer a much better view of the chest and abdominal contents in a far quicker and less invasive way. Increasingly, however, positron emission tomography (PET) which uses radiolabelled substrates taken up preferentially by cancer cells is being combined with CT scanning (PET-CT) to pick up even the smallest of metastases which were previously not seen by CT scans alone.

A chest and abdominal CT is performed on Mrs Crabbe. It confirms a mass in the descending colon that does not appear to have invaded beyond the bowel wall. No obvious masses are apparent in any adjacent structures, and the liver and lungs look normal. A small degree of prolapse is noted in her intervertebral disc at L4/L5 which is not impinging on either nerve root and is therefore likely to be an incidental finding. She is diagnosed with colorectal cancer that is provisionally staged as T2N0M0 (Dukes' A) and is referred to the colorectal surgeons. She receives a laparoscopic left hemicolectomy and is back home within a few days. Five years later, she remains free of recurrence.

19

Short cases

Mr Tanner is a 27-year-old lorry driver who has come to see his GP regarding long-standing constipation. He often fails to open his bowels for an entire week and this makes him irritable. The problem has been ongoing for many years, but he has finally come to see his GP to see if there is any medication that can help.

Mr Tanner has not had any pain or blood per rectum. His stools are often hard and his urine is always yellow in colour. He has not noticed any weight loss, change in appetite, heat intolerance, or lethargy. He occasionally uses a salbutamol inhaler for his asthma but his past medical and drug history is otherwise unremarkable. There is nil of note in his family history. He smokes a pack of cigarettes every day but drinks only the occasional pint of beer at weekends. On a typical day he eats white toast and jam with coffee for breakfast; a Mars bar half way through the morning; a sandwich (white bread) and packet of crisps for lunch; and meat with potatoes or chips for dinner. He rarely eats fruit or vegetables (other than potatoes). He drinks about six cups of coffee a day and rarely exercises.

On examination, Mr Tanner is overweight. His abdomen is soft and non-tender, with no masses or organomegaly. A digital rectal examination reveals a rectum loaded with hard faeces, normal anal tone, a normal feeling prostate, and no masses.

What are the most likely causes of Mr Tanner's constipation? How can it be managed?

The most likely cause of Mr Tanner's constipation is the most common aetiology: a combination of **lack of fibre** in the diet, **dehydration**, and a degree of **immobility**. Management can include the following options, introduced incrementally until the problem is solved:

- **Lifestyle changes:** this is likely to have the greatest long-term effect. Increase fluid intake and fibre intake. Explain the benefits of a high-fibre diet beyond improving constipation (it *may* reduce the risk of coronary heart disease and colon cancer). Exercise is also useful (e.g. jogging).

- **Bulk producers:** fibre helps constipation by providing bulk (which activates stretch receptors in the bowel and triggers peristalsis) and by retaining water (which makes faeces softer). Simple dietary changes such as eating a fibre-rich cereal and changing from white to wholemeal bread could make a lot of difference to Mr Tanner. Various fibre supplements exist for patients who cannot achieve sufficient bulk by modifying their diet alone (e.g. methylcellulose tablets, ispaghula husk).

- **Stool softeners:** liquid paraffin and arachis oil enemas can be used to soften stool. They should only be used in the short term as they can lead to unpleasant side-effects such as steatorrhoea and anal seepage.

- **Osmotic laxatives:** lactulose or magnesium salts act by retaining fluid in the bowel, thus causing a mild osmotic diarrhoea. These should only ever be used as a short-term remedy as they can cause dehydration and tolerance without addressing the underlying cause.

- **Peristalsis stimulants:** glycerol suppositories, bisacodyl, or senna can all be used to stimulate peristalsis.

- **Phosphate enemas:** these should only be used as a last resort.

Miss Pope is a 22-year-old lady complaining of a change in bowel habit. She is not sure how long it has been going on as it seems to have 'crept up on me gradually over many months'. With hindsight, she is sure that she used to open her bowels every day but now she only goes maybe once or twice a week. When she does go, she does not have to strain and there is no pain, blood, or tenesmus. She says her weight has been increasing despite the fact that she is eating less than before, although she no longer goes to the gym as she feels very tired all the time and her hands often hurt. When asked to expand on her hand symptoms, she explains she often gets a numbing, tingling feeling in her hands that she tries to shake off. She has not felt especially cold of late, although it is obvious she hasn't felt hot either to judge by the thick jumper she is wearing indoors. She does mention that her periods have been rather heavy lately, despite being on the combined oral contraceptive pill, which is the only medication she takes.

Miss Pope's past medical history and family history are unremarkable. She works in a call centre and lives with her boyfriend.

On examination, Miss Pope looks tired and has a heart rate of 60 bpm, regular. Phalen's test is performed and is positive. Examination of her cardiovascular, respiratory, and abdominal systems is unremarkable.

What is the likely diagnosis? What investigations would you order to confirm this? How is it managed?

Miss Pope describes reduced frequency of bowel motions along with lethargy, reduced appetite, weight gain, and what sounds very much like carpal tunnel syndrome. There is also a suggestion of cold intolerance. On examination, her heart rate is on the low side for an adult who is not very athletic and prolonged wrist hyperflexion reproduces the hand symptoms (positive Phalen's test for carpal tunnel syndrome). This is all highly suggestive of **hypothyroidism**. The most likely cause for hypothyroidism in a woman of this age is chronic autoimmune thyroiditis, also known as Hashimoto's hypothyroidism.

Hypothyroidism is easily confirmed by a blood test revealing a high TSH level, which is due to the lack of sufficient thyroxine to negatively feed back on its production. If this is Hashimoto's hypothyroidism, one will also find high antithyroid peroxidase antibodies.

Management is by daily oral levothyroxine and prognosis is very good (all symptoms should resolve), although patients have to remain on levothyroxine for life.

19

Mr Laporte is a 46-year-old retail manager suffering with constipation. He describes only opening his bowels twice a week for the past 2 months, although he previously opened his bowels almost daily. Defecation is not painful, but he has been getting aches and pains all over his body recently which he cannot explain. He has not noticed any blood in his faeces or on wiping. He has been passing a lot of urine lately but says this is probably because he has been drinking a lot of water. He feels very thirsty all the time, to the extent that he will wake up at least once every night and drink a pint glass of water. He has not noticed any change in his weight or appetite and does not feel unusually sensitive to heat or cold. His past medical history, drug history, and family history are unremarkable. He does not smoke or drink alcohol. He eats a healthy and varied diet that is rich in vegetables and fruit. He is an amateur triathlete who trains four times a week, although he admits he has not been keeping this up recently as he feels tired and low in mood after work. On examination, you find nothing remarkable. A quick capillary glucose measurement is done in the clinic to exclude diabetes mellitus, because of the polyuria and polydipsia, and it reads 5.1 mM.

What is the likely aetiology for Mr Laporte's symptoms based on his history? What tests will you arrange?

Mr Laporte describes constipation, but also polydipsia (excessive thirst), polyuria, aches and pains, and symptoms of depression (lethargy, low mood). This is all quite suggestive of **hypercalcaemia**, which produces a constellation of symptoms often described as 'moans, groans, bones, and stones' referring to the depression, aches and pains, and renal stones often found in this condition. Polidipsia and polyuria are also common, with the classic (but rarely seen) hypercalcaemia patient waking up at night to down a glass or two of water.

Hypercalcaemia is confirmed by checking serum calcium. The underlying cause can be ascertained by checking the blood results (Table 19.2).

Table 19.2 Underlying causes of hypercalcaemia

	Alkaline phosphatase (ALP)	Parathyroid hormone (PTH)	Phosphate
Bone metastases	High	Low	High
Myeloma	Normal	Low	High
Hyperparathyroidism (primary/tertiary)	Normal/High	Normal/High	Low
Vitamin D overdose	Low	Low	High

- Bone metastases cause increased turnover of bones, hence the high ALP. This releases both calcium and phosphate from the bones.
- Myeloma causes a similar picture to bone metastases. However, in myeloma, osteoclasts are activated and osteoblasts are inhibited. As ALP comes from osteoblasts, it remains normal.
- In primary and tertiary hyperparathyroidism, PTH causes increased bone turnover; hence you also get high ALP (although this can be normal if the bone turnover is slow). Bone turnover releases both calcium and phosphate,

but as PTH increases renal excretion of phosphate, this is low. Note that PTH levels are often in the 'normal range' but that this is actually abnormal as they should be low in the presence of high calcium (remember that PTH release is normally inhibited by high calcium levels).

- Vitamin D causes increased gut absorption of both calcium and phosphate. As there is no increased bone turnover, ALP is low, and because calcium levels are high, PTH is suppressed and also low.

Mr Laporte was found to have a serum calcium of 3.2 mM, phosphate of 0.6 mM, ALP 309 U/L, and PTH of 7.5 pM suggesting primary hyperparathyroidism. This is usually caused by a solitary, benign parathyroid adenoma, although parathyroid hyperplasia, parathyroid carcinoma, or PTH-secreting ectopic tumours also occur. Mr Laporte was referred to an experienced surgeon who ordered a ^{99}Tc-sestamibi scan to localize all parathyroid tissue and undertook a minimally invasive parathyroidectomy to remove the offending gland. The pathologist later confirmed that the removed tissue was indeed consistent with a benign parathyroid adenoma.

19

Mrs Doherty is a 78-year-old inpatient receiving palliative care for advanced, metastatic breast cancer affecting her bones and liver. She has recently become constipated, having opened her bowels only once in the past 5 days. Despite having deep bone pains over her back and arms, she denies any abdominal pain or any new symptoms since her admission several weeks ago. The nurses say that when she did open her bowels, the faeces looked normal. Mrs Doherty also has hypertension, for which she takes amlodipine. For her breast cancer she takes pamidronate (to reduce bone turnover caused by the metastatic deposits), paracetamol and morphine sulphate (for the bone pain), and metoclopramide (for the nausea caused by morphine). Her appetite has been low for some months, although she still manages at least one decent meal a day. Her fluid intake and urine output have both been adequate since her admission. Examination of Mrs Doherty reveals nothing other than some long-standing tenderness over a few ribs, caused by the metastatic bone disease. Her peripheral nervous system is normal and her abdomen is soft and non-tender with no masses or organomegaly. A digital rectal examination reveals normal anal tone and a rectum full of soft faeces.

There are many reasons for Mrs Doherty to be constipated – what are they?

Mrs Doherty's case is not unusual and constipation is commonly seen in such patients. Her constipation is most likely multifactorial, with the following contributing factors:

- **Medications,** particularly opiates which reduce gut motility, but her calcium-channel blocker may be contributing.
- **Hypercalcaemia** from bone metastases.
- **Immobility.** Mrs Doherty is elderly and unwell, and therefore likely to be fairly immobile.
- **Weakness.** Again as she is elderly and unwell, she is likely to find it that much more difficult to strain.
- **Poor diet and dehydration.** Patients with cancer often lose their appetite and it is likely that her fibre intake is inadequate. Her fluid intake might also be low.
- **Megarectum.** Patients with chronic constipation can develop a dilated rectum that is susceptible to constipation.

Given Mrs Doherty's malignancy, one might also consider the possibility of the constipation being due to either spinal cord or cauda equina compression, although this is less likely to be the case given the normal peripheral neurological examination.

A reasonable first step would be to trial her on stimulant laxatives (to counteract the effect of the opiates) such as bisacodyl or senna, in addition to an osmatic laxative such as lactulose. If standard laxatives do not work, one might consider trying the newer agent methylnaltrexone, which has been developed specifically for opioid-induced constipation.

19

Mr Nikolaidis is a 68-year-old gentleman who is referred to his local hospital by his GP because of his constipation. On arrival, he relates to the junior doctor that he often finds it hard to open his bowels, but that things are different this time: he has been unable to open his bowels for 2 days and he has developed severe, 'crampy' pains all over his lower abdomen which are worse after any food or cups of tea. He denies feeling sick, but admits he has probably not passed any wind for the last 48 hours either. His past medical history is remarkable for bilateral hip replacements and a right inguinal hernia, which was repaired 2 years ago. He is otherwise fit and well and does not take any regular medications.

On examination, Mr Nikolaidis has dry lips, a heart rate of 110 bpm (regular), a blood pressure of 115/78 mmHg, respiratory rate of 15/min, and temperature of 36.8°C. His abdomen is distended, tympanic to percussion, and bowel sounds are present, albeit high pitched. No masses or organomegaly are palpable. A digital rectal examination reveals an empty rectum. His cardiovascular and respiratory examinations are unremarkable and his neurological system appears grossly intact.

The junior doctor arranges for an abdominal radiograph of Mr Nikolaidis, which is shown in Fig. 19.2.

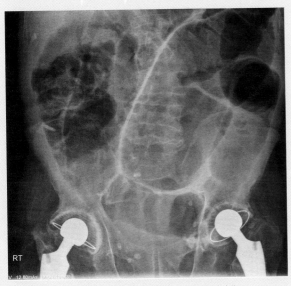

Figure 19.2 Abdominal radiograph for Mr Nikolaidis.

What is the most likely diagnosis? How will Mr Nikolaidis be managed?

19

Mr Nikolaidis has presented with most of the clinical features of bowel obstruction:

- Absolute constipation (no faeces or flatus passed)
- Colicky abdominal pain
- Distended abdomen
- Nausea and vomiting (this is mainly seen in *small* bowel obstruction)

The best way to confirm bowel obstruction is a plain abdominal radiograph. Small bowel loops with a diameter >3 cm, or large bowel loops with a diameter >6 cm, indicate bowel obstruction. Large bowel loops with a diameter >9 cm indicate risk of imminent perforation and the need for urgent surgery. Mr Nikolaidis' abdominal radiograph shows dilated loops of large bowel, confirming **large bowel obstruction**. This is usually due to mechanical obstruction by a colorectal tumour, sigmoid volvulus (twisting of the sigmoid colon), or inflamed diverticula (diverticulitis), but can be due to functional causes (e.g. hypothyroidism). Mr Nikolaidis' radiograph shows the 'coffee bean' sign (an enormous, dilated loop of bowel, shaped like a coffee bean and extending from the pelvis up to the diaphragm), caused by the sigmoid portion of the bowel twisting on itself. Thus, Mr Nikolaidis has **sigmoid volvulus**.

Management of sigmoid volvulus involves:

- **'Drip and suck'.** The patient is placed nil by mouth, a nasogastric tube is inserted, and intravenous (IV) fluids are given, all in an effort to rest the bowel and replace the fluids and electrolytes that are building up in the obstructed bowel.

- **Remove the obstruction.** In sigmoid volvulus, this is done using a sigmoido-scope with a long, soft flatus tube to untwist the bowel, or surgery if this is unsuccessful or the patient is peritonitic. In colorectal cancer, a metallic stent can be used to relieve the obstruction until the tumour is removed surgically. In diverticulitis, reduction of the inflammation with bowel rest and antibio-tics may be enough to reduce the obstruction, although surgical resection is occasionally necessary.

19

Viva questions

What are the main advantages and disadvantages of the following methods for visualizing colon masses?

(1) Rigid sigmoidoscopy

(2) Flexible sigmoidoscopy

(3) Colonoscopy

(4) CT colon

(5) CT colonography ('virtual colonoscopy' or 'CT pneumocolon')

(6) DCBE

1) Rigid sigmoidoscopy
   - **Advantages**: quick, can be performed on the wards with minimal expertise and allows both visualization of the rectum and biopsy taking.
   - **Disadvantages**: will only visualize the rectum, thus missing many masses.

2) Flexible sigmoidoscopy
   - **Advantages**: allows visualization as far as the splenic flexure, which is not bad given that 75% of sporadic, non-familial colorectal cancers will be in the left colon.
   - **Disadvantages**: will obviously miss 25% of sporadic colorectal cancers and a greater proportion of familial ones.

3) Colonoscopy
   - **Advantages**: allows visualization and biopsy of the entire colon.
   - **Disadvantages**: uncomfortable as it requires the bowel to be filled with gas (gas insufflation) and has a risk of 1/500 for GI bleeding, 1/1000 for bowel perforation, and 1/10,000 for death. Requires 2 days of special diet ('bowel preparation') to empty the bowel of its contents. Limited visibility if bowel preparation is inadequate.

4) CT colon
   - **Advantages**: rapid and non-invasive visualization of the entire colon. Does not involve any bowel preparation and is thus suitable for frail patients.
   - **Disadvantages**: does not allow for biopsies and has a poorer sensitivity at detecting lesions than CT colonography because of the lack of bowel preparation (it can be hard to distinguish a malignant lesion from faeces).

5) CT colonography (aka virtual colonoscopy/CT pneumocolon)
   - **Advantages**: quick. Because it visualizes all the organs of the abdomen (rather than just the bowel lumen), it allows one to assess the degree of invasion of any bowel masses and look for masses in other organs, therefore allowing one not only to identify a cancer (e.g. colon, ovarian) but also assess how far it has spread (staging) all in one go.
   - **Disadvantages**: does not allow for biopsies. Also requires uncomfortable bowel preparation and gas insufflation. The radiation probably *contributes* to fatal cancer in about 1/2000 patient scans (0.05%). This may sound like a lot, but fatal cancer is so common (20%) that this would only increase the risk from 20% to 20.05%.

6) DCBE
   - **Advantages**: readily available in many hospitals.
   - **Disadvantages**: does not allow for biopsies. Less specificity and sensitivity for picking up colon cancer unless the lesion is large.

Why is constipation very common after surgery?

The combination of anaesthesia, opiate analgesia, and (in abdominal surgery) bowel manipulation often sends the bowel into a state of paralysis called *ileus*. Electrolyte disturbances (e.g. hypokalaemia, hypomagnesae-mia) can further exacerbate this situation. On top of this, patients may find it difficult to pass faeces because of pain or the embarrassment of having to use a 'commode' on the public wards.

Post-operative ileus is usually self-limiting, with normal peristalsis returning 24–72 hours after surgery. However, whilst the bowel is in a state of paralysis, it continues to secrete fluid into its lumen but fails to reabsorb it. The consequence is that fluid remains trapped in a 'third space' and for this reason, patients often require IV fluids post-operatively to ensure a urine output of at least 0.5 mL/kg/hour (but not so much fluid that one causes oedema or shortness of breath). After 24–72 hours, the bowel usually starts working again, the 'third space' fluid is reabsorbed, and there is often a sudden diuresis by the patient.

The risk of post-operative ileus can be minimized by: using local/epidural anaesthesia where possible; minimizing opiate analgesia (e.g. by using more local anaesthetics); minimizing bowel manipulation; and encouraging early mobilization of patients.

What staging classifications do you know for colon cancer?

Cancers are often staged using the international TNM **classification** which, at its most basic, stands for:

Tumour size: scored from 1–4 depending on either size or local invasion.

Nodes: scored from 0 (none) to 3 (many and distant) depending on the lymph nodes affected by the cancer.

Metastasis: scored either 0 (none) or 1 (present) depending on spread of cancer in other organs.

Some cancers also have specific staging systems. For colon cancer, the older **Dukes' classification** is still often used:

Dukes' A	No spread into muscularis propria
Dukes' B	Tumour invading beyond muscularis propria
Dukes' C	Tumour spread to lymph nodes
Dukes' D	Tumour metastasized to other organs (although curiously, there was no stage D in the original Dukes' classification).

How is Dukes' staging system used for guiding management and prognosis?

Dukes' A

- 90% survival at 5 years.

- Such patients are offered **surgical removal** of the tumour-affected portion of bowel, together with its enveloping blood vessels, adipose tissue, and lymph nodes. This was traditionally done via a laparotomy but is increasingly done laparascopically as studies have shown this is just as effective but has fewer complications in expert hands. Indeed, patients having a laparoscopic colectomy are often walking and eating with 24 hours of surgery. Some studies suggest that the use of pre-operative **radiotherapy** may further improve survival rates if the cancer is *rectal* but note that radiotherapy is not done if the tumour is proximal to the rectum as there is then a risk of damaging the highly radiosensitive small bowel.

Dukes' B and C

- Approximately 65% and 30–45% survival at 5 years, respectively.
- Such patients will get **surgical removal** of the tumour plus multidrug adjuvant **chemotherapy**. Some patients with *rectal* tumours may also get pre-operative **radiotherapy**. Multiple chemotherapy agents are needed because colon cancers are intrinsically very resistant to chemotherapy. This is a reflection of their adaptation to constant exposure to toxins in the diet (e.g. they naturally express multidrug efflux pumps such as P-glycoprotein).

Dukes' D

- Approximately 5–10% survival at 5 years.
- Treatment in such patients is largely **palliative**. Patients may have surgical resection of the tumour and larger metastases (e.g. liver), chemotherapy (standard or experimental), stenting of the tumour if the patient is unfit for resection surgery, and/or palliative radiotherapy.

Patients often ask what can be done to reduce the risk of colon cancer when one of their family members has been diagnosed with this condition. Do you know of any key studies that have investigated modifiable risk factors for colorectal cancer?

- **Smoking**: the **Physicians Health Study**[1] and the **Women's Health Initiative**[2] study both found that smoking was an important, independent risk factor for colorectal cancer.
- **Exercise and obesity**: the observational, prospective **Nurses Health Study**[3] found that people who exercise regularly (>4 hours a week) and are not obese were about 40% less likely to develop colorectal cancer than people who are sedentary (<1 hour of exercise a week) and obese. The link appears to be independent of healthy lifestyle factors often associated with people who regularly exercise and are not obese (e.g. they are less likely to smoke).
- **Fibre**: there is a transatlantic split on this topic. The **European Prospective Investigation into Cancer (EPIC) trial**[4] was an observational, prospective trial looking at the effect of lifestyle factors on cancer in 500,000 Europeans over 10 years. The trial concluded that a high-fibre diet (>35 g/day) could reduce the risk of colon cancer by up to 40% compared with a low-fibre diet (<15 g/day). However, critics claim that the authors did not account for a significant confounder: exercise patterns in patients. Patients who eat lots of fibre may well be those who exercise regularly, and exercise has been shown to reduce the risk of colon cancer. The **Nurses Health Study** and **Health Professional Follow-Up Study**,[5] which prospectively looked at the role of diet and colorectal cancer in 135,000 people over a 16-year period *did* take into account exercise patterns and found no significant *independent* link between dietary fibre and the risk of colorectal cancer. But before you stop recommending a fibre-rich diet to your patients, note that the Nurses Health Study (and others) *did* find a significant protective effect of a fibre-rich diet on the incidence of cardiovascular disease.
- **Other dietary factors**: many studies have looked at the relationship between other details of dietary intake (e.g. red meat, saturated fats, fresh vegetables) and colorectal cancer. The short answer is that the data from these studies are contradictory. This probably reflects the fact that people's diets are complex and that the contribution of any one type of food to colorectal cancer may be too small to detect using an observational study. In lung cancer, the contribution of smoking is sufficiently large to avoid being confounded in observational studies. However, in colorectal cancer, the contribution of

19

red meat or saturated fats may be small and therefore easily masked by other confounding factors (e.g. people who eat less red meat may eat more soya products, and both may increase the risk of colorectal cancer by a similarly small amount).

- **Aspirin.** The **BDAT** and **UKTIA** studies were randomized controlled trials investigating the role of *high-dose* daily aspirin in the prophylaxis of cerebrovascular thrombosis (TIAs and strokes). A meta-analysis of their data by Flossmann and Rothwell[6] incidentally found that patients on high-dose aspirin were about 50% less likely to develop colorectal cancer. However, the massive **Women's Health Study**[7] and **Physicians Health Study**[8] failed to find any association between *low-dose* aspirin and colorectal cancer.

[1] Sturmer, T, Glynn RJ, Lee IM, Christen WG, Hennekens CH (2000). Lifetime cigarette smoking and colorectal cancer incidence in the Physicians' Health Study I. *J Natl Cancer Inst*, **92**: 1178–1181.

[2] Paskett ED, Reeves KW, Rohan TE, Allison MA, Williams CD, Messina CR *et al.* (2007). Association between cigarette smoking and colorectal cancer in the Women's Health Initiative. *J Natl Cancer Inst*, **99**: 1729–1735.

[3] Wolin KY, Lee IM, Colditz GA, Glynn RJ, Fuchs C, Giovannucci E (2007). Leisure-time physical activity patterns and risk of colon cancer in women. *Int J Cancer*, **121**: 2776–2781.

[4] Bingham SA, Day NE, Luben R, Ferrari P, Slimani N, Norat T *et al.* (2003). Dietary fibre in food and protection against colorectal cancer in the European Prospective Investigation into Cancer and Nutrition (EPIC): an observational study. *Lancet*, **361**: 1496–1501.

[5] Michels KB, Fuchs CS, Giovannucci E, Colditz GA, Hunter DJ, Stampfer MJ, Willett WC (2005). Fiber intake and incidence of colorectal cancer among 76,947 women and 47,279 men. *Cancer Epidemiol Biomarkers Prev*, **14**: 842–849.

[6] Flossmann E, Rothwell PM (2007). Effect of aspirin on long-term risk of colorectal cancer: consistent evidence from randomised and observational studies. *Lancet*, **369**: 1603–1613.

[7] Cook NR, Lee IM, Gaziano JM, Gordon D, Ridker PM, Manson JE et al. (2005). Low-dose aspirin in the primary prevention of cancer: the Women's Health Study: a randomized controlled trial. *J Am Med Assoc*, **294**: 47–55.

[8] Gann PH, Manson JE, Glynn RJ, Buring JE, Hennekens CH (1993). Low-dose aspirin and incidence of colorectal tumors in a randomized trial. *J Natl Cancer Inst*, **85**: 1220–1224.

For a range of Single Best Answer questions related to the topic of this chapter go to http://www.oxfordtextbooks.co.uk/orc/ocms/

19

Diarrhoea

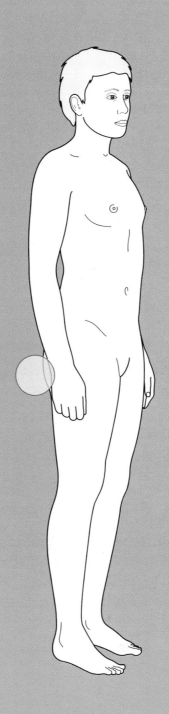

Core case

! *Read through the sections in red, covering up the sections in white that follow so that you don't see the answer. At the end of each red section, try to answer the question before reading on.*

Miss Bowles is an 18-year-old university student referred by her general practitioner (GP) to the local hospital because of diarrhoea which has been going on for 3 days. The word 'diarrhoea' means different things to different patients.

What is the clinical definition of diarrhoea? What are the main causes of diarrhoea?

Strictly speaking, diarrhoea is an increase in the amount of stool passed daily to over 300 g of stool per day. This is usually accompanied by increased frequency and loosening of the stools. However, many patients will talk of 'diarrhoea' when they actually have *haematochezia* (bright red stools from frank blood), *melaena* (dark, tarry stools from digested blood), *steatorrhoea* (pale, floating stools from undigested lipid), or simply *loose stools* (soft faeces but no increase in frequency or quantity).

Diarrhoea can be caused by:

- Infection of the bowel (infectious diarrhoea)
- Inflammation of the bowel (e.g. inflammatory bowel disease (IBD), diverticular disease)
- Increased bowel motility (e.g. hyperthyroidism, anxiety, irritable bowel syndrome (IBS))
- Malabsorption of lipids (e.g. coeliac disease, pancreatic insufficiency)
- Obstruction overflow (e.g. colon cancer, ovarian cancer)
- Medications (e.g. laxatives, digoxin, metformin, thiazides, some antibiotics, etc.)

The GP referral letter explains that for the last 3 days, Miss Bowles has been going to the toilet 5 times a day and passing soft, watery faeces that do not contain blood and are of normal colour.

What is your differential diagnosis for diarrhoea in a patient of this age? Try organizing your differential in order of likelihood.

For a young adult with acute diarrhoea, the most likely diagnoses are:

> Infective diarrhoea
> Irritable bowel syndrome (IBS)
> Coeliac disease
> Crohn's disease
> Ulcerative colitis (UC)
> Medications (e.g. antibiotics, laxatives)
> Hyperthyroidism

20

> Would your differential diagnosis look different if the patient was 64 years old?

Yes, it would. In elderly patients, neoplastic disease (villous polyps, colonic adenocarcinoma, pancreatic cancer), diverticular disease, ischaemic colitis, microscopic colitis, and bacterial overgrowth (e.g. in patients with diabetes mellitus) are much more likely, whereas immune-related diseases such as coeliac disease and UC are less likely to present for the first time (as they tend to present in younger patients). Curiously, Crohn's disease has a second incidence peak at ages 50–80.

> The fact that the GP has referred a patient with diarrhoea to the hospital suggests that they feel the patient is ill enough to warrant in-hospital management and investigations.
>
> Given the 3-day history of diarrhoea, how will you manage this patient before taking a history? Is there anything in particular you are concerned about?

- **Airway, Breathing, and Circulation (ABC):** always, always, always start the management of a patient with ABC. Whilst the ABCs will be obviously normal in a large number of patients presenting in a non-emergency setting, you should always keep it in mind when admitting patients to hospital. Note that hypotension is a late and worrying sign in young patients.

- **Dehydration:** in a patient with a 3-day history of diarrhoea, one should be concerned about the possibility of dehydration (hypovolaemia). Dehydration is the main cause of morbidity and mortality in this patient group, so check the heart rate (tachycardia?), the blood pressure (narrow mean arterial pressure or low blood pressure?), mucous membranes (dry lips?), and whether the patient feels thirsty.

- **Electrolyte or pH disturbance:** these can occur either due to excessive loss of ions (e.g. K^+, HCO_3^-) in the faeces, or secondary to the hypovolaemia and ischaemia of tissues (e.g. hyperkalaemia in response to a metabolic acidosis caused by ischaemia). If the patient appears to be *in extremis*, the quickest way to obtain information on both electrolytes and pH is an arterial or venous blood gas.

20

> Miss Bowles looks very unwell: she has dry, pale lips and looks tired. Her airways are clear (she can talk) and her breathing is deep and sighing (Kussmaul) at 12/min. Her heart rate is 110 bpm (regular), her blood pressure is 95/70 mmHg, and her temperature is 36.8°C. Arterial blood gas shows a pH = 7.32, arterial partial pressure of oxygen (P_aO_2) = 13 kPa, arterial partial pressure of carbon dioxide (P_aCO_2) = 4.2 kPa, HCO_3^- = 17 mM, Na^+ = 134 mM, K^+ = 3.1 mM, Cl^- = 101 mM, glucose = 6.1 mM.
>
> How would you interpret these clinical and biochemical findings?

Miss Bowles has:

- **Shock (tachycardic and hypovolaemic).** Whilst it is possible that the tachycardia is due to anxiety or a systemic inflammatory response, and it is possible that she has naturally low blood pressure, it is safe to assume that this patient is dehydrated given the 3-day history of diarrhoea.

- **Acidosis (pH <7.35).** Her CO_2 is low (P_aCO_2 <4.5 kPa) suggesting she is trying to compensate for the acidosis by blowing off CO_2, thus shifting the following equation to the left in an attempt to reduce the amount of H^+:

$$CO_2 + H_2O \leftrightarrow H^+ + HCO_3^-$$

  This is therefore a **metabolic** acidosis (if it was respiratory, the CO_2 would be high and driving the acidosis). In broad terms, metabolic acidosis can be due to either gain of acid (H^+), loss of base (HCO_3^-) or both. Her anion gap ($Na^+ + K^+ - Cl^- - HCO_3^-$) is elevated (>18 mM) suggesting the presence of extra acids (e.g. lactic acid? aspirin? ketone bodies?). It is likely that this patient's tissues are ischaemic due to the hypovolaemia and therefore relying on anaerobic glycolysis for energy, producing lactic acidosis.

- **Hypokalaemia.** This patient probably has hypokalaemia due to K^+ loss in the faeces. It is common for patients with diarrhoea to lose multiple electrolytes in their faeces and thus have low K^+, low Na^+, low Cl^-, and low HCO_3^-. All that is needed to correct these imbalances if the patient's kidneys are functioning adequately is fluid rehydration.

How will you manage this patient acutely?

This patient is essentially **dehydrated** due to her ongoing diarrhoea. She therefore needs a cannula placed, bloods taken (so you don't have to bleed her again later), and fluids given. One way to administer fluids is orally, but the fact that she is hypovolaemic after 3 days suggests she is not managing to hydrate orally. The alternative is therefore intravenous (IV) fluids. At this stage, one could give a 'fluid challenge' of 250 mL normal saline and then reassess the patient's blood pressure after 30 minutes. If her blood pressure remains low, she needs more fluids. If her blood pressure has improved you can switch to providing maintenance fluids IV or orally.

The metabolic acidosis and electrolyte disturbances will all self-correct with adequate restoration of fluid balance, assuming her kidney function is normal.

20

Miss Bowles responded well to a 250 mL fluid challenge, with her blood pressure rising to 105/75 mmHg.

What would you like to know about Miss Bowles' history? It is tempting to ask a broad and comprehensive set of questions but instead, think of your differential diagnosis and ask questions that will provide important clues pointing you towards or away from each diagnosis.

Characterize the stool

- **Are the faeces bloody?** If so, can the patient describe their faeces?
  - If the blood is only on the paper when they wipe, or the faeces are streaked with blood, it suggests anal pathology (e.g. anal fissure, haemorrrhoids, vigorous wiping secondary to the diarrhoea).
  - If the blood is red and mixed in with the faeces it suggests colorectal pathology (e.g. UC, dysentery, colorectal carcinoma).

- **Are the faeces mucoid or jelly-like?** This classically suggests infection by *Salmonella* or villous polyps in the colon, but can be seen in any disease causing inflammation of the bowel wall.
- **Are they foul smelling and floating?** This suggests malabsorption, due to coeliac disease, pancreatic duct obstruction (pancreatic cancer, cystic fibrosis), or biliary insufficiency (e.g. recent cholecystectomy).
- **Are the faeces unusually pale?** This suggests lack of bile salts in the faeces due to obstruction of the biliary or pancreatic ducts (e.g. chronic pancreatitis, gallstones).

Ask about her bowel habit

- **Is there nocturnal diarrhoea?** If so, this suggests an 'organic' aetiology (rather than a 'functional' aetiology as in IBS).
- **Does she ever find herself having to rush to the toilet to pass motions?** Urgency to defecate is suggestive of infectious diarrhoea or IBD.
- **After passing motions, does she ever feel that she hasn't fully evacuated her bowel?** This sensation is called tenesmus and is suggestive of a space-occupying lesion in the rectum (e.g. carcinoma).
- **Has she had a variable bowel habit?** Both IBS (in younger patients) and colorectal cancer (in older patients) can present as alternating habit that varies from diarrhoea to normal stools to constipation.
- **How often does she suffer from diarrhoea?** Infectious diarrhoea is typically a one-off event (although we will nearly all have had this at some point), whereas other pathologies are usually recurrent. However, remember that chronic diseases still have to present for the first time!

Ask about associated symptoms

- **Has there been any vomiting?** This suggests an infectious gastroenteritis.
- **Has there been any abdominal pain?**
  - Pain in the right iliac fossa associated with diarrhoea is suggestive of terminal ileum inflammation (e.g. Crohn's disease, *Yersinia enterocolitica* infection).
  - Pain in the left iliac fossa associated with diarrhoea is suggestive of diverticular disease.
  - Pain relieved by passing motions is suggestive of IBS.
- **Has she noticed any (significant) weight loss?** Try to quantify this in terms of amount over which time period. Significant weight loss over months suggests a chronic pathological process, e.g. IBD, rather than an acute pathology, e.g. infection.
- **Has she had any eye problems, joint pains, or skin rashes?** Uveitis (painful red eye with loss of vision), scleritis (painful red eye with no loss of vision), episcleritis (uncomfortable red eye with no loss of vision), enteric arthritis, erythema nodosum (painful, dark red nodules on shins), and pyoderma gangrenosum (ulcers with a surrounding purple halo) are all associated with IBD (UC and Crohn's disease).

20

Ask about risk factors for causes of diarrhoea

- **Has she been abroad recently? Has she eaten anything unusual? Does she know other people with similar symptoms?** Foreign travel and eating certain types of meals (e.g. barbeques, kebabs...) are significant risk factors for infectious diarrhoea. Knowing other people with similar symptoms at the same time is also suggestive of an infectious aetiology.

- **Has she been stressed as of late? What is her diet like?** Stress and a low-fibre diet are associated with IBS.

- **What medications does she take? Have these changed recently?** Remember that diarrhoea is one of the commonest side-effects of all oral medications. Look out in particular for antibiotics and proton-pump inhibitors (PPIs), which are associated with *Clostridium difficile* diarrhoea.

Ask about her family history

- **Family history of bowel disease?** Is there a family history of Crohn's disease, UC, coeliac disease, or rarer conditions such as hereditary non-polyposis colorectal cancer (HNPCC)?

The questions above can help to narrow your differential diagnosis. However, it is also helpful for management to find out whether the patient is still eating and drinking and what medications they have tried for their diarrhoea (e.g. loperamide? oral rehydration salts?).

20

Miss Bowles is in her first year of university, where she is studying French and Spanish. She says the course is going well. It is the first time she has been away from home but she is not finding it hard. Her main concern is that she will have some illness that will stop her from playing lacrosse with the university team, of which she is vice-captain.

Four days ago she developed pain in her abdomen. The pain was dull and started in the right lower quadrant of her abdomen, before becoming more generalized and giving her cramps that were bad enough to make her curl up in bed. The diarrhoea also came on 3 days ago and has persisted since. She has been passing watery faeces about five times a day. She has had five similar episodes of abdominal pain and diarrhoea over the past year, although they have always been milder and resolved within 2 days. She has been well between episodes, but this episode has left her feeling 'very ill and run down'. She has not vomited, has not noticed any weight loss (although she is fairly slim), and her diarrhoea has always been watery, but never bloody, mucoid, or particularly foul smelling. Passing faeces or wind does not relieve her abdominal pain, which she recalls often starts in her lower right quadrant. She cannot recall eating anything unusual before her symptoms started, and she is a vegetarian who usually cooks for herself. Nobody else in her house or group of friends has been affected at any stage. She has not felt hot or hungry (if anything, she feels 'cold and sleepy'). She has not had any eye problems other than being short-sighted and has not had any joint pains. She has noticed 'a few red marks on my shins when I shave my legs' but thought these were either knocks from lacrosse training or a rash from the shaving cream. She is single and has not been sexually active in the past year.

Miss Bowles has never been to hospital before, and until today, had only ever gone to her GP for 'the usual checks and vaccines'. She takes echinacea drops diluted in hot water when she has a cold but otherwise uses no regular medications. She is not allergic to anything as far as she knows. Her parents and two older brothers are all alive and well, although she thinks her father (aged 52) may have angina. One of her grandmothers is alive but has 'arthritis'; her other grandparents all died of 'old age'.

This history is not suggestive of any one diagnosis in particular, but it does make some pathologies more likely and some less likely.

Try rearranging your original differential diagnosis in order of likelihood given Miss Bowles' history.

Irritable bowel syndrome (IBS) (there is no suggestion of anxiety or depression in the history but this is nonetheless the most common cause of recurrent diarrhoea in young females)

Coeliac disease

Crohn's disease (a strong possibility given the right iliac fossa pain and the suggestion of shin marks which may be erythema nodosum)

Ulcerative colitis (UC) (less likely in the absence of bloody diarrhoea)

Infective diarrhoea (less likely given the relapsing/remitting symptoms over past year)

Hyperthyroidism (less likely as her symptoms are relapsing/remitting)

Medications (very unlikely as she takes no medications)

Is there anything in particular you will look for during your examination of Miss Bowles?

Figure 20.1 shows the features to look for on examination of a patient with diarrhoea.

- **Clubbing?** Crohn's disease, UC, hyperthyroidism, and coeliac disease are causes of nail clubbing although in practice this association is rarely seen as few patients in the Western world with these diseases get unwell enough for long enough to develop clubbing.

- **Iritis** (aka anterior uveitis)**? Episcleritis? Scleritis?** Look for signs of these eye diseases, which are associated with both Crohn's disease and UC.

- **Mouth ulcers?** Crohn's disease produces ulcers anywhere in the gastrointestinal (GI) tract – from mouth to anus.

- **Erythema nodosum?** Both Crohn's disease and UC are systemic inflammatory diseases that can manifest in the skin in the form of erythema nodosum (tender, raised, red nodules) or, less commonly, pyoderma gangrenosum (necrotic ulcers). However, bear in mind that the combined oral contraceptive pill is also a common cause of erythema nodosum in young women.

- **Dermatitis herpetiformis?** Coeliac disease is often associated with an itchy rash known as dermatitis herpetiformis. The rash is typically found over the extensor surfaces of the limbs and over the scalp. The rash is very itchy, so its papules are usually raw or crusted from the patient scratching them.

20

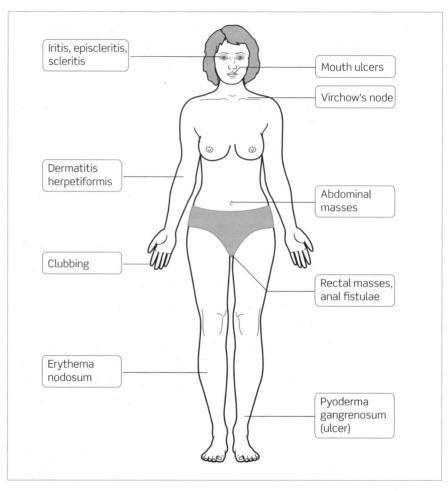

Figure 20.1 Features to look for on examination of a patient with diarrhoea.

- **Virchow's lymphadenopathy?** The stomach, and small and large bowel all have lymphatic drainage that travels via the central thoracic duct and joins the venous system in the left subclavian vein. Lymphadenopathy in the left supra-clavicular fossa (Troisier's sign) is strongly suggestive of bowel malignancy that has spread.

- **Abdominal masses?** A mass in the right lower quadrant is often found in Crohn's disease (due to inflammation of the terminal ileum). Masses else-where in the abdomen, in particular the left lower quadrant, could indicate a malignancy.

- **Anal ulcers or fistulae?** Crohn's disease can cause both ulcers and fistulae around the anus, and the patient may well be unaware of these so be sure to inspect for them.

- **Digital rectal examination.** This is part of any abdominal examination and should be performed in the presence of a chaperone. You are looking for caus-es of obstruction that could lead to overflow diarrhoea: a malignant rectal car-cinoma, or an enlarged prostate (in a man). You are also looking at the faeces themselves: are they mucoid or bloody?

On examination, Miss Bowles has no clubbing, no red eyes, and no mouth ulcers. Her shins do have a few red marks that are slightly raised and tender to touch, suggesting they may be erythema nodosum. Her abdomen is tender to palpation throughout but no masses are palpable. A digital rectal examination reveals an empty rectum with no palpable masses, and there are no anal ulcers or fistulae.

Given this examination, what first-line investigations will you arrange? Think of investigations that can help rule in or exclude items on your differential diagnosis list.

Blood tests

- **Full blood count (FBC):** coeliac disease, Crohn's disease, and UC can all cause anaemia from malabsorption of iron, folate, or vitamin B_{12}; from GI blood loss caused by the disease (especially UC); or from the chronic disease process *per se*. They can also cause a high platelet count as this is an inflammatory marker.

- **Erythrocyte sedimentation rate (ESR):** Crohn's disease and UC are systemic inflammatory diseases and usually lead to elevated ESR.

- **C-reactive protein (CRP):** infectious diarrhoea, Crohn's disease, and UC can all cause a rise in CRP levels.

- **Tissue transglutaminase (TTG) and IgA levels:** a positive result has a sensitivity and specificity of over 90% for coeliac disease. You should always check the IgA levels, too, as IgA deficiency can cause false negative results. Anti-endomysial antibodies can be used instead of TTG but are more susceptible to IgA deficiency causing false negatives. Antigliadin antibodies have been used to test for coeliac disease but are less sensitive and specific.

- **Thyroid function tests (TFTs):** a low thyroid-stimulating hormone (TSH) and a high tri-iodothyronine/thyroxine (T_3/T_4) level would strongly suggest hyperthyroidism.

- **Urea and electrolytes (U&Es):** the patient may be dehydrated or suffering electrolyte disturbances from the diarrhoea itself (loss of ions) or secondary to acidaemia caused by hypoperfusion and ischaemia.

- **Albumin:** this will be low in patients with chronic diarrhoea and malabsorption, e.g. IBD.

- **Capillary glucose:** a simple bedside blood glucose test will tell you if this patient is diabetic. Whilst diarrhoea would be an unusual presenting complaint for diabetes mellitus, it is easy to exclude.

Faeces tests

- **Faecal occult blood test (FOBT):** the patient may not have overt blood in the faeces, but may have blood detectable using a FOBT. This would point towards infection or UC, and away from hyperthyroidism, coeliac disease, and IBS. However, this should only be requested after stopping any drugs that can cause bleeding (e.g. aspirin, warfarin), as these will give a false positive result. If they cannot be stopped, a positive result does not help the diagnosis and therefore you should not order the test.

20

- **Faeces microscopy and culture:** infection is still a possibility and should be excluded by the microbiologists. Pus cells may be visible and can indicate inflammation in IBD. Remember that *Giardia* can be very hard to visualize under the microscope even if it is present (i.e. false negative).

- ***C. difficile* toxin test:** The patient has no history of antibiotic use that would predispose her to *C. difficile* infection. However, if the patient did have recent antibiotic use, you should consider testing for *C. difficile* toxin.

Miss Bowles is admitted to hospital for fluid resuscitation and observation. Her blood tests on admission reveal Hb = 10.8 g/dL, MCV = 98 fL, WCC = 8.9×10^9 cells/L, platelets = 300×10^9 cells/L, ESR = 45 mm/h, Na = 135 mM, K = 3.2 mM, negative anti-endomysial antibodies, TSH = 2 mU/L (normal), T_4 = 8 µg/dL (normal) and glucose = 5.2 mM. Her faecal occult blood test is negative. Stool is sent off for microscopy and culture.

  (Hb, haemoglobin; MCV, mean corpuscular volume; WCC, white cell count)

What is the most likely diagnosis in light of these results? What investigations could be arranged to confirm the diagnosis?

Whilst infection is still a possibility (pending the results of the stool sample), the raised ESR implies chronicity. Combined with the anaemia and erythema nodosum, this is most consistent with a diagnosis of **IBD** (either Crohn's disease, UC, or indeterminate colitis). The blood tests helped rule out hyperthyroidism and coeliac disease. IBS is largely a diagnosis of exclusion, which although statistically the most common cause of recurrent diarrhoea in young females, would not usually cause a diarrhoea severe enough to warrant hospitalization for fluid resuscitation.

In Miss Bowles' case, the lack of bloody diarrhoea and the fact that the abdominal pain often starts in her right lower quadrant are suggestive of **Crohn's disease**. In UC, the pain is usually diffuse and the diarrhoea is often bloody. In addition, patients with Crohn's disease are more likely to suffer with weight loss and failure to thrive between attacks, whereas patients with UC are more likely to be relatively well between acute attacks.

Crohn's disease is believed to be due to mutations in genes responsible for clearing up phagocytosed bacteria. The inability of macrophages to correctly clear the bacteria they ingest leads to them secreting cytokines that make the immune system try to 'wall off' the aberrant situation, forming a granuloma (a situation analogous to what happens in tuberculosis, where macrophages also have difficulty clearing the mycobacteria). The granuloma leads to chronic inflammation. Locally, this leads to diarrhoea, ulcers, strictures of the bowel, and fistulae between the bowel and other compartments (or the outer world). Associated systemic complications include inflammation of the eyes (iritis, episcleritis, scleritis), the joints (arthritis), and the skin (erythema nodosum); as well as anaemia (either through malabsorption or chronic inflammation *per se*), weight loss, and fatigue.

The next step is to refer Miss Bowles to the gastroenterology team. They can then arrange for **second-line investigations** to confirm or exclude Crohn's disease, such as:

- **Abdominal (plain) radiograph:** this may show signs of bowel inflammation. If localized to discrete areas (skip lesions), this would be in keeping with Crohn's disease. Abdominal radiographs are essential for patients with severe

UC as they are at risk of toxic megacolon (which can perforate), and this can be detected as a large bowel loop that is >6 cm in diameter.

- **DCBE radiograph:** this may show discrete lesions and strictures in the colon, suggestive of Crohn's disease.

- **Colonoscopy:** this can help visualize the discrete, interrupted lesions of Crohn's disease (or the diffuse, erythematous inflammation of UC) and allows for biopsies to be taken in search of non-caseating granulomas in the bowel mucosa (the hallmark of Crohn's disease).

Miss Bowles' care was taken over by the gastroenterology team. A colonoscopy was arranged and performed during the same admission, and revealed several discrete linear ulcers in the ascending and transverse colon. Histology of biopsies taken at the time of colonoscopy confirmed the presence of non-caseating granulomas and a diagnosis of Crohn's disease was made.

What types of drugs to you think Miss Bowles will be placed on to help manage her Crohn's disease? Will Miss Bowles be able to continue playing lacrosse?

The symptoms of Crohn's disease are due to chronic activation of the immune system in various tissues (e.g. the bowel wall). Because of this, immunosuppressant medications are used to treat the symptoms of the disease. Medications such as sulfasalazine (a sulfa drug of unknown mechanism) and budesonide (a steroid) are both poorly absorbed immunosuppressants whose action is therefore greatest in the intestine, and both drugs are good at achieving remission from an acute attack of Crohn's disease. The disease can then often be kept at bay using immunosuppressants such as methotrexate (a folate antagonist), azathioprine (a purine synthesis inhibitor), or newer medications such as anti-tumour necrosis factor-α (anti-TNFα) monoclonal antibodies (e.g. infliximab). A large proportion of Crohn's patients ultimately require surgery to resect the most affected portions of their bowel, although the emphasis is on managing the disease medically because surgery is only a temporary solution and other portions of bowel will ultimately become affected, too.

Miss Bowles can continue to play lacrosse. Indeed, provided her disease becomes well managed, it is likely that she will be able to lead her usual active lifestyle.

20

Short cases

Miss Latham is a 25-year-old research scientist who presents to her local A&E at 6 a.m. on a Sunday morning. The previous night she attended a wedding reception and consumed a wide and varied assortment of foods. Within an hour of getting home she was vomiting. She spent all night on the toilet and came in because she feels very unwell. Her only previous episodes of diarrhoea that she can remember were as a child, but she has otherwise been fit and well until today. She looks pale and clammy, but her heart rate is 80 bpm and her blood pressure is 120/90 mmHg.

What is the most likely diagnosis? What management is required?

The history of a single, acute episode of sudden-onset diarrhoea and vomiting after a meal that was potentially undercooked or allowed to stay warm for long periods of time is highly suggestive of an **infectious diarrhoea** (due to the presence of pathogens) or **food poisoning** (due to the presence of toxins). The onset of symptoms within hours of consuming the meal suggests the pathogen had a pre-formed toxin that can affect the bowel, making *Staphylococcus aureus* or *Bacillus cereus* likely candidates.

For the vast majority of infectious diarrhoeas, the only management that is required is isolation and adequate **rehydration**. Isolation involves putting the patient in a separate side room with the appropriate infection control measures (e.g. gown and gloves on entering the room, hand washing with soap rather than alcohol gel). Rehydration can be achieved by encouraging the patient to drink water with dissolved **oral rehydration salts**, obtainable at any pharmacy and to be taken 'little and often'. You should emphasize to the patient that these are much better than water because they also contain the electrolytes lost in the diarrhoea, and glucose which helps reabsorb water faster (the glucose importer in the gut co-imports Na^+, which in turn drives water absorption by osmosis). Consider IV fluids if the patient becomes severely dehydrated or unable to tolerate oral fluids. Most infectious diarrhoeas resolve within 48 hours, and only if they persist should microbiological analysis of the faeces and antibiotics be considered.

Miss Webb is a 22-year-old lady who presents for the fourth time in 3 months to her GP practice complaining of recurrent diarrhoea and abdominal pain. You are the locum GP and have never met this patient, so she explains that for the past year she has had bouts of diarrhoea and abdominal crampy pain every couple of weeks. The abdominal pain is diffuse and hard to localize, appearing in different places at different times. It is relieved on defecation. These bouts of diarrhoea and pain are interspersed by weeks where her faeces are often small and hard to pass. Her medical notes reveal that recent investigations have found a normal thyroid function, negative anti-endomysial antibodies, a normal FBC and ESR, and no weight loss in the past year. Miss Webb appears anxious and when asked if anything else is wrong, she admits she is finding it hard to get over a break-up with a long-term boyfriend.

What is the most likely diagnosis? How will you manage this patient?

The most likely cause of recurrent diarrhoea in an anxious female patient in the absence of other obvious pathology is **IBS**. The pathophysiology of IBS is unclear, although it is clearly linked to stress, anxiety, and depression. The diagnosis is largely one of exclusion, avoiding over-investigation of the patient and emphasizing that you expect any investigations undertaken to be normal, as they are done to *exclude* other pathologies rather than to diagnose IBS. Diagnosis of IBS is based on the ROME III criteria:

- At least 3 months, with onset at least 6 months previously of recurrent abdominal pain or discomfort associated with two or more of the following:
  - Improvement with defecation; and/or
  - Onset associated with a change in frequency of stool; and/or
  - Onset associated with a change in form (appearance) of stool.

There is no known cure for IBS. Management consists of:

- **Reassurance:** patients benefit greatly from reassurance that they do not have any serious bowel pathology.

- **Antispasmodics:** medications that decrease smooth muscle activity in the bowel (e.g. mebeverine, hyoscine) can alleviate symptoms of IBS. Loperamide is a particularly strong inhibitor of smooth muscle activity in the bowel and should be reserved only for acute episodes of diarrhoea.

- **Antidepressants:** tricyclic antidepressant medications have been found to slow colonic transit time and alleviate symptoms of IBS at doses that are lower than those required for their antidepressive effect, suggesting their effect in IBS is independent of any effect on depression. It is important that the patient understands that using medications that are given at higher doses to other patients for depression does not imply they are depressed.

- **Diet and herbal remedies:** many patients report improvement by avoiding certain foods (e.g. beans that cause bloating), increasing the fibre content in their diet, or by using certain herbal drinks (e.g. peppermint tea).

20

Mrs Adams is an 82-year-lady who is on a general medical ward at her local hospital, receiving antibiotics for community-acquired pneumonia. She has had a diagnosis of Alzheimer's disease for the past year and broke her right neck of femur 4 months ago, which was repaired by the orthopaedic surgeons by pinning it *in situ* with a dynamic hip screw. The nurse has called you to inform you that Mrs Adams is suffering from 'explosive diarrhoea' and they are having to change her bed hourly. When you arrive, you find a frail old lady who appears delirious. Her lips are dry, her eyes are sunken, her pulse is 100 bpm and her blood pressure is 105/70 mmHg.

What diagnosis should you be worried about? How will you manage this patient?

An elderly (and therefore inevitably immunosuppressed to some extent) patient receiving antibiotics is a high-risk candidate for letting the *Clostridium difficile* that naturally populates our guts grow out of control, become pathogenic, and start producing its toxin. You should be worried that this patient may have developed ***C. difficile* colitis**. Early management is essential and should include:

1) **ABC:** this lady's blood pressure is low for an elderly patient and her mucous membranes are dry, suggesting she is indeed hypovolaemic, which is unsurprising if the nurses are having to change her bed every hour due to diarrhoea. She needs IV fluid resuscitation urgently (e.g. 250 mL boluses of IV normal saline until clinical signs and blood pressure suggest she is no longer hypovolaemic).

2) **Faeces analysis:** send a stool sample off immediately to microbiology for microscopy, culture, and analysis for *C. difficile* toxin.

3) **Isolation:** an obvious, effective, and simple solution to preventing the spread of pathogenic *C. difficile* on the wards, but one that is often hard to implement in many overcrowded and under-resourced hospitals.

4) **Meticulous hygiene:** all staff and visitors should 'glove and gown' and hands must be washed between patients using warm water and soap (alcohol gels will *not* inactivate *C. difficile* which forms highly durable spores).

5) **Antibiotics:** if the faeces analysis is positive for *C. difficile* toxin, you should start appropriate antibiotic therapy without delay. The choice of antibiotic will depend on local guidelines, which you should always consult.

Mr Singh is a 22-year-old webpage designer who presents to A&E complaining of bloody diarrhoea. He has had some discomfort in his left iliac fossa over the past 2 days but, since this morning, he has found himself rushing to the toilet four times and then passing 'lots of blood'. He also describes having to remain on the toilet for some time to 'get it all out'. Despite the dramatic nature of his faeces, he admits he feels relatively well, with no fever, malaise, nausea, or vomiting. He has not lost any weight recently, has not travelled abroad, and does not know anybody else who is also suffering from diarrhoea at the moment. He does not smoke or drink alcohol. Examination of the patient is remarkable only for fresh blood in the rectum on digital rectal examination. His observations are heart rate 90 bpm regular, blood pressure 115/80 mmHg, temperature 36.8°C. His initial blood results are shown below:

Hb	14.3 g/dL
RBC	5.8×10^{12} cells/L
WCC	9.2×10^{9} cells/L
Platelets	185×10^{9} cells/L
MCV	98 fL
Urea	5.1 mM
Creatinine	42 µM
Na	136 mM
K	4.1 mM
Prothrombin time	13.5 seconds
APTT	34 seconds
ESR	78 mm/h

Blood is sent off for cultures and stool is sent off for microscopy and culture. A colonoscopy is arranged for the next day and reveals a uniformly inflamed rectum and descending colon, with a clear cut-off point between inflamed and normal bowel at the level of the splenic flexure. Biopsies of the inflamed bowel are taken and histology reports 'inflamed crypts, full of fibrin and PMNs [polymorpho-nuclear leucocytes]'.

What is the likely diagnosis and why? What other conditions are associated with this disease? How is the disease managed?

It is likely that Mr Singh is suffering from **UC**. This is a form of IBD whose aetiology is unknown. The GI tract is affected in a distal to proximal fashion (i.e. from the rectum upwards) and shows gross, uniform inflammation with a clear cut-off point between abnormal and normal bowel. Patients typically present with painless, bloody diarrhoea.

UC, like Crohn's disease, is actually a systemic inflammatory disease that simply happens to manifest most prominently in the bowel. Like Crohn's disease, the systemic inflammation can affect joints (arthritis, sacroiliitis), eyes (uveitis, scleritis, episcleritis), skin (erythema nodosum), and blood (anaemia of chronic disease). Unlike Crohn's disease, UC has a much stronger association with colonic adenocarcinoma (1% risk per year); primary sclerosing cholangitis (obstructive jaundice and liver failure), and cholangiocarcinoma (cancer of the common bile duct).

Management of UC involves three approaches:

1) **Medical therapy:** UC is a systemic inflammatory disease that responds well to anti-inflammatories. Salicylate derivatives (e.g. sulfasalazine, mesalazine),

20

methotrexate, azathioprine, corticosteroids, and anti-TNF antibodies (e.g. infliximab) can all be used to control the inflammation.

2) **Disease monitoring:** due to the high rates of colonic adenocarcinoma in UC, patients are monitored with colonoscopy for early signs of cancer on a regular basis.

3) **Surgical therapy:** surgery for UC involves removing the portion of affected bowel. This approach is potentially curative as it removes the main symptomatic focus of the disease and eliminates the risk of colonic adenocarcinoma. However, the removal of the rectum has traditionally resulted in a lifelong end ileostomy which put many patients off the idea of surgery. The development of the ileal pouch-anal anastomosis (IPAA), whereby a pouch of ileum is used to fashion a rectum and connected to the anus to allow almost normal defecation, has been an important development in surgery for UC patients.

Mrs Thompson is a 78-year-old lady who is currently an inpatient at a geriatric psychiatry unit, where she is being managed for her Lewy body dementia. The nurses have reported to the junior psychiatrist on call that Mrs Wilkinson has become incontinent of faeces over the past few days, with her uncontrolled motions being extremely liquid in nature. Nobody else in the unit is affected with diarrhoea.

Mrs Thompson is unable to give a coherent history or explain how she feels due to her advanced dementia. You look in the notes and see that she has hypertension and osteoporosis for which she is taking bendroflumethiazide, alendronate, vitamin D, and calcium. Her past medical history is remarkable for hip replacements 3 and 5 years ago, and for osteoarthritis of the right knee. Examination reveals a thin, cachectic-looking woman. Her abdomen is soft and non-tender but there is a palpable mass in her left iliac fossa that is roughly cylindrical and extends a few centimetres longitudinally. Virchow's node is not palpable. Bowel sounds are present. A digital rectal examination reveals a mass of irregular surface on the posterior wall of the rectum and triggers a gush of fluid faeces and flatus. The faeces are positive for blood when tested with a disposable Hemoccult® kit.

What is the likely diagnosis? How does that explain her liquid faeces? What key investigations should Mrs Thompson receive?

Mrs Thompson is an elderly lady suffering with incontinence of liquid faeces. Despite her incontinence, her left iliac fossa (i.e. descending colon/sigmoid colon) feels full to palpation and a digital rectal examination reveals a rectal mass. Tellingly, the digital rectal examination causes a gush of fluid faeces and flatus. Mrs Thompson is most likely suffering from **overflow diarrhoea**. This is caused by an obstruction that allows only fluid and air to bypass, causing a liquid diarrhoea that is hard to control. The obstruction may be due to a mass within the lumen (e.g. solid, impacted faeces due to dehydration and lack of fibre); a mass within the bowel wall (e.g. colonic adenocarcinoma), or a mass outside the bowel wall (e.g. a large ovarian tumour compressing the bowel).

Mrs Thompson's age, the presence of a mass in her rectum on examination, and positive test for occult blood in her faeces should all alert you to the possibility of rectal carcinoma. Mrs Thompson should be investigated by either flexible sigmoidoscopy or rigid proctosigmoidoscopy looking for rectal masses that can be biopsied. She may also be offered a double-contrast barium enema (DCBE), which may reveal an 'apple core sign' in the rectal lumen due to the tumour, or CT colonography which has the advantage of being non-invasive and visualizing the surrounding organs for tumour spread. If a tumour is identified and a CT has not been done, a pelvic MRI and liver ultrasound are usually performed to stage the spread of the cancer beyond the bowel wall (e.g. to the liver) using the Dukes' staging system.

20

Mr Cox is a 42-year-old zoology researcher who attends his GP complaining of diarrhoea. For the past few weeks, he has found himself going to the toilet up to six times a day and passing fairly loose (albeit not liquid) motions. He used to open his bowels only once a day and his faeces were 'more solid'. He reports being otherwise well although very busy with work. The GP notices that he is wearing only a T-shirt and has come with no jumper or jacket, despite the fact that it is a cold autumn day outside. When asked about weight loss, Mr Cox says he hadn't noticed any but that he has had to wear his belt tighter despite eating rather a lot recently. His past medical history is unremarkable and he takes no medications. He does not smoke and only drinks the occasional pint of ale when socializing with friends. He lives with his wife and their child, who has cystic fibrosis.

The GP asks Mr Cox to take off his T-shirt so that he can be examined. His heart rate is 110 bpm and regular. A resting tremor is noticed when Mr Cox holds his arms out. His eyes look normal but when asked to follow the GP's finger with his eyes, as it descends in front of him, an obvious lid lag is noted. The neck is normal to palpation and the rest of the examination is normal.

What diagnosis should be suspected? What investigations should the GP arrange?

Mr Cox has presented with increased frequency and softer consistency to his stools. He appears to have heat intolerance and may have lost some weight recently, to judge by him wearing his trousers tighter than usual. He has an obvious lid lag and is tachycardic. Feeling hot, losing weight despite increased appetite and eating, increased frequency of bowel motions, tachycardia, lid lag (due to the eyelids trying to remain wide open when the patient looks down), and a possibility of hyperactivity ('very busy at work') are all suggestive of excessive sympathetic stimulation throughout the body. The likeliest cause is **hyperthyroidism**, as thyroid hormones make tissues more sensitive to sympathetic stimulation.

The GP should take a blood sample and check Mr Cox's TSH, and T_3 and T_4 levels. In hyperthyroidism, one finds elevated T_3 and T_4 but decreased TSH (due to negative feedback by T_3/T_4 on TSH secretion). If hyperthyroidism is confirmed, one should seek a cause. The most common aetiology is Graves' disease, which can be investigated by looking for a raised antithyroid peroxidase (which is not pathogenic but usually correlates with the presence of the pathogenic thyroid-stimulating antibodies) and a raised ESR in the blood. It is unusual to look for the pathogenic thyroid-stimulating antibodies because of the high cost of the test, but this may be requested in pregnant women with hyperthyroidism because these antibodies can cross the placenta, resulting in a thyrotoxic foetus that would require special care at the time of delivery. If these antibody tests are negative, one should arrange for a scan using radiolabelled iodine or technetium, which may reveal one or more nodules in the thyroid gland. Cold nodules are more likely to be malignant thyroid tumours than hot nodules, although both are still more likely to be benign than malignant.

20

Viva questions

Patients with IBD (Crohn's disease or UC) can experience a number of complications outside the bowel. What are these complications?

- **Nails:** clubbing of finger nails
- **Eyes:** inflammation leading to iritis (anterior uveitis), episcleritis, or scleritis
- **Skin:** erythema nodosum (inflammation of subcutaneous fat nodules leading to raised, red nodules) or pyoderma gangrenosum (inflammatory ulceration and necrosis of the skin)
- **Joints:** inflammation leading to enteric arthritis
- **Blood:** iron-deficiency anaemia (from blood loss in the bowel, especially in UC), folate or vitamin B_{12} deficiency anaemias (from malabsorption due to irritation of the bowel)
- **Biliary system:** primary sclerosing cholangitis (associated with UC), cholesterol gallstones (due to reduced reabsorption of bile salts by the inflamed bowel, leading to precipitation of insoluble cholesterol)
- **Kidneys:** kidney stones, because fat malabsorption leads to (fat-soluble) Ca^{2+} being sequestered in the bowel. The lack of Ca^{2+} (which usually binds to oxalate in the blood) allows oxalate to precipitate and form stones
- **Bones:** the lack of Ca^{2+} (due to malabsorption of fat) can lead to osteomalacia or even osteoporosis
- **Amyloidosis:** chronic systemic inflammatory disorders can lead to deposition of serum amyloid A protein in multiple organs

Why should patients with UC be offered regular colonoscopies?

Patients with UC are at increased risk (five-fold) of colon cancer, and for this reason they are offered regular colonoscopic studies looking for early signs of malignancy. If malignancy is detected, the usual procedure is to excise the entire colon (colectomy). Traditionally, this resulted in the patient needing a permanent colostomy but modern surgical techniques allow for the creation of a new rectum and preservation of anorectal function by performing an ileo-rectal anastomosis with an ileal pouch.

A common symptom of hyperthyroidism is increased bowel movements, often resulting in frank diarrhoea. Why does hyperthyroidism cause diarrhoea?

T_3 is a hormone that results in cells expressing more adrenergic receptors and modifying the components of the adrenergic response pathway so that they are more sensitive to catecholamine stimulus. The net result is that cells become more sensitive to catecholamines such as adrenaline and noradrenaline, and therefore more sensitive to sympathetic stimulation. Many physiology textbooks claim that sympathetic stimulation of the bowel results in constipation, but as many students nervous before exams will testify, the prolonged effect of catecholamines on the bowel is to increase bowel movements.

What are the most likely infective organisms in each of the following diarrhoea scenarios?

1) An outbreak of vomiting and diarrhoea in an old persons' nursing home
2) An outbreak of bloody diarrhoea at a local primary school
3) A university student with watery diarrhoea a few days after a barbeque
4) A group of guests with sudden-onset diarrhoea a few hours after a wedding reception
5) An 82-year-old gentleman in hospital receiving antibiotics for pneumonia
6) A young woman who has just returned from Ghana and has right iliac fossa pain and diarrhoea

The reality is that it is often hard to predict the pathogenic organism in cases of infectious diarrhoea and microbiological culture often reveals the pathogen to be multiple organisms or an unexpected organism. However, certain patterns are typical for certain pathogens and these are frequently asked about in exams and vivas. Hence:

1) Outbreaks of vomiting and diarrhoea in institutions are usually due to viruses of the small structured round virus (SSRV) type, such as **Norovirus**.

2) Outbreaks of dysentery (bloody diarrhoea) are often associated with bacteria of the *Shigella* species or with *Escherichia coli* strain O157.

3) In truth, this could be due to a multitude of organisms, but in exams and vivas the answer is that *Campylobacter jejuni* would be a good candidate for a post-barbeque case of diarrhoea.

4) Rapid-onset diarrhoea after a meal suggests that the meal was contaminated with bacteria that have excreted active toxins, hence the rapid onset of symptoms. When the diarrhoea is caused by the pathogen's growth in the bowel, the onset of symptoms is usually much slower. *Staphylococcus aureus* and *Bacillus cereus* are both bacteria that grow on warm food and produce toxins that result in rapid-onset diarrhoea.

5) The diarrhoea could be caused by a multitude of organisms or even the antibiotics *per se*, but in elderly patients receiving antibiotics you should always be wary of *Clostridium difficile*.

6) Again, the diarrhoea could be simple 'traveller's diarrhoea' caused by an enterotoxigenic strain of *E. coli* but the right iliac fossa pain should make you suspicious of *Yersinia enterocolitica*.

20

What is the most important aspect in the management of any of the infectious diarrhoeas mentioned above?

Fluid balance. Patients with infectious diarrhoea are at risk of dehydration due to the constant watery faeces they pass, and it is dehydration which most commonly kills patients with infective diarrhoea worldwide. Maintaining adequate hydration **with oral rehydration salts** in patients with diarrhoea is more important than establishing the identity of the pathogen or treating it with antimicrobial agents.

What is the difference between (1) a fluid challenge, (2) maintenance fluids, and (3) replacement fluids?

1) **Fluid challenge:** this is an IV bolus of 250–500 mL of normal saline given over 30 minutes to a patient who is hypovolaemic (thirsty, dry mucous membranes, tachycardic, and with a narrow and/or low blood pressure). After the fluid challenge is given, one must reassess the patient. Three outcomes are possible:
   - **No response:** blood pressure remains low. The patient has not received enough fluids or they weren't actually hypovolaemic to begin with. Reassess the patient clinically (to double check they really are hypovolaemic) and repeat a fluid challenge.
   - **Transient response (increase) in blood pressure:** the patient was indeed hypovolaemic but you either haven't given them enough fluids *or* they are losing them very rapidly (e.g. haemorrhage). Give them more fluids and consider possible explanations for continuing fluid loss.
   - **Sustained response (increase) in blood pressure:** the patient was indeed hypovolaemic and you have restored them to normal fluid balance.

2) **Maintenance fluids:** the average, normal adult loses about 2.5 L of fluid every day in urine (1.5 L/day), faeces (200 mL/day), and 'insensible losses' (i.e. those you aren't aware of such as sweating and respiration, 800 mL/day). Lost fluids contain dissolved electrolytes and so the average, normal adult also loses about 100 mM of Na^+ and about 70 mM of K^+ every day. Fluids and electrolytes must be replaced daily to maintain fluid balance, and this is normally achieved by drinking about 2 L of fluids a day and eating normally. If a patient cannot drink, they need maintenance IV fluids to restore their 2.5 L fluid, 100 mM Na^+, and 70 mM K^+ a day. This is usually achieved on the wards by prescribing:
   - Bag 1: 1 L of normal saline (=1 L of H_2O, 154 mM Na^+, 154 mM Cl^-) plus 20 mM K^+, IV over 8 hours.
   - Bag 2: 1 L of 5% dextrose (=1 L of H_2O, 50 g of dextrose), plus 20 mM K^+, IV over 8 hours.
   - Bag 3: 1 L of 5% dextrose (=1 L of H_2O, 50 g of dextrose), plus 20 mM K^+, IV over 8 hours.
   - Total: 3 L of H_2O, 154 mM Na^+, 60 mM K^+ over 24 hours.

(Note that the above prescription is not precise – it gives slightly too much Na^+ and slightly too little K^+. However, the exact requirements vary depending on a patient's weight and current electrolyte concentrations, and thus the requirement figures given are a guideline only. Indeed, the above formula is increasingly recognized as a cause of hyponatraemia in some patients, hence it is increasingly common to prescribe two or three bags of normal saline a day rather than the traditional single bag.)

3) **Replacement fluids:** maintenance fluids (see above) will maintain fluid balance in many patients. However, some patients have conditions that result in abnormally high fluid loss and therefore they need extra fluids on top of their maintenance fluids to replace the extra losses. Examples of patients requiring extra, replacement fluids are:
   - **Fever:** febrile patients need an extra 500 mL of fluid for every 1°C above 37°C.
   - **Burns patients:** patients with burns need extra fluids and this can be calculated using the Parkland formula:
   $$\text{Fluids (mL)} = 4 \times \text{weight (kg)} \times \text{\% surface area burnt}$$
   - **Stoma patients:** patients with intestinal stomas lose fluids because these exit the bowel before fluids can be reabsorbed. Small bowel stomas obviously result in greater fluid loss than large bowel stomas as more fluid will have been reabsorbed by the time faeces exit a large bowel stoma than a small bowel stoma. The only way to calculate how much excess fluid is being lost is by *measuring and recording* how much fluid a stoma drains, keeping in mind that normal faecal loss of fluid is only 200 mL/day.

20

- **Third spacing:** traditionally, fluid found in the vasculature is said to be in the 'first space' whereas fluid found in interstitial tissue space is said to be in the 'second space', as both of these 'spaces' contain volumes of fluid that are variable (intracellular fluid is usually fairly constant). The 'third space' refers to areas of the body that accumulate fluid only in disease, thus draining, fluids away from the first and second spaces. Thus, patients may have fluid in their peritoneal cavity (for example due to ascites in liver cirrhosis or inflammatory exudate around the pancreas in pancreatitis), fluid in their intrapleural space (pleural effusion as in parapneumonic effusions for example), build-up of excess fluid in their GI tract (for example in small bowel obstruction), etc. Estimating how much fluid has been 'third spaced' in a patient is difficult, and one usually relies on trial and error (giving replacement fluids and then assessing the patient) to work out how much replacement fluid to give.

What must you always do (and mention in Objective Structured Clinical Examinations!) with any patient who is receiving IV fluids of any sort?

If a patient is receiving IV fluids, you must always **document fluid input/output** and **always reassess** the patient clinically and biochemically. That is why, on ward rounds, patients on IV fluids get examined clinically and have bloods taken for (amongst other things) electrolyte levels.

Clinical examination may reveal a patient who is still thirsty, with dry mucous membranes, tachycardia, a narrow pulse pressure, and a urine output <30 mL/h despite IV fluids, suggesting they are not receiving enough fluids. Alternatively, it may reveal a the patient who looks puffy (oedematous), has crackles in the bases of their lungs, and a raised jugular venous pressure, suggesting they are receiving too much fluid.

Blood biochemistry may reveal a patient who is hyponatraemic (they may need more normal saline and less 5% dextrose) or hyperkalaemic (they may need less K^+ supplementation in their fluids).

For a range of Single Best Answer questions related to the topic of this chapter go to
www.oxfordtextbooks.co.uk/orc/ocms/

20

Rectal bleeding

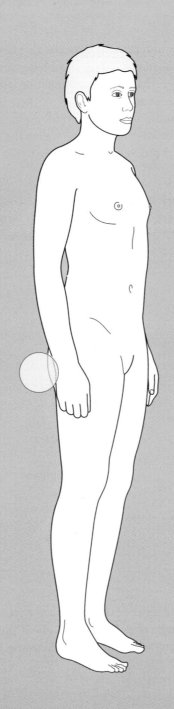

Core case

!
♦

Read through the sections in red, covering up the sections in white that follow so that you don't see the answer. At the end of each red section, try to answer the question before reading on.

Mr McCarthy is a 62-year-old butcher who presents to his local accident and emergency (A&E) department because he has passed blood per rectum.

What is your first priority when assessing Mr McCarthy?

As with all acute patients, always start by assessing ABCDE: Airways, Breathing, Circulation, Disability, and Exposure. In a patient with acute gastrointestinal (GI) haemorrhage (whether upper or lower), assessing their circulation (i.e. haemodynamic status) is a priority. If there are clinical features to suggest haemodynamic instability – such as hypotension, tachycardia, cool peripheries, tachypnoea, or decreased consciousness – then the immediate priority is to resuscitate the patient before proceeding to a thorough history and examination.

You run through the ABCDE algorithm of assessment, and establish that Mr McCarthy is haemodynamically stable. The next stage is to take a full history of the presenting complaint. Before doing so you should have a mental list of differential diagnoses in mind.

What is your differential diagnosis for rectal bleeding? You may wish to construct your list anatomically.

Table 21.1 Differential diagnosis for rectal bleeding

Anorectal	Colonic	Ileo-jejunal	Upper GI
• Haemorrhoids	• Diverticular disease	• Peptic ulceration (including Meckel's diverticulum)	• Peptic ulcer
• Rectal tumour (benign or malignant)	• Angiodysplasia	• Angiodysplasia	• Gastritis/duodenitis
• Anal tumour (benign or malignant)	• Colitis (inflammatory, ischaemic, infective)	• Arteriovenous malformation	• Varices
• Anal fissure	• Colonic tumour (benign or malignant)	• Crohn's disease	• Tumour
• Anal fistula	• Iatrogenic (endoscopic biopsy, anastomotic leakage)	• Coeliac disease	• Mallory–Weiss tear
• Solitary rectal ulcer	• Vasculitis	• Aorto-enteric fistula	• Osler–Weber–Rendu syndrome
• Radiation proctitis		• Small bowel tumours	• Aorto-enteric fistula
• Rectal varices			• Dieulafoy lesion
• Trauma			

The differential diagnosis for rectal bleeding is shown in Table 21.1. There are a couple of points to note about this differential diagnosis. GI haemorrhage may present as *overt* or *occult* bleeding. This table, and the indications of prevalence

21

within it, refers to *overt* rectal bleeding as *occult* rectal bleeding will not be noticed by the patient. The second point to note is that upper GI sources of haemorrhage may occasionally present with rectal bleeding alone. Whilst it is more likely that such upper GI sources will also present with haematemesis, you should note that large volumes of blood in the GI tract can act as a cathartic (stimulant of peristalsis) and the resultant rapid transit through the intestine leads to the passage of red blood per rectum.

What questions would you like to ask specifically about the history of the presenting complaint?

---

* **How much blood has been passed?** This question is directly relevant to your initial haemodynamic status survey. Ask the patient to quantify approximately how much blood they have passed – familiar measures such as a teaspoon, egg cup, or wine glass may be easier for the patient than asking them to provide an estimate in millilitres. Note, however, that it is very easy to overestimate volumes of blood loss if, for example, blood has mixed with water in the toilet bowl. You should additionally enquire about symptoms of hypovolaemia – any postural hypotension, light-headedness, or collapse?

* **What is the duration and frequency of the symptoms?**

* **What did the blood look like?** Generally speaking, the fresher the blood, the more distal the bleed.[†] Substantial bleeding from lesions proximal in the GI tract may present with melaena (jet black liquid stool caused by bacterial oxidation of haem) or may present as frank blood (haematochezia) if transit times are sufficiently rapid. You may need to specifically ask the patient about melaena.

* **What is the relationship of blood with stool?** This is the key question with regard to potentially localizing the source of bleeding.[†] There are four scenarios:
  - **Blood is mixed with the stool:** this suggests that the lesion is proximal to the sigmoid colon. Stool in the proximal colon is soft (thus facilitating mixing with blood) and there is sufficient transit time to enable mixing.
  - **Blood streaked on stool:** suggests a sigmoid or anorectal source of bleeding.
  - **Blood is separate from the stool:** if the blood is passed immediately after stool, the likelihood is that this is an anal condition such as haemorrhoids. If, however, blood is passed on its own, this implies that there has been sufficient bleeding to dilate the rectum and produce a defecation stimulus. Such bleeding is most likely to occur with diverticular disease, angiodysplasia, inflammatory bowel disease, or sometimes a rapidly bleeding cancer (upper GI haemorrhage is another small-print cause).
  - **Blood is only seen on the toilet paper:** this implies relatively minor bleeding from the anal canal, most likely due to haemorrhoids or an anal fissure.

21

[†] But note, as discussed under the differential diagnosis, that rapid intestinal transit times can produce a confusing picture.

+ **Is there any pain or prolapse when opening the bowels?** Most of the conditions resulting in rectal bleeding are non-painful. The most notable exception is an anal fissure, which produces intense/tearing pain during defecation and perhaps lasting for several hours post-defecation; such patients may also complain of an itch or perianal irritation. Colitis may be associated with abdominal cramping, and lower anal cancers may present with pain. Haemorrhoids are not typically associated with pain unless they have thrombosed, but patients may have noticed prolapse.

+ **Is there any tenesmus (sensation of incomplete evacuation)?** This question is most specific for rectal cancer, where a luminal mass in the rectum can cause the feeling of incomplete bowel evacuation *after* defecation. It can also be a symptom of colitis.

+ **Has there been any change of bowel habit?** The passage of blood per rectum may be associated with diarrhoea (such as with colitis) or mucus (think of colitis, proctitis, rectal cancer, and villous adenomas of the rectum). Extensive haemorrhoids may also be associated with the passage of mucus per rectum.

+ **Has the patient lost weight?** In older patients in particular you must retain a high index of suspicion for cancer. Note that rectal cancer may lead to substantial weight loss even in the absence of metastatic spread.

+ **Are there any symptoms of anaemia?** The current overt bleed may represent an occult bleed that has been unmasked, for example by anticoagulant drugs. Hence it is useful to ask about symptoms of anaemia such as lethargy and shortness of breath.

> As shown in the differential diagnosis in Table 21.1, diverticular disease, angiodysplasia, haemorrhoids, colitis, anal fissures, and lower GI tumours are the most common causes of rectal bleeding.
>
> Construct a 4 × 2 table that shows how these top diagnoses typically present in terms of (a) relationship of blood and stool and (b) pain or not.

21

Table 21.2 4 × 2 table for rectal bleeding diagnosis

	Pain	No pain
Blood mixed with stool	Colitis	Colonic tumour Colitis
Blood streaked on stool	Anal tumour	Rectal tumour
Blood separate from stool	Colitis	Haemorrhoids Diverticular disease Angiodysplasia Rapidly bleeding colonic or rectal tumour Colitis (+ mucus)
Blood on toilet paper	Anal fissure	Haemorrhoids

What is the specific relevance of past medical/surgical history?

There are a number of relevant features in the past medical/surgical history:

- **Previous rectal bleeding?** If so, were these episodes investigated and what was the outcome?
- **Ulcerative colitis?** Increases the likelihood of colonic malignancy…or a flare-up of their ulcerative colitis!
- **Recent bowel trauma?** For example bowel surgery, colonoscopy, double-contrast barium enema (DCBE), or other anorectal procedure such as trans-rectal prostate biopsy. All may result in rectal bleeding.
- **Aortic surgery?** Non-trivial GI bleeding in a patient who has had previous aortic surgery should make you suspect an aorto-enteric fistula until proven otherwise.
- **Radiotherapy to the rectum?** Can induce proctitis.
- **Bleeding tendency?** For example warfarin, haemophilia, platelet dysfunction. In a patient with a known bleeding tendency the degree of blood loss may be disproportionate to that normally expected from a particular lesion.
- **Past medical history that predisposes to upper GI bleeds?** Many diseases that can cause an upper GI bleed (e.g. peptic ulcer disease, chronic liver disease) can also present as rectal bleeding.

Why is a detailed drug history of particular importance when investigating rectal bleeding?

The drug history is vital as drugs may contribute towards rectal bleeding in four ways:

1) **Increased risk of bleeding.** Anticoagulant and antiplatelet medications can accentuate bleeding from established lesions (a previously occult bleed may become overt). Long-term anticoagulation (such as may occur following insertion of a prosthetic heart valve) makes any existing angiodysplasia more likely to bleed. Non-steroidal anti-inflammatory drugs (NSAIDs) are known to increase the likelihood of bleeds from diverticular disease.

2) **Increased risk of peptic ulcers.** NSAIDs, steroids, and bisphosphonates predispose to peptic ulceration.

3) **Increased risk of infectious colitis.** Antibiotic use may predispose to *Clostridium difficile* colitis, as may use of proton-pump inhibitors.

4) **Decreased heart response to hypovolaemia.** β-Blockers can stop patients from mounting the usual tachycardic response to hypovolaemia.

Mr McCarthy describes passing 'about a pint' of bright red blood per rectum an hour ago. There was no pain associated with the bowel motion. He says that it looked as if he was passing pure blood – with very little stool mixed in. He was alarmed at the appearance of the toilet bowl and decided to drive straight to his local hospital.

21

There have been no previous episodes of rectal bleeding. Mr McCarthy has not experienced any tenesmus or recent change in bowel habit. He has not lost weight recently, and reports no symptoms of lethargy or general malaise. Mr McCarthy states that he is otherwise fit and well. He has had no previous operations, no recent bowel trauma, and no radiotherapy to the rectum. His past medical history is unremarkable. He takes simvastatin for his hypercholesterolaemia, and has no known drug allergies. He smokes 10 cigarettes a day, and enjoys approximately 20 units of beer each week.

Mr McCarthy will need to be examined.

What are the relevant aspects of the physical examination?

You may wish to consider the examination in three stages: general, abdominal, and rectal.

General examination

- Is Mr McCarthy still **haemodynamically stable?** You must continue to assess Mr McCarthy's pulse and blood pressure for signs of continuing or new bleeding.
- Are there any features suggestive of **chronic blood loss** (signs of anaemia such as pallor or koilonychia) or **malignancy** (such as cachexia or obvious lymphadenopathy)?

Abdominal examination

- You should examine the abdomen for any **focal tenderness** or **masses** – principally looking for signs of GI malignancy (left supraclavicular lymphadenopathy (Virchow's node), palpable lesions of the colon, hepatomegaly, ascites etc).

Rectal examination

- The first step is to **inspect the anus** – you may see an anal fissure ± associated skin tag ± 'sentinel pile', haemorrhoid, or fistula (perhaps associated with inflammatory bowel disease). **All patients presenting with rectal bleeding should have a digital rectal examination (DRE).** The only times that a DRE may be omitted are in the presence of a painful anal fissure or abscess. While performing the DRE you should be feeling for **palpable masses**, and then inspecting for **blood on the withdrawn gloved finger**. Note that you should not expect to palpate haemorrhoids during a DRE unless they are either prolapsed or thrombosed.

21

Mr McCarthy is still haemodynamically stable. His pulse is 92 bpm regular, blood pressure 132/87 mmHg, and respiratory rate 14/min. Abdominal examination is unremarkable. A DRE reveals blood in the rectum but no palpable masses.

What are the first-line investigations that you would like to request?

Bloods

- **Full blood count (FBC):** you want to know if the patient is anaemic (due to chronic blood loss) or has low platelets.
- **Clotting:** you want to know if the patient has a bleeding tendency.

- **Group and save** (or cross-match if needed urgently): if there is a suspicion that the patient may need blood replacement or may go to theatre. Mr McCarthy is haemodynamically stable and there is no current indication to request an urgent cross-match. If, however, he was unstable and/or showed signs of continued bleeding a cross-match would be more appropriate.

- **Urea:** a rise in urea is consistent with a recent upper GI bleed (urea is a breakdown product of digested red blood cells).

Endoscopy

- **Proctoscopy ± rigid sigmoidoscopy** should be performed in all such patients unless there are painful anal lesions such as an anal fissure. But note that the view of the rectum may be unsatisfactory if there is a lot of blood. Proctoscopy ± rigid sigmoidoscopy will enable the identification of bleeding haemorrhoids or a rectal cancer, and can be performed at the bedside in A&E.

A blood sample is taken from Mr McCarthy and intravenous (IV) fluids are prescribed. Proctoscopy and rigid sigmoidoscopy are performed at the bedside but do not reveal a source of haemorrhage. Mr McCarthy is still haemodynamically stable and there has been no further passage of blood per rectum.

The blood results are reported as:

Hb	13.6 g/dL
RBC	4.8×10^{12} cells/L
WCC	9.3×10^9 cells/L
Platelets	320×10^9 cells/L
MCV	84 fL
PT	12.9 seconds
APTT	36 seconds

(Hb, haemoglobin; RBC, red blood cell [count]; WCC, white cell count; MCV, mean corpuscular volume; PT, prothrombin time; APTT, activated partial thromboplastin time)

How would you proceed to establish the source of haemorrhage?

There are four further main investigations for *acute* lower GI haemorrhage (frank blood per rectum) that may be considered in stable patients in the following order (Fig. 21.1 shows a potential algorithm for the investigation of acute rectal bleeding):

1) **Colonoscopy**
   - During an acute bleed it is difficult to achieve a good view of the bowel lumen without copious lavage. If, however, it is possible to fully prepare the bowel, colonoscopy is the investigation of choice in the stable patient.
   - In addition to being diagnostic, colonoscopy affords therapeutic options of controlling local haemorrhage by means of adrenaline injection, argon plasma coagulation, diathermy, or clipping.

21

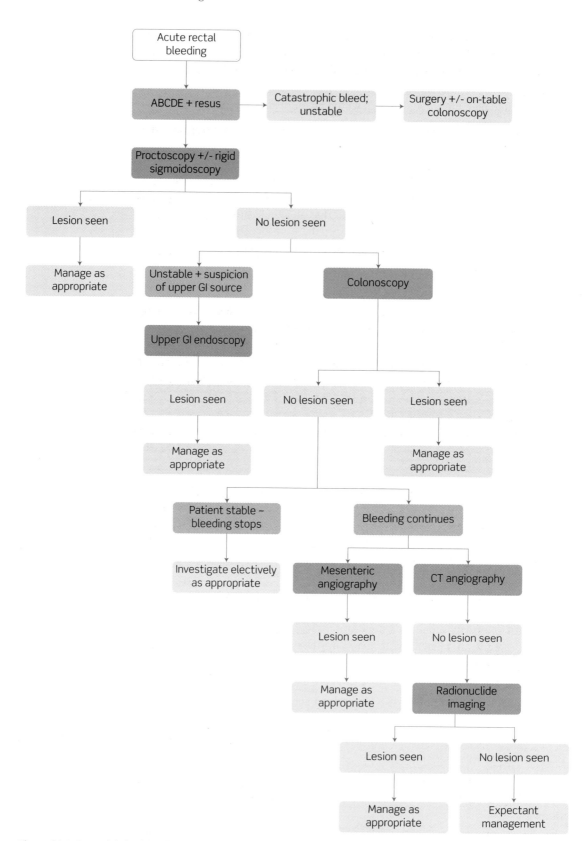

Figure 21.1 Potential algorithm for the investigation of acute rectal bleeding.

- There is an additional role for on-table colonoscopy in those patients who present with profuse haemorrhage and proceed straight to theatre. The colon can be irrigated via a caecal catheter to maximize visualization.

2) **Mesenteric angiography (if available)**
   - Useful if haemorrhage obscures the view with colonoscopy, or colonoscopy is not possible. Hence it is often used if patients bleed, then stop, and then rebleed.
   - Rarely available in smaller hospitals or out of hours.
   - Mesenteric angiography is particularly useful for detecting angiodysplasia, as evidenced by early filling of vessels and/or bleeding during the capillary phase. In order to demonstrate active bleeding there must be blood loss of >0.5–1 mL/min.
   - Embolization of the bleeding vessel can be performed during the procedure.

3) **Computed tomography (CT) angiography**
   - Gaining popularity as an alternative to conventional mesenteric angiography, particularly as multislice CT can now detect even relatively minor bleeds.
   - Involves venous access thus fewer potential complications than mesenteric (arterial) angiography. In addition, it provides rapid imaging and enables other abdominal pathology (either related or incidental to the rectal bleeding) to be visualized by CT.
   - On the downside, there is a lack of therapeutic capability, thus patients with bleeding lesions identified by CT angiography will need to proceed to mesenteric angiography or laparotomy.

4) **Technetium-99m-labelled red blood cell scintigraphy (if available)**
   - Useful in patients for whom other investigations have failed to identify a source – typically these will be patients who have short-lived intermittent bleeds (such as from a Meckel's diverticulum).
   - Rarely available in smaller hospitals or out of hours.
   - Lacks the specificity of colonoscopy and mesenteric angiography but is non-invasive. It may be useful if the other two techniques have failed to localize the lesion.
   - Can detect bleeding at >0.1 mL/min, and can also be used to detect bleeding lesions up to 24 hours after tracer administration, but has no therapeutic potential (its main role is in guiding surgical resection).
   - Also has the advantage of requiring no bowel preparation.

Upper GI endoscopy? Some surgeons would advocate upper GI endoscopy in many patients with lower GI haemorrhage, and would certainly do so if there is any indication of haemodynamic compromise. As we have already stated, upper GI haemorrhage may occasionally present as rectal bleeding. Not only is upper GI haemorrhage more common than lower GI haemorrhage (**80% of acute GI haemorrhage is upper**), it is less likely to stop spontaneously and thus more life-threatening.

Gastric lavage? Some surgeons occasionally advocate gastric lavage via a nasogastric tube to exclude an upper GI source of bleeding. If the gastric aspirate is bilious and there is no blood you can effectively rule out an upper GI source. If, however,

21

the aspirate is negative for both bile and blood you will still need to rule out an upper GI source since the negative aspirate result may simply reflect spasm of the pylorus (which would prevent blood from, for example, a duodenal ulcer entering the stomach).

Small bowel visualization by enteroscopy or video capsule endoscopy? These imaging modalities have limited application in the context of *acute* lower GI haemorrhage. They are only really used if other imaging modalities have failed to find a source of haemorrhage in patients with repeated episodes of haemorrhage.

It is worth noting that the investigations may all come back negative, either because the source of bleeding cannot be found (yet there is evidence of bleeding) or because the bleeding has stopped. Angiodysplasia and a Dieulafoy lesion (a ruptured submucosal artery, most commonly at the oesophagogastric junction, but also in the small bowel and rectum) are two 'classic' causes of intermittent bleeds that may be very difficult to visualize.

Mr McCarthy passes another ~200 mL of bright red blood per rectum. His observations are still stable, but the Registrar rings the blood bank to check on the status of Mr McCarthy's cross-match as a precaution.

Proctoscopy does not reveal any obvious source of bleeding. Rigid sigmoidoscopy is not done as the ongoing bleeding would obscure the view. The endoscopist on call performs an oesophagogastroduodenoscopy because of a suspicion of possible upper GI bleeding, but it shows no stigmata of haemorrhage in the upper GI tract. The endoscopist decides that colonoscopy is likely to give inadequate views of the bowel lumen due to the continued rectal bleeding. A mesenteric angiogram is therefore performed and shows an actively bleeding area of angiodysplasia in the ascending colon which is successfully embolized by the radiologist.

What is angiodysplasia?

Colonic angiodysplasia is a submucosal arteriovenous malformation that is believed to be acquired. The cause of these lesions is unknown, but the predominance of lesions in the right colon raises the possibility that high wall tension may be a contributory factor. Typically, lesions are less than 1 cm in diameter, but they can bleed out of proportion to their size. In contrast to haemorrhage from colonic diverticular disease (which is arterial, from the vasa recta), angiodysplasia results in venous blood loss. Angiodysplasia produces a characteristic 'cherry red spot' appearance at endoscopy (although blood will frequently obscure the field of view during acute haemorrhage). The diagnosis has become more common since the advent of mesenteric angiography. It may present with frank rectal bleeding or may result in occult blood loss and subsequent anaemic symptoms. Treatment options include embolization, surgical resection, or endoscopic laser electrocoagulation.

Short cases

Mr Barnes is a 37-year-old gardener who presents to his GP following an episode of rectal bleeding. On further questioning, Mr Barnes describes that this is his first and only episode of rectal bleeding. He says that he passed a stool a few hours earlier in the day. After wiping his rear, he noticed fresh blood on the toilet paper. Upon inspecting the toilet bowl he saw drips of blood lining the side of the bowl. He describes blood in the water, but estimates that the amount was very small. To the best of his knowledge, his stool was not bloodstained. He has not experienced any abdominal or rectal pain, and has not noticed any prolapse. There has not been a change in bowel habit and he is otherwise fit and well. He has not experienced anything similar before and has no significant past medical history.

General and abdominal examination of Mr Barnes is unremarkable. He consents to a DRE. There are no perianal lesions on inspection. DRE reveals no palpable masses in the anal canal, but the gloved finger is streaked with blood when it is withdrawn.

Mr Barnes is referred to the general surgeons, who subsequently perform proctoscopy and rigid sigmoidoscopy. Proctoscopy revealed two smooth lesions in the anal canal below the dentate line – at positions corresponding to 3 o'clock and 7 o'clock when viewed with Mr Barnes in the left lateral position. Rigid sigmoidoscopy was unremarkable.

What is the diagnosis and what management options exist for Mr Barnes?

Mr Barnes is suffering from **internal haemorrhoids**.[†]

There are a variety of treatment strategies, including conservative, medical, and surgical management:

Lifestyle modification

- Increased dietary fibre, which may soften faeces and minimize straining at stool (although study evidence is somewhat lacking)
- Keep well hydrated
- Avoid straining at stool

Medical management

- Local anaesthetic creams can be used to relieve soreness and itching
- Steroidal creams/suppositories can be used to reduce local inflammation
- Evidence of efficacy for both is limited

Surgical management

There are numerous surgical options, the suitability of which may differ according to patient and the haemorrhoid characteristics:

- Rubber band ligation
- Injection sclerotherapy

21

[†] You should note, however, that the presence of haemorrhoids does not exclude the possibility of an additional and more proximal – and more sinister – culprit lesion (see viva questions).

- Infrared coagulation/photocoagulation
- Haemorrhoidectomy
- Stapled haemorrhoidopexy
- Doppler-guided haemorrhoidal artery ligation and recto-anal repair (DG-HAL-RAR)

Dr Sloane is a 63-year-old retired psychiatrist who presents to her GP complaining of rectal bleeding. She reports that she has noticed small amounts of blood on the toilet paper over the last couple of months, and that the toilet water is sometimes bloodstained. Until recently, there has never been enough blood for her to worry. However, over the past few weeks there has been more blood than normal for her. Direct questioning reveals that this blood is not bright red, but it is not melaena either. Dr Sloane remarks that she 'may not remember much from her days as a junior doctor, but I'd never forget the sight or smell of melaena!'. Instead, the blood is dark red and is mixed with the stool. The passage of blood has not been associated with any pain, and Dr Sloane denies any tenesmus. She has, however, noticed a change in her bowel habit, with looser motions over the past 6 weeks. On direct questioning, she concedes she has lost a little weight recently and has been feeling rather 'washed out'.

Dr Sloane says she has suffered with haemorrhoids since the birth of her second child 30 years ago, for which she was treated with rubber band ligation on two occasions. However, she says that neither of these treatments has been particularly successful, and she still suffers from intermittent anal itching and minor bleeds. There is no other remarkable past medical history. She takes no regular medications and has no allergies. She has never smoked, but drinks approximately 14 units of wine with meals each week.

On examination, Dr Sloane is in sinus tachycardia (107 bpm, regular). Abdominal examination reveals no masses or tenderness. A DRE reveals a small amount of dark red blood, but no masses. The GP sends bloods for FBC, urea and electrolytes (U&E), and clotting.

Her blood results are as follows:

Hb	9.1 g/dL
RBC	4.1×10^{12} cells/L
WCC	7.6×10^9 cells/L
Platelets	278×10^9 cells/L
MCV	72 fL
Urea	6.2 mM
Creatinine	71 µM
Na	136 mM
K	4.1 mM
PT	13.7 seconds
APTT	39 seconds
Ferritin	8 µg/L
CRP	6 mg/L

(CRP, C-reactive protein)

What is the most likely diagnosis? How would you proceed to investigate Dr Sloane?

While it is possible that a recurrence of her haemorrhoids could account for the blood which is streaked onto the toilet paper and dripping into the toilet pan, haemorrhoids would not account for the appearance of dark red blood which is mixed with the stool. Given the additional details of a 6-week history of altered bowel habit and weight loss you should have **colorectal carcinoma** at the top of your differential diagnosis. Dr Sloane is also suffering from iron-deficiency anaemia (microcytic red blood cells, and a low ferritin), most likely caused from occult bleeding in her GI tract.

Short case

21

She should **urgently** be referred to the colorectal surgeons where she will be investigated using proctoscopy, rigid sigmoidoscopy, and colonoscopy. In addition, it would be useful to request additional blood tests that give some insight into the possibility of liver or bone metastases: liver enzymes (although Dr Sloane's pro-thrombin time is normal), calcium, alkaline phosphatase.

21

Mr Potter is a 72-year-old retired factory worker who attends A&E following the passage of 'profuse' amounts of blood per rectum. He is immediately assessed and is deemed to be haemodynamically stable.

On further questioning, Mr Potter reports that he felt the urge to defecate while gardening at home. He went to the toilet but realized that he was not passing anything solid. On inspecting the toilet bowl he realized that he had passed 'bright red' blood and what looked to him like a few clots. His vague estimate was that a pint of blood had been passed. There was no pain associated with the bowel movement, and Mr Potter reports that he has felt very well recently. He is specifically asked about any previous episodes of rectal bleeding, tenesmus, change in bowel habit, or weight loss – and denies any of these symptoms.

Regarding his past medical history, Mr Potter suffered an ischaemic stroke 4 years ago and has hypertension, atrial fibrillation, and osteoarthrosis of the wrist. He takes warfarin, bisoprolol, atorvastatin, bendroflumethiazide, diclofenac, and omeprazole. He is a non-smoker and is teetotal.

The A&E team keep Mr Potter under observation and restrict him to his bed, fearing that if he gets up to go to the toilet he may pass more blood and collapse. The colorectal surgeons take over Mr Potter's care. They arrange for his bowel to be prepared for colonoscopy, which takes place the following day. Colonoscopy reveals mural out-pouchings throughout the left colon, with stigmata of haemorrhage (but no active bleeding) within such lesions in the sigmoid.

What is the most likely diagnosis? How would you like to manage Mr Potter?

The history of a relatively large, non-painful, bright red rectal bleed with no other associated symptoms is most suggestive of either diverticular disease or angiodysplasia. The colonscopy findings confirm that Mr Potter is indeed suffering from **diverticular disease**. The absence of any previous episodes of left iliac fossa pain, a characteristic feature of diverticulitis, is not surprising given that diverticulitis does not increase the risk of bleeding diverticular disease and it is rare for the two pathologies to coexist. Colonic diverticula are most common in the left colon and sigmoid, but it is notable that right-side diverticula (which are usually only seen when left-sided lesions are also present) have a greater propensity to bleed.

The first priority when managing Mr Potter is to establish that he is haemodynamically stable. Once this has been confirmed you can think about stopping the bleeding and preventing recurrence. Bleeding stops spontaneously in as many as 75% of patients with symptomatic diverticular disease, but there is a ~25% chance of a second bleed. In the case of Mr Potter, his haemorrhage stopped spontaneously, but his chance of future bleeds can be substantially reduced by stopping his diclofenac. NSAIDs are known to increase the risk of diverticular haemorrhage, and thus he may wish to discuss other means of controlling his arthritis with his GP. In all likelihood Mr Potter's warfarin will have been stopped following his admission to hospital. Whether to restart warfarin should involve discussion with a cardiologist.

If the rectal bleeding had not stopped, Mr Potter would likely have been taken to theatre where the portion of colon affected by bleeding diverticula would have been removed. Traditionally, patients undergo a Hartmann's procedure to resect the abnormal bowel. Some centres now advocate primary anastomosis at the time of resection (see Fig. 21.2).

21

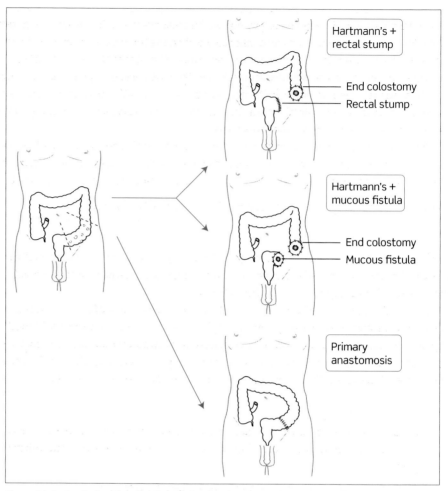

Figure 21.2 Surgical options for diverticular disease.

Mrs Chapoutier is a 26-year-old nursery nurse who presents to her GP complaining of rectal bleeding. She describes how she has noticed bright red blood on the toilet paper after wiping her rear. This has happened after every bowel motion for the past week. She adds that it is exquisitely tender for her to wipe herself and thus she does so with great care. She says defecation produces a tearing sensation in her back passage that may take up to an hour to subside. On further questioning, she says she has not noticed any blood in the toilet bowl, and has had no previous episodes of bleeding. There has been no change of bowel habit and no other symptoms.

She is otherwise fit and well, with no significant past medical history and no medications or allergies.

The GP examines Mrs Chapoutier in the left lateral position. A small, posterior, midline anal crack is visible. The examination is painful for Mrs Chapoutier and the GP does not attempt a DRE.

What is the likely diagnosis? What options exist for treating Mrs Chapoutier?

The history of a persistent tearing pain following defecation, accompanied by fresh red blood on wiping and examination findings of a posterior midline crack, indicate that Mrs Chapoutier has an **anal fissure**.

Most anal fissures are shallow and will heal spontaneously within a few weeks. Deep fissures have poor healing because sphincter spasm impairs the anal blood supply. The main aim of treatment is to relieve anal sphincter spasm and tearing of the anal mucosa, in addition to promoting healing. This can usually be achieved with medical therapy, although surgery may be needed for refractory cases:

Medical management

- A high-fibre diet coupled with laxative and non-constipating analgesics (e.g. avoid opioids) may prevent further damage (caused by hard stool) and relieve pain.
- Topical anaesthetics (e.g. lidocaine gel) can help with the pain.
- Topical glyceryl trinitrate (GTN) may increase local blood flow and relax the internal anal sphincter, thus promoting healing, but GTN often causes headaches. Topical diltiazem (calcium-channel blocker) has been advocated for use when topical GTN has been ineffective, but the evidence base is weak.
- Botox injections into the anal sphincter can relieve spasm and promote healing in patients with chronic fissures.

Surgical management

- Lateral internal sphincterotomy is very effective at reducing sphincter spasm in those patients who have failed to respond to medical therapies. The integrity of the external anal sphincter must be checked with an ultrasound scan before surgery because cutting the internal sphincter in the presence of a damaged external sphincter (e.g. due to childbirth) would cause disastrous faecal incontinence. Indeed, previously, both anal sphincters used to be manually dilated under general anaesthetic but this is no longer done as, unsurprisingly, it resulted in anal incontinence for many patients.
- Anal advancement flap is also used by some specialists.

21

Viva questions

What is the anatomical definition of 'lower' GI haemorrhage?

'Lower' GI haemorrhage refers to bleeding that arises distal to the ligament of Treitz at the duodeno-jejunal junction.

How do you classify internal haemorrhoids?

The most commonly used grading system for internal haemorrhoids reflects the degree of prolapse and reducibility, but does not necessarily reflect symptom severity:

- First degree: bleed but do not prolapse
- Second degree: prolapse but reduce spontaneously
- Third degree: prolapse and do not reduce spontaneously, but can be manually reduced
- Fourth degree: prolapse and are irreducible

What is the anatomical significance of the dentate line?

The dentate or pectinate line represents an anatomical watershed that separates zones of different epithelial cell types, arterial supply, venous drainage, lymphatic drainage, and nervous supply (see Fig. 21.3 and Table 21.3):

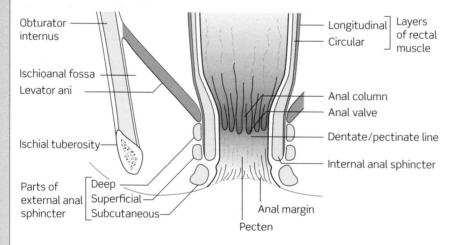

Figure 21.3 Anatomy of the anal canal.
From Monkhouse WS, *Clinical Anatomy*, p. 138, Fig. 11.37. Churchill Livingstone.

Table 21.3 Zones of the anal canal

	Above dentate line	Below dentate line
Epithelium	Columnar (mucosa)	Stratified squamous (skin)
Arterial supply	Branches of inferior mesenteric, e.g. superior rectal artery	Branches of internal iliac, e.g. inferior rectal artery
Venous drainage	Portal circulation via inferior mesenteric veins	Systemic circulation via internal iliac veins
Lymphatic drainage	Mesenteric nodes	Inguinal nodes
Innervation	Autonomic (stretch only)	Somatic (normal skin sensation)

What is the difference between diverticulosis, diverticular disease, and diverticulitis?

- Diverticulosis refers to the presence of diverticula (out-pouchings of the mucosa) in the intestine
- Symptomatic diverticulosis (e.g. bleeding, producing pain) is referred to as diverticular disease
- Diverticulitis refers to diverticular inflammation

[As an aside, colonic diverticula are not actually 'true' diverticula (out-pouchings covered by all layers of the bowel wall, as in a Meckel's diverticulum). Since colonic diverticula lack the outer coat of muscularis propria they are 'false' diverticula.]

A patient presents to you with a known diagnosis of haemorrhoids. He is now suffering acute anal pain. What is your differential diagnosis?

Uncomplicated haemorrhoids are not normally painful, thus acute pain in the anal region suggests either a complication of haemorrhoids or an additional pathology. The differential diagnosis includes:

- Thrombosed external haemorrhoid
- Anal fissure
- Proctalgia fugax (a poorly understood stabbing/cramp-like sensation in the anus, that may last up to 30 minutes, and is more common at night)
- Anal abscess
- Lower anal cancer

21

What are the known risk factors for colorectal carcinoma?

The risk factors with the strongest evidence base include:

- Increasing age
- Male sex (only for rectal carcinoma)
- Central obesity
- Colorectal disease:
  - Inflammatory bowel disease (especially ulcerative colitis, but also Crohn's)
  - Previous history of colorectal cancer
  - Colorectal polyps
  - Colorectal irradiation
- Familial conditions including:
  - Familial adenomatous polyposis (FAP)
  - Hereditary non-polyposis colorectal cancer (HNPCC)
  - Peutz–Jeghers
  - Juvenile polyposis
  - Cowden's disease
  - MYH-related polyposis
- Sedantary lifestyle (lack of regular exercise)

Dietary factors such as red meat, high fat, and low fibre may also be risk factors, but the evidence base for these is weaker (see Viva questions in Chapter 19).

How do serum ferritin and total iron-binding capacity (TIBC) help distinguish between iron-deficiency anaemia and anaemia of chronic disease? What is the role of CRP?

Ferritin is an acute-phase reactant and may be elevated by infection, inflammation, or malignancy, and is also increased by excess alcohol consumption. By requesting CRP in addition to ferritin you can establish the significance of a raised ferritin level. The only way of identifying iron-deficiency anaemia in the presence of a raised CRP level is by also looking at the TIBC.

Table 21.4 Summary of ferritin, TIBC, and CRP in anaemias

	Ferritin	TIBC	CRP
Iron-deficiency anaemia	Low	High	Normal
Anaemia of chronic disease	High	Low	Normal or High
Iron-deficiency anaemia + inflammation/infection	High	High	High

A 61-year-old patient presents to their GP with rectal bleeding, and internal haemorrhoids are identified as a probable culprit lesion. Should the patient also be referred for colonoscopy with a view to excluding colorectal carcinoma?

The presence of haemorrhoids does not exclude the possibility of an additional and more sinister culprit lesion such as malignancy, but the dilemma is in deciding which patients warrant further investigation. The National Institute for Health and Clinical Excellence (NICE) has published guidelines (2005) for the urgent referral of patients with suspected lower GI malignancy. Although these guidelines were intended for use by GPs, they also serve as a useful reference for investigation of inpatients. It is recommended that patients are referred for urgent specialist investigation in the following instances:

- Aged 40 years and older, reporting rectal bleeding with a change of bowel habit towards looser stools and/or increased stool frequency persisting 6 weeks or more.
- Aged 60 years and older, with rectal bleeding persisting for 6 weeks or more without a change in bowel habit and without anal symptoms.
- Aged 60 years and older, with a change in bowel habit to looser stools and/or more frequent stools persisting for 6 weeks or more without rectal bleeding.
- Any age with a right lower abdominal mass consistent with involvement of the large bowel.
- Any age with a palpable rectal mass (intraluminal and not pelvic; a pelvic mass outside the bowel would warrant an urgent referral to a urologist or gynaecologist).
- Men of any age with unexplained iron-deficiency anaemia (Hb ≤11 g/dL).[†]
- Non-menstruating women with unexplained iron-deficiency anaemia (Hb ≤10 g/dL).[†]

[†] Unexplained in this context means a patient whose anaemia is considered on the basis of a history and examination in primary care not to be related to other sources of blood loss (for example, ingestion of NSAIDs) or blood dyscrasia.

 For a range of Single Best Answer questions related to the topic of this chapter go to www.oxfordtextbooks.co.uk/orc/ocms/

21

Poor urinary output

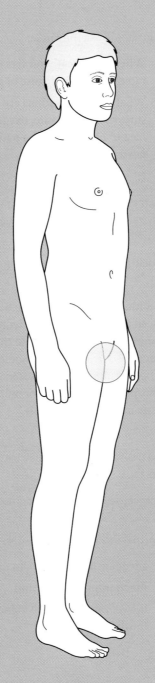

Core case

! *Read through the sections in red, covering up the sections in white that follow so that you don't see the answer. At the end of each red section, try to answer the question before reading on.*

Mr Chowdhury is a 68-year-old gentleman who is recovering from surgery. You have been bleeped at 1 a.m. and informed by the duty nurse that Mr Chowdhury has not passed any urine into his catheter bag in the last 3 hours.

What should you ask the nurse whilst they are on the phone?

You should ask the nurse:

* Whether the catheter has been checked for blockage by flushing it. This is a rapidly reversible cause of poor urinary output.

* What the observations are for the patient. Ask for the heart rate, blood pressure, respiratory rate, oxygen saturations, and temperature, so you can get an idea of how unwell the patient is. This will help you prioritize how soon you need to see the patient.

The nurse confirms that the urinary catheter is not blocked. The patient is stable, with a heart rate of 70 bpm, respiratory rate of 12/min, temperature of 36.8°C, blood pressure of 115/65 mmHg, and oxygen saturations of 97% on air.

How much urine should Mr Chowdhury be passing? Why does he need your attention?

Healthy adults have a urine output of about 1 mL/kg/hour. **Oliguria** refers to a reduced urine output and is defined variously as <400 mL/day, <0.5 mL/kg/hour or <30 mL/hour. **Anuria** refers to the complete absence of urine output.

Decreased urine output should be taken very seriously as it may be the first (and only) sign of impending acute renal failure. Untreated, patients may die from hyperkalaemia, profound acidosis, or pulmonary oedema due to the kidneys not performing their usual physiological role.

As you walk over to the surgical ward to see Mr Chowdhury, you run through the possible diagnoses causing poor urine output.

What are the possible causes for poor urine output?

Normal urine output requires:

* adequate blood supply to the kidneys;

* functioning kidneys; and

* flow of urine from the kidneys, down the ureters, into the bladder, and out via the urethra.

Pathology affecting any of these requirements can result in poor urine output, which is why the differential diagnosis for poor urinary output is often classified as shown in Table 22.1.

Table 22.1 Differential diagnosis for poor urinary output

Pre-renal (i.e. inadequate blood supply to the kidneys)	Renal (i.e. damage resulting in impaired kidney function)	Post-renal (i.e. obstruction to urinary flow)
• **Hypovolaemia** (e.g. dehydration, haemorrhage) • **Heart failure** • Reduced local perfusion of kidneys (e.g. dissecting aneurysm, renal emboli) • Decreased systemic vascular resistance (e.g. sepsis, pancreatitis)	Tubular • **Acute tubular necrosis** Glomerular • Glomerulonephritis Interstitial • Interstitial nephritis (usually caused by drugs, e.g. NSAIDs, antibiotics) Vascular • Vasculitides • Haemolytic uraemic syndrome • Thrombocytic thrombocytopenic purpura • Disseminated intravascular coagulation • Malignant hypertension • Scleroderma Infectious • Malaria • Legionnaires' disease • Leptospirosis Complex mechanism • Multiple myeloma	Ureters • Abdominal/pelvic mass (e.g. tumour) compressing ureters • Complication of pelvic surgery • Bilateral calculi • Retroperitoneal fibrosis Bladder • **Neuropathic bladder** • Anticholinergic or sympathomimetic drugs • Bladder stones or tumour • Uterovaginal prolapse (women) Urethra • **Benign prostatic hyperplasia (BPH)** • Blocked catheter • Prostate cancer • Urethral stricture • Posterior urethral valve • Trauma • Infection (e.g. herpes simplex making it painful to pass urine)

22

In practice, as a junior doctor **you want to diagnose and treat the pre-renal and post-renal causes**. If you come to the conclusion that it is a renal cause (by exclusion), call the renal physicians for an expert opinion.

> You arrive on the ward and find Mr Chowdhury fast asleep and with stable observations. You decide to look at Mr Chowdhury's notes before waking him up.
>
> **What clues in the notes might help you establish the cause of Mr Chowdhury's poor urinary output?**

Fluid balance chart

This is *crucial* in determining the diagnosis:

- **Adequate intake?** Remember that an adult of average size will require about 3 L of fluid intake per 24 hours (30–50 mL/kg/day). Febrile patients will require an extra 500 mL for every 1°C above 37.0°C to compensate for increased loss of fluids from evaporation and increased respiratory rate.

- **Positive balance?** Ensure that there is at least as much fluid going into the patient (orally or via intravenous (IV) fluids) as there is coming out (urine, fluid faeces, nasogastric (NG) tubes, vomit, stomas, drains). Don't forget to look through the notes carefully for charts because fluid balance is often documented in various separate places (e.g. NG tube output is sometimes documented separately).

Surgical operative notes

- **Type of surgery?** Pelvic surgery may result in damage to the urinary tract. Surgery to the urinary tract itself can cause damage (e.g. urethral strictures after a cystoscopic procedure). Laparotomies (especially those of long duration) can result in dehydration by evaporation of water from the open peritoneal cavity and this loss of volume will not be recorded in the fluid balance charts.

- **Blood loss?** Inadequately replaced blood loss may cause a patient to be sufficiently hypovolaemic that their kidneys cannot filter blood properly. Blood loss that has been adequately replaced may nonetheless have resulted in temporary ischaemic damage to the underperfused kidneys (ischaemic acute tubular necrosis) so that the kidneys no longer function properly.

- **Anaesthesia?** A patient with an epidural catheter delivering a local anaesthetic for post-operative pain may not be able to pass urine as the lumbosacral nerve roots may be anaesthetized. Fortunately, such patients will routinely return from theatre with a urinary catheter *in situ*. It may also be useful to check the anaesthetic chart for documentation of intraoperative fluids and fluid output – the surgical notes may state nothing more than 'haemostasis achieved', whilst the anaesthetic chart may reveal that several units of transfused blood were necessary before this was achieved.

Drug chart

- **Nephrotoxic drugs?** Some drugs are potentially damaging to the kidneys, in particular non-steroidal anti-inflammatory drugs (NSAIDs) and some antibiotics (e.g. gentamicin, vancomycin). Be prepared to stop these drugs if you conclude that there is a renal cause for the poor urinary output. Consider switching to an alternative antibiotic if appropriate.

- **Antimuscarinics? Sympathomimetics?** The parasympathetic nervous system promotes urination (detrusor contraction, internal sphincter relaxation)

The surgical notes show that Mr Chowdhury underwent an emergency splenectomy 36 hours ago after a road traffic accident. There was no external blood loss (the bleeding was intraperitoneal due to a ruptured spleen). The procedure lasted 45 minutes and the estimated blood loss was 2.5 L. The patient received 2 L of Hartmann's in accident and emergency (A&E) and 1 unit (500 mL) of O-negative blood during the operation. An indwelling urinary catheter was placed in theatre during induction of anaesthesia.

The nursing notes contain Mr Chowdhury's fluid chart (Table 22.2).

Table 22.2 Mr Chowdhury's fluid chart

Name: Janesh Chowdhury Hospital number: 13265844
Date: 01/03/2010
Nil by mouth? YES/NO   Previous day's balance:

Time	INTAKE (mL) Oral Vol. given	Oral Running total	Intravenous Vol. given	Intravenous Running total	OUTPUT (mL) Urine Vol. measured	Urine Running total	Other Vol. Measured	Other Running total
0100								
0200								
0300								
0400								
0500								
0600								
0700								
0800								
0900								
1000								
1100								
1200								
1300								
1400								
1500			1000	1000	550	550		
1600								
1700					200	750		
1800								
1900								
2000								
2100					200	950		
2200								
2300					50	1000		
2400								
TOTAL								

22

whereas the sympathetic nervous system does the opposite. Check if the patient is on antimuscarinic (i.e. antiparasympathetics such as tolterodine) or sympathomimetic medications (e.g. ephedrine).

Past medical history

From notes and previous investigations.

- **Renal function?** The patient may have long-standing renal impairment so you should compare the pre-operative creatinine and urea and electrolytes with the current results.

- **Other comorbidities?** Patients with pre-existing cardiac disease, for example, may be more vulnerable to developing acute renal failure. This can provide clues as to the aetiology (e.g. more likely to be pre-renal in patients with heart failure).

> The drug chart shows that Mr Chowdhury is on 1 g paracetamol q.d.s. [four times a day] and 100 mg tramadol p.r.n. [as needed] for analgesia. He has also been prescribed compression stockings for both legs to prevent deep vein thrombosis.
>
> Mr Chowdhury is now awake despite the late hour as the nurse has just given him his paracetamol with a cup of water. You ask the nurse how much water he has been drinking and she estimates that he has probably had one full glass of water since arriving on the wards. The bag of normal saline has about 50 mL of fluid left in it.
>
> **What is Mr Chowdhury's fluid balance status? What has happened to his urinary output over time?**

Mr Chowdhury's fluid intake/output can be tabulated as follows:

Input	Output
2 L Hartmann's	2.5 L of blood loss (estimated)
500 mL blood	1 L urine
950 L normal saline	
100 mL of oral water (rough estimate)	
Total: 3550 mL	Total: 3500 mL

It would appear that Mr Chowdhury has a positive fluid balance of 3550 – 3500 = 50 mL. Whilst this is positive, it is not great if one considers that the blood loss and the oral intake are both rough estimates. Do not be surprised by the fact that Mr Chowdhury's limited oral intake has not been documented in the fluid balance chart: it is hard to find perfectly kept charts on any busy ward.

22

Mr Chowdhury's urinary output has been dropping over time, suggesting a gradual onset of pathology (e.g. gradual dehydration) rather than a sudden one (e.g. bladder stone blocking the outlet, blood clot blocking the catheter):

Time period	Output	Rate
13:00–14:30 (2.5 hours)	550 mL	220 mL/hour
14:30–17:00 (2.5 hours)	200 mL	80 mL/hour
17:00–21:00 (4 hours)	200 mL	50 mL/hour
21:00–23:00 (2 hours)	50 mL	25 mL/hour (oliguria)
23:00–01:00 (2 hours)	0 mL	0 mL/hour (anuria)

What questions will you ask Mr Chowdhury?

Remember that it is 3 a.m. and the patient is likely to be sleepy, so keep your questions to a targeted minimum. A good approach is to think of questions which might identify some of the more likely diagnoses from the above.

Pre-renal disease (e.g. hypovolaemia, heart failure)

- **Does he feel thirsty?** A symptom of dehydration and hypovolaemia.
- **Does he feel short of breath? If yes, did he feel like this before the operation? Is it worse when exercising or lying down?** Symptoms of heart failure.

Renal disease (e.g. nephrotoxic drugs, glomerulonephritis)

You have already looked at the drug chart for nephrotoxic medications.

- **Does he have any pre-existing renal disease?** This may not be in the notes and it is worth asking.

Post-renal obstruction (e.g. BPH, blocked catheter)

He is catheterized, making post-renal obstruction very unlikely. Indeed, rather than asking the (uncatheterized) oliguric patient questions that are not that sensitive or specific, once you have excluded pre-renal causes you would catheterize them to see if obstruction was the problem.

However, were the patient not catheterized, you might expect (and ask about) lower urinary tract symptoms (LUTS), e.g. hesitancy, frequency, strangury, poor stream, terminal dribbling.

22

Mr Chowdhury says he is thirsty. He has pain around the surgical incision but not down by his bladder. He has never stopped passing urine before.

You must examine Mr Chowdhury to establish the cause of his poor urinary output.

What would you look for on examination?

- **Check the catheter bag:** you are looking to see if there has been any more urine output since the last entry in the fluid balance chart, and also for blood in the bag which would suggest the possibility of clot retention.

- **Signs of dehydration:** dry lips, mouth, and tongue; sunken eyes. Dark urine (check the urinary catheter bag). If the patient is becoming hypovolaemic, you may also find tachycardia, a narrow pulse pressure, and eventually a low blood pressure. A lying versus standing blood pressure showing a significant postural drop is another important clue suggesting hypovolaemia. It is important to be aware of the signs of intravascular hydration status versus extravascular hydration status – the former is the critical parameter in this instance, and the relevant markers are pulse, blood pressure, capillary refill time, and jugular venous pressure (JVP). Remember that it is perfectly possible for a patient to be overloaded with fluid in the extravascular compartment, but to be fluid depleted intravascularly, e.g. septic shock. You may also see an increased respiratory rate, particularly in children.

- **Signs of heart failure (i.e. fluid overloaded):** raised JVP; displaced apex beat; gallop rhythm (third heart sound); bilateral and basal lung crepitations; dependent oedema (sacrum if in bed). Beware oedematous patients though, as their intravascular volume may be depleted, with the potential for renal hypoperfusion.

- **Signs of urinary retention due to post-renal obstruction:** palpable, distended bladder that is dull to percussion (as it is filled with fluid). Pressing may stimulate the urge to urinate.

- **Digital rectal examination:** compulsory in anyone not catheterized with poor urinary output. Check for a colon loaded with faeces and for an enlarged prostate.

(In women with poor urinary output, you might consider a bimanual vaginal examination to check for pelvic masses that may be compressing the ureters or urethra.)

On examination, Mr Chowdhury is obviously tired. The urinary catheter bag contains very dark urine from earlier in the day. His lips are moist (as he has just had water to take his medication). His eyes do not appear sunken although his skin turgor shows some loss of elasticity. His heart rate is 110 bpm, regular. His blood pressure is 115/85 mmHg. His JVP is not raised and his apex is undisplaced. He does not have any dependent oedema but there are faint crackles in the bases of both lungs. His abdomen is tender around the subcostal incision but his bladder is neither palpable nor tender.

What do your findings suggest so far?

22

- **Hypovolaemia.** Mr Chowdhury has experienced a gradual decrease in urinary output. He is only just in positive fluid balance, if one assumes the estimates of blood loss are accurate. His urine is very dark, his skin turgor is reduced, he is tachycardic, and has a narrow pulse pressure. This all suggests that Mr Chowdhury has become progressively dehydrated and hypovolaemic, and this may well account for his gradual decrease in urinary output.

- **?Heart failure.** Mr Chowdhury has bilateral basal lung crackles. Whilst these could be due to heart failure, there is no other evidence for this. It is more likely that they are due to post-operative atelectasis: small areas of alveolar collapse that are common after surgery.

> You suspect that Mr Chowdhury has reduced urinary output due to hypovolaemia, a fairly common scenario in post-operative patients.
>
> **What investigations will you arrange?**

- **Check that the catheter has been flushed.** It is possible that Mr Chowdhury's urinary catheter has become blocked. Although this would typically cause a sudden drop in urinary output (rather than a gradual one as is the case here) you should always check that the urinary catheter is patent. Using aseptic technique, gently flush 100 mL of normal saline up the catheter. You should not meet any resistance – if you do, it suggests a blockage and you should replace the catheter.
- **Venous blood gas:** this is a quick way of getting his electrolyte balance (particularly potassium), acid–base status, and haematocrit.
- **Bloods:** you are mainly interested in the markers of renal function: urea and creatinine. If the urea is raised, it suggests hypovolaemia. If the creatinine is also raised, it suggests renal injury (e.g. acute tubular necrosis). You are also interested in the electrolytes and glucose so that you can calculate the serum osmolarity. You should interpret the results in the context of previous investigations.
- **Fluid challenge:** if you suspect the cause of oliguria/anuria is hypovolaemia, give the patient a bolus of 250 mL normal saline, stat (i.e. under gravity, fast flowing). Monitor the urine output and basic observations (pulse, blood pressure etc.) carefully. If his observations and urine output improve over the next hour and stay like that, you have solved the problem. If they improve but fall back again, the patient was indeed hypovolaemic but needs even more fluids – try another fluid challenge. If it does not increase, consider the possibility that the patient is not hypovolaemic. If the patient becomes short of breath and his JVP rises, it suggests fluid overload, i.e. congestive heart failure.
- **Urine versus serum concentrations:** comparing urinary versus serum concentrations of Na^+ or creatinine, for example, can sometimes be useful in distinguishing pre-renal from renal causes. However, these investigations often yield an intermediate value that is of no diagnostic value:
  - Pre-renal: if the patient is hypovolaemic but the kidneys are still working, the urine will be very concentrated relative to the serum; and the urinary Na^+ will be low as the kidneys desperately try to reabsorb Na^+ and water to combat the hypovolaemia.
  - Renal: if the kidneys are failing, they will be unable to concentrate urine effectively by reabsorbing Na^+ and water. The urine osmolality will therefore be dilute relative to the serum, but will have high Na^+.

In patients who are not catheterized (i.e. not Mr Chowdhury), you should consider an **ultrasound** to exclude post-renal causes.

22

Mr Chowdhury's catheter can be easily flushed with 100 mL of normal saline, suggesting no obstruction at all. His venous blood gas and urinalysis are unremarkable. You take bloods and send a sample of urine off to the labs for osmolality and urine Na^+. Meanwhile, you start Mr Chowdhury on a 250 mL bolus of normal saline, stat. You ask the nurse to kindly record his observations and urine output every 30 minutes. You return to assess Mr Chowdhury an hour later and see from his fluid chart that he passed 40 mL of urine during the first 30 minutes and 20 mL of urine during the next half hour. Mr Chowdhury still has reduced skin turgor but his heart rate is now 90 bpm and his blood pressure is 115/70 mmHg. The blood results are now available and show:

Na	134 mM
K	3.6 mM
Cl	102 mM
Urea	19 mM
Creatinine	125 mM
Glucose	5.8 mM

What is the reason for Mr Chowdhury's poor urinary output? How will you manage him?

Mr Chowdhury has experienced a gradual decrease in urinary output that responds transiently to a fluid bolus. In addition, he has shown clinical signs of hypovolaemia and has a raised urea. This suggests that the reason for Mr Chowdhury's poor urinary output is **pre-renal hypovolaemia**, probably due to insufficient fluid replacement. This case illustrates the importance of always assessing and reassessing the patient clinically when working out fluid balance in a patient, rather than relying on fluid charts which can be helpful but often incorrect (due to estimations and inadequate clerking).

The fact that the fluid bolus corrected the situation only transiently suggests Mr Chowdhury is still dehydrated. You should correct the dehydration with further fast IV fluids until his observations normalize and remain so. You then need to remember to keep him on maintenance fluids. Convention is to give 3 L over 24 hours, comprising 1 L of normal saline (+20 mM K^+) and 2 × 1 L of 5% dextrose (+20 mM K^+). This should provide 3 L of water and the correct amount of electrolytes, but you will obviously have to adjust this for individual patients based on the urea and electrolyte (U&E) results.

Mr Chowdhury's urine output remained adequate for the next few days and he was eventually discharged home.

22

Short cases

> Mr Garcia is a 76-year-old retired teacher who presents to his local hospital complaining that he has been unable to pass any urine for the last 8 hours. He has the urge to pass urine intermittently every half hour or so, and his lower abdomen is very painful. He is not constipated, having opened his bowels once a day regularly up to and including last night. He has had a poor stream and frequency for many months but never sought help as he assumed it was just him 'getting old'. On examination, his bladder is palpable and tender in the suprapubic area of the abdomen. An enlarged, smooth, symmetrical prostate with a central sulcus can be palpated on digital rectal examination and his rectum contains some soft faeces.
>
> **What is the likely diagnosis? How should Mr Garcia be managed?**

Mr Garcia has presented with a painful desire but inability to urinate: **acute urinary obstruction**. You know it is acute or acute-on-chronic as he has pain, and chronic obstruction is painless. This is almost certainly due to his enlarged prostate, which is probably **BPH** given its smooth and symmetrical nature. However, prostate cancer is also a possibility.

Management of Mr Garcia will consist of:

1) **Catheterization and IV fluids:** if you cannot pass a standard 16G urinary catheter due to an enlarged prostate, try gently with a larger and more rigid catheter. Catheterization will void the bladder (the patient will be very grateful) and give you a clue about the pathogenesis: if the volume voided is >1 L, it suggests this is an acute-on-chronic urinary retention, as acute retention alone rarely gets to such a large volume. IV fluids should be set up in advance to compensate for the expected diuresis that often follows relief of the urinary obstruction and which can otherwise lead to substantial hypotension.

2) **Assess renal function:** assess renal function by monitoring blood urea, creatinine, and electrolytes, and by monitoring urine output over the subsequent 12–48 hours with the catheter. If the creatinine is raised you should anticipate a diuresis.

3) **Assess cause of obstruction:** the most likely cause is BPH, as Mr Garcia is not constipated. Prostate cancer should be kept in mind, particularly since the digital rectal examination revealed an enlarged prostate. Suspected prostate cancer should be investigated with a prostate-specific antigen (PSA) test and a urology referral where relevant.

4) **Trial without catheter (TWOC):** if the patient voided <1 L upon catheterization and has normal renal function, they are suitable for a TWOC. The patient is started on an α-blocker (to relax the internal urinary sphincter) and given a single dose of antibiotics (to prevent urinary tract infection after the catheter is removed) and then one simply waits to see if the patient can urinate.
   - If they can urinate, they are discharged on an α-blocker or 5α-reductase inhibitor but warned that the risk of recurrence is very high (up to 70% over a year).
   - If they cannot urinate, they are discharged with an indwelling or intermittent catheter and booked for a surgical solution to their problem, most likely a transurethral resection of the prostate (TURP).

22

Mrs Janeway is a 52-year-old lady who is well known to her local A&E. She has attended 125 times over the last 10 years, usually because of back pain or other musculoskeletal pain and demanding opioid analgesia. She is the principal carer for her husband, who is disabled due to multiple sclerosis.

Mrs Janeway was lifting her husband out of bed the day before when she suddenly developed lower back pain. The pain was excruciating at first but gradually became more bearable as the day went by and she took some ibuprofen and paracetamol. However, she has not been able to pass any urine for 12 hours. She has a strong urge to go and finds her bladder painful. She last opened her bowels before the onset of back pain but usually only passes faeces a few times a week anyway. She has not noticed any loss of sensation or power in her lower limbs.

On examination, the range of movement in Mrs Janeway's lower spine is severely restricted due to pain. Her lower limbs have reduced power (4/5 on the MRC power scale) and reduced knee and ankle reflexes. Her plantar reflexes are downgoing, and both coordination and sensation in the lower limbs appear normal. On digital rectal examination there is marked perianal numbness and lax anal tone. Throughout the clerking, Mrs Janeway begs for Entonox (nitrous oxide gas and air) for the pain and for something to 'let her pee'. A urinary catheter is placed and she voids 560 mL of urine, much to Mrs Janeway's relief.

Which diagnosis should you be worried about? What should the next step in management be?

Mrs Janeway has presented with lower back pain, urinary retention (it would be difficult to voluntarily retain >500 mL of urine), signs of a lower motor neuron lesion affecting both lower limbs, perianal numbness, and lax anal tone. Until proven otherwise radiologically, this is **cauda equina syndrome**. This is a medical emergency whereby the lumbosacral nerve roots that form the cauda equina in the spinal canal become compressed (usually by a centrally prolapsing intervertebral disc). This results in a lower motor neuropathy affecting the bladder sphincters, bowel sphincters, and lower limbs.

Cauda equina syndrome needs urgent attention from neurosurgeons. Mrs Janeway needs an urgent magnetic resonance imaging (MRI) scan of her back to investigate the possibility of cauda equina compression and, if this is confirmed, she will need an urgent surgical intervention to decompress the affected nerve roots (Fig. 22.1). The longer treatment is delayed, the less likely she is to recover any loss of function.

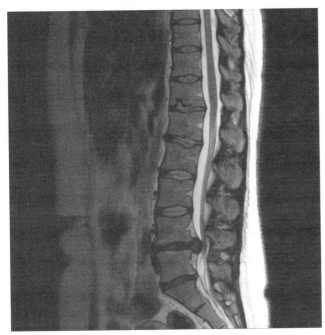

Figure 22.1 Magnetic resonance imaging (MRI) scan showing cauda equina syndrome due to an intervertebral disc prolapse.
With kind permission from Dr J. Teh.

22

Mr Bodden is 64-year-old gentleman who presents to his GP because of problems passing urine. For some months now, he has noticed his urine 'spraying' when he goes to the toilet. However, for the past few weeks he has found it hard to pass urine, having to spend minutes at a time in the toilet as his urine painfully drips out slowly. He is worried that this is related to his bladder cancer. He has not noticed any discharge from his urethra and declares that he otherwise feels fit and well.

His medical notes reveal that he has had transitional carcinoma of the bladder, papillary type, for the last 6 years. For this, he receives regular cystoscopies to resect the low-grade tumour and to inject Bacille Calmette–Guérin (BCG) into the bladder. His last cystoscopy was 6 weeks ago.

What is the likely diagnosis? What is the next step?

It is likely that Mr Bodden has developed a **urethral stricture** due to the repeated trauma to his urethra over the years of cystoscopies. The next step is to refer Mr Bodden to the urological surgeons and visualize the actual stricture if it exists (using, ironically, cystoscopy). If a urethral stricture is found, treatment options include dilating the urethra, a urethral stent, a cystoscopic urethrotomy (a small incision to relieve the stricture), or surgery to remove the affected portion of urethra altogether.

Mrs Jackson is a 32-year-old lady recovering on an obstetric ward from emergency surgery for heavy post-partum haemorrhage. You have been called because her urine output has consistently been <20 mL/hour since the operation. The operative notes estimate that she lost 2 L of blood but she received four units (~2 L) of blood during the operation and a further 2 L of Hartmann's solution over the last 16 hours on the ward.

Mrs Jackson looks pale and lethargic, with stable observations and a catheter in place that has been flushed. She denies any urge to pass urine, although she still has an epidural anaesthetic *in situ*. She is not thirsty and does not feel short of breath. Her heart rate is 80 bpm and her blood pressure is 130/80 mmHg. Her JVP is visible at about 6 cm above the manubriosternal angle and there are faint crackles at the bases of her lungs.

The latest bloods (taken post-operatively) for Mrs Jackson reveal:

Na	131 mM
K	4.8 mM
Cl	104 mM
Urea	11.4 mM
Creatinine	280 mM
Glucose	5.5 mM

What is the likely diagnosis? What is the next step?

Pre-renal cause of oliguria?

A pre-renal cause of oliguria (e.g. hypovolaemia, heart failure) is unlikely. Mrs Jackson is currently fluid overloaded (high JVP, pulmonary oedema) and is very young for heart failure.

Post-renal cause of oliguria?

A post-renal cause of oliguria (e.g. ureter damage, urinary tract obstruction) is unlikely in this case, as Mrs Jackson is catheterized and has passed some urine since the operation, although it must be ruled out. If a post-renal cause is suspected, Mrs Jackson should be referred to the urological surgeons.

Renal cause of oliguria?

A renal cause of oliguria (e.g. nephrotoxic medications, acute tubular necrosis due to previous hypovolaemia) is very likely in Mrs Jackson by default, given that pre-renal and post-renal causes appear unlikely. If a renal cause is suspected, Mrs Jackson should be referred to the renal physicians.

Next steps?

- **Stop her IV fluids.** She is already fluid overloaded.
- **Check her drug chart** for nephrotoxic drugs that can be stopped (e.g. NSAIDs).
- **Renal tract ultrasound** or **CT scan** to confirm intact ureters and rule out hydronephrosis due to obstruction. Small kidneys with poor corticomedullary differentiation suggest this is actually a long-standing kidney failure that may have suddenly deteriorated.

22

- **Assess the need for dialysis.** Hyperkalaemia, a large rise in the urea, severe acidosis, and intractable fluid overload are indications for urgent dialysis.
- **Urine analysis.** Haematuria may suggest renal tract damage. Its absence makes a glomerulonephritis less likely. A raised urine albumin:creatinine ratio can suggest nephrotic syndrome.
- **Blood tests:** A low Ca^{2+} and high inorganic phosphate (P_i) are suggestive of chronic renal failure, but can sometimes occur in acute renal failure, too.

Ultimately, the most likely cause of renal failure in Mrs Jackson is **acute tubular necrosis** due to the prolonged renal ischaemia that followed from her post-partum haemorrhage. Most patients with acute tubular necrosis recover 80% of their kidney function (in terms of creatinine clearance) over the next 2–8 weeks.

Viva questions

What are the main complications of urethral bladder catheterization?

- Urethral trauma (pain, bleeding)
- Urethral scarring and stricture (slow-flowing micturition, painful micturition, urinary retention)
- Creation of a false passage in the urethra (pain, infection)
- Urinary tract infection (dysuria, confusion, pyelonephritis), particularly with *Proteus mirabilis* which is a highly motile bacterium that can swim up the catheter
- Bladder perforation (pain, bleeding, peritonitis)

What are the main complications of chronic urinary retention?

- Urinary incontinence due to overflow. The patient may not be able to void the bladder completely but will 'dribble' small amounts of urine uncontrollably
- Urinary tract infection (upper or lower) due to urinary stasis in the bladder
- Bladder stones due to urinary stasis
- Hydronephrosis (dilatation of the ureters and kidney calices)
- Renal failure (secondary to the hydronephrosis)
- Acute-on-chronic urinary retention (painful, unlike chronic urinary retention)
- Bladder wall hypertrophy (trabeculation) and out-pouchings (diverticula)

What are the principal physiological mechanisms for regulating serum volume and serum osmolarity?

Volume is primarily regulated by the **renin–angiotensin–aldosterone** axis. Renin is released by the kidneys in response to signals from the body that circulating volume is low. Amongst other effects, it stimulates the production of angiotensin I in the liver and its conversion to angiotensin II by the angiotensin-converting enzyme (ACE) produced in the lungs. Angiotensin II has many effects (aimed at increasing blood pressure), including vasoconstriction and stimulating the release of aldosterone from the adrenal cortex. Aldosterone acts on the distal tubule to increase sodium (and hence water) uptake into the blood.

Osmolarity is primarily regulated by **antidiuretic hormone** (ADH, vasopressin), released by the posterior pituitary. ADH increases water (but not sodium) reabsorption in the distal tubule, concentrating the urine and diluting the serum.

Which nerves, neurotransmitters, and receptors are responsible for bladder control and micturition? How is this applied in the pharmacological treatment of continence problems?

Urine is continuously produced but its release (micturition) is controlled by the bladder. The first urge to void is normally felt at around 200 mL (total bladder capacity is 300–500 mL), conveyed by afferent stretch fibres in the bladder wall. These relay information to the pons, which is responsible for the micturition reflex.

The sympathetic, parasympathetic, and somatic nervous systems are all involved in bladder control (Fig. 22.2):

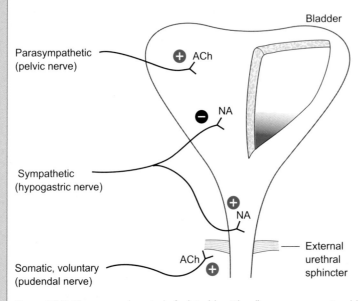

Figure 22.2 The neuronal control of micturition. The diagram represents a bladder with a section missing to show urine inside.

- The smooth muscle (detrusor) of the bladder wall is under joint control of the parasympathetic and sympathetic nervous systems. The parasympathetic system, via the pelvic nerve and muscarinic acetylcholine receptors, stimulates detrusor muscle contraction. Antimuscarinics, e.g. tolterodine and oxybutynin, are used in individuals with incontinence due to an overactive bladder. The sympathetic system, via a branch of the hypogastric nerve and using noradrenaline as a neurotransmitter, inhibits the detrusor muscle.

- The internal urethral sphincter is made of smooth muscle and is therefore under sympathetic control, mediated by the action of noradrenaline on alpha receptors. The input arises from another branch of the hypogastric nerve. α-Adrenergic blockers, e.g. doxazosin and prazosin, act on these receptors to block sphincter contraction and so are used to alleviate outflow obstruction.

- The external urethral sphincter is made of striated muscle and is under voluntary control, i.e. the somatic nervous system, via the pudendal nerve. The neuromuscular junction contains nicotinic acetylcholine receptors.

- The pelvic floor and striated muscle of the urethra are also under voluntary control.

Micturition occurs when bladder pressure exceeds urethral pressure.

Which drugs commonly cause urinary retention?

Any drug with antimuscarinic effects can cause urinary retention, particularly:

- Antihistamines (e.g. chlorpheniramine, cetirizine)
- Tricyclic antidepressants (e.g. amitryptilline, imipramine)
- Drugs used to treat urinary incontinence (e.g. tolterodine, oxybutynin)

What are the indications for dialysis in the acute setting (e.g. at 3 a.m.)?

If the patient is in acute renal failure (i.e. oliguria or anuria with deranged renal function) and has any or all of the following, they are a candidate for dialysis:

- Severe hyperkalaemia ≥ 6.5 mM
- Severe acidosis pH ≤ 7.2
- Severe pulmonary oedema
- Urea ≥ 30 mM and creatinine ≥ 1000 μM
- Uraemic encephalopathy

Otherwise the patient can wait for an urgent (same day) inpatient renal referral.

A 55-year-old man requests that his prostate-specific antigen (PSA) levels be tested to check whether he has prostate cancer. Is the PSA test any good for screening for prostate cancer in asymptomatic men?

When considering whether to offer PSA testing to asymptomatic men, there are two main issues to consider:

1) How good is the test?
2) Is there an effective treatment?

How good is the test?

A lot of patients will enquire about the usefulness of the PSA test for detecting prostate cancer. Figure 22.3 shows what would happen if you screened a population of 1000 asymptomatic men aged 50–70 using the PSA test.

22

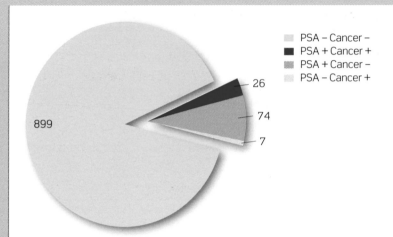

Figure 22.3 Incidence of prostate-specific antigen (PSA) test positives and true cancers in men aged 50–70 years.

As you can see, the vast majority of those with a raised PSA will *not* have prostate cancer on transrectal biopsy of the prostate. The vast majority of men with a raised PSA will actually have either BPH or prostatitis. However, the usefulness of the PSA test for diagnosing prostate cancer can be increased somewhat by setting various cut-off values, rather than simply reporting 'positive' or 'negative':

PSA <3 ng/mL	Very low risk of prostate cancer (~0.7%)
PSA 3–10 ng/mL	Moderate risk of prostate cancer
PSA >10 ng/mL	High risk of prostate cancer
PSA >40 ng/mL	High risk of metastatic prostate cancer
PSA >100 ng/mL	Almost certainly metastatic prostate cancer

Thus, the PSA test is useful if it is <3 ng/mL (prostate cancer unlikely, but still possible) or >10 ng/mL (prostate cancer likely). Unfortunately, most patients with a positive PSA lie in the 3–10 ng/mL range and will need referring according to local/national guidelines (which are often age related). For these patients, one needs to keep in mind that:

- The majority of patients with a PSA of 3–10 ng/mL will *not* have prostate cancer.
- Finding out which of them have cancer involves a transrectal prostate biopsy. This involves a rectal probe that inserts several (up to 12) needles through the rectal wall, into the prostate. The procedure is uncomfortable, often painful, and can cause prostatitis, sepsis, rectal bleeding, and (very rarely) death.

So, is the PSA test useful for detecting prostate cancer?

- **YES,** if the patient has possible **symptoms** of prostate cancer (prostatism, bone pain) as a diagnosis of prostate cancer will then dictate treatment that can help with symptoms.
- **YES,** if the PSA turns out to be **>10 ng/mL** as a diagnosis of prostate cancer is then likely and detecting prostate cancer at an early stage improves prognosis.
- **NO,** if the PSA turns out to be 3–10 ng/mL as the patient will then be anxious about prostate cancer, may undergo a significant procedure (biopsy), and may be diagnosed with a prostate cancer that would never have caused any problems (as a significant proportion of prostate cancers cause no problems).

Is there an effective treatment for prostate cancer?

Prostate cancer is *very* common (60% of men over 80 years), usually asymptomatic (90% of cases), and usually not fatal (75% of cases). The management of prostate cancer depends on the stage and grade of the prostate cancer. At present, National Institute for Health and Clinical Excellence (NICE) guidelines suggest the management strategy shown in Table 22.1.

Table 22.1 NICE guidelines for the management of prostate cancer

Prostate cancer	Preferred treatment	Alternatives
In situ, low Gleeson grade	Active surveillance[†]	Prostatectomy[‡]
In situ, high Gleeson grade	Prostatectomy *or* radiotherapy + LHRH analogues	Brachytherapy
Locally invasive	Prostatectomy *or* radiotherapy + LHRH analogues	
Metastatic	LHRH analogues, antitestosterones, oestrogens	

LHRH, luteinizing hormone-releasing hormone.

[†] Active surveillance involves regular (every 3 months) review of symptoms, PSA testing, and digital rectal examination, as well as a transrectal ultrasound ± biopsy every few years.

[‡] A recent trial suggested that prostatectomy offers a survival advantage over active surveillance in this group of patients [Bill-Axelson A *et al.* (2008). *J Natl Cancer Inst*, **100**: 1144-1154].

For a range of Single Best Answer questions related to the topic of this chapter go to
www.oxfordtextbooks.co.uk/orc/ocms/

22

Polyuria

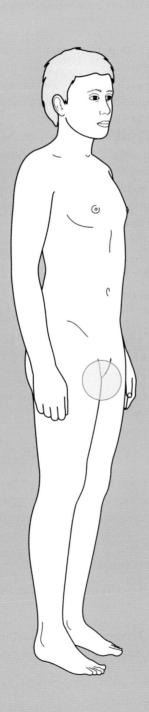

Core case

! *Read through the sections in red, covering up the sections in white that follow so that you don't see the answer. At the end of each red section, try to answer the question before reading on.*

Mr George is a 74-year-old retired taxi driver who presents to his general practitioner (GP) complaining that he is going to the toilet 'all the time'.

What would you ask to work out whether this is polyuria or high urinary frequency?

In both polyuria and high urinary frequency the patient will be passing urine more often than before. But in polyuria, patients will pass **large volumes** of clear urine each time. In urinary frequency, the volume voided each time will be normal or reduced. The only way of knowing objectively whether this is the case is by collecting a 24-hour urine sample (>3 L = polyuria). As this is usually impractical outside of hospital, one must rely on the patient's recall, with the caveat that many patients find it difficult to estimate urine output. In the history, then, ask them whether they feel they are passing a larger volume every time they go to the toilet.

Remember that it is important to be as sure as you can that you are dealing with polyuria and not urinary frequency or nocturia, as the differential diagnoses are quite distinct.

You ask Mr George and his responses indicate he has polyuria.

What is the differential diagnosis for polyuria?

Diabetes mellitus (type 1 or type 2)
Diuretics
Diabetes insipidus (cranial or nephrogenic)
Primary polydipsia
Hyperuricaemia

Chronic renal failure and hypercalcaemia (e.g. due to bone metastases) cause polyuria by inducing nephrogenic diabetes insipidus. Similarly, steroids and Cushing's syndrome can cause polyuria by causing diabetes mellitus, but this is rare.

The history can help to separate out some of the causes above.

What questions in the history will narrow down the differential?

- **Temporal pattern of urine output** (number of times in the day and at night), especially **nocturia**. At night, the kidneys concentrate urine in order to retain fluid (as intake is zero), removing the need to urinate during sleep. Thus nocturia (in the absence of other causes of nocturia, e.g. benign prostatic hyperplasia (BPH)) is often one of the earliest signs of a loss of concentrating ability. This symptom makes primary polydipsia less likely.

- **Fatigue, weight loss, recurrent infections**. All can be features of diabetes mellitus.

- **Lower urinary tract symptoms (LUTS)**, e.g. frequency, urgency, hesitancy, terminal dribbling, incomplete voiding. These symptoms indicate pathology in the bladder or the outflow tract, e.g. prostatism in men, detrusor instability and prolapse in women. Not strictly speaking polyuria.

- **Pain, frequency, change in urine colour and smell**. These are all symptoms suggestive of a urinary tract infection (UTI), which would cause increased *frequency* but not polyuria.

- **Past medical history**. Look for any history of renal problems or conditions that may precipitate chronic renal failure (e.g. vasculitides, hypertension, chronic urinary retention). In older patients, ask about cancer and known bony involvement, as this is one of the most common causes of hypercalcaemia. Primary polydipsia is more common in patients with a history of psychiatric disorders (although hyponatraemia from polydipsia may itself cause mania).

- **Drug history**. Diuretics are a potential and obvious cause of polyuria.

- **Family history**. There is a hereditary component to diabetes mellitus and some forms of cancer. Familial forms of diabetes insipidus (both nephrogenic and cranial) present very early in life.

Mr George tells you he has been passing urine on average 10 times a day for the past week, and has to get up three or four times every night to pass urine, which is bothering his wife (Ms Bungle). He has not been particularly fatigued, had any weight loss, or recent infections.

His past medical history is notable for chronic back pain over the past 18 months and occasional heartburn, for which he takes diclofenac and omeprazole (he finds his heartburn returns if he stops the omeprazole). He takes no other medications and has no drug allergies. His parents both died in their 80s but he cannot remember what from. His brother is alive and well, and Mr George knows of no conditions running in his family.

As examination rarely reveals anything about the cause of polyuria, the GP moves straight to investigations.

What investigations should the GP request?

23

First and foremost the GP should perform:

- **Capillary blood glucose**, to look for diabetes mellitus.
- **Urinalysis** with a dipstick, to exclude a UTI. This would give urinary frequency without polyuria, but it is important to exclude given the different management pathways and the fact that patients often confuse urinary frequency with polyuria. Urinalysis can also detect glucosuria and ketonuria, other signs of diabetes mellitus.

As a next step, the GP should request the following investigations:

- **Fasting plasma glucose**. If the capillary blood glucose is towards the upper limit of normal (or indeed above), the GP should request a fasting plasma glucose to exclude diabetes mellitus. This also allows you to calculate serum osmolarity.

- **Urine osmolality**. There are two different mechanisms that lead to polyuria, with differing effects on urine osmolality:
  - Inability to reabsorb solutes by the kidneys. The solutes (e.g. glucose, urea) remain in the urine and keep water with them, leading to *high urine osmolality* (>300 mOsm) and volume.
  - Inability to reabsorb water due to distal tubule pathology or a deficient antidiuretic hormone (ADH) pathway. This results in *low urine osmolality* (<250 mOsm).

- **Electrolytes**. In primary polydipsia, the serum sodium will be dilute due to the excessive water intake. In all other pathologies, the serum sodium will be concentrated as the patient is dehydrated. These abnormalities will be mirrored in the other electrolytes. You will also need the potassium if you want to calculate serum osmolarity.

- **Urea, creatinine, and estimated glomerular filtration rate (eGFR)**. This will help you exclude chronic kidney failure.

- **Serum calcium**. Although Mr George's clinical picture doesn't suggest hypercalcaemia, it is still worth excluding with a simple blood test.

The GP tests Mr George's capillary blood glucose, which is 5.2 mM. Urinalysis is unremarkable. He then proceeds to request a fasting plasma glucose, urine osmolality, serum sodium, and serum calcium. The results come back:

Glucose (fasting)	5.4 mM
Na	144 mM
K	3.7 mM
Ca (corrected)	2.51 mM
Urea	7.2 mM
Creatinine	130 µM
eGFR	110 mL/minute
Urine osmolality	242 mOsm

What is the most likely diagnosis? How does this cause the diuresis?

23

The polyuria, absence of symptoms of diabetes mellitus, and normal blood and urine glucose suggest this is not diabetes mellitus. The low urine osmolality and normal serum sodium indicate that the kidney is failing to reabsorb water. The most likely diagnosis is a problem with the ADH pathway: **diabetes insipidus**. As a result the kidneys do not concentrate the urine and the patient, unable to retain fluid, passes large quantities of urine.

The next step is to determine which subtype of diabetes insipidus Mr George is suffering from.

What is the difference between the subtypes of diabetes insipidus?
What test can you use to distinguish them, and what are the principles behind this test?

There are two subtypes of diabetes insipidus that have a different underlying mechanism:

1) **Cranial**. ADH secretion is either reduced or absent due to a defect in the hypothalamic–pituitary axis. Consequently the signal to the kidneys to concentrate the urine is weak or absent. Causes include head injury (particularly whiplash injuries in car accidents), pituitary tumours, craniopharyngiomas or metastases, surgery, a vascular lesion, and meningitis.

2) **Nephrogenic**. The kidneys become less sensitive to ADH, and therefore do not respond to signals to concentrate the urine. This insensitivity may follow renal damage caused by low potassium, high calcium, drugs such as lithium, pyelonephritis, hydronephrosis, or may be inherited.

The **water deprivation test** can be used to distinguish between these two. As the name implies, the patient is fluid restricted. The normal response to water deprivation is release of ADH from the pituitary causing the kidneys to concentrate the urine. In diabetes insipidus, the urine remains abnormally dilute. However, if desmopressin, an artificial ADH analogue, is given, those with cranial diabetes insipidus (but normal kidneys) will be able to concentrate their urine. Those with nephrogenic diabetes insipidus will continue to have dilute urine. This is a very labour-intensive test, so before you start, you should confirm there is *true polyuria* by ensuring a 24-hour urine collection is >3 L. The test is also potentially dangerous in patients with diabetes insipidus as the deprivation of water intake can cause hypovolaemia, so patients must be weighed throughout and the test must be stopped if there is body weight loss of >3%.

The approach to the patient with polyuria outlined above is summarized in the flow chart in Fig. 23.2.

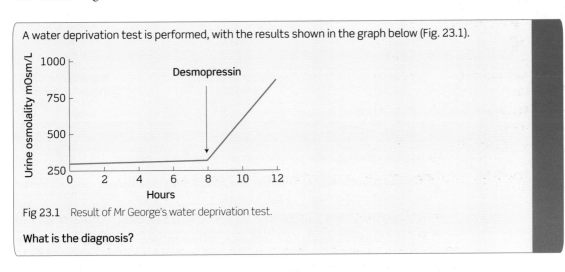

A water deprivation test is performed, with the results shown in the graph below (Fig. 23.1).

Fig 23.1   Result of Mr George's water deprivation test.

What is the diagnosis?

23

Mr George has diabetes insipidus, as indicated by his inability to concentrate urine despite water deprivation. The correction on administration of the ADH analogue desmopressin demonstrates that this is due to a lack of ADH, i.e. he has cranial diabetes insipidus.

Given Mr George's diagnosis, how should he be managed?

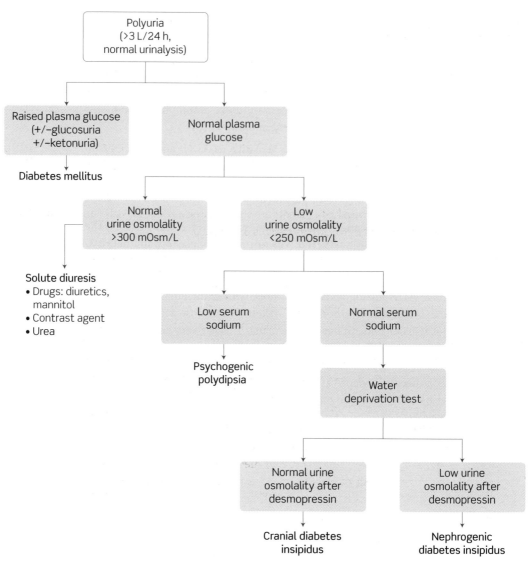

Fig 23.2   The diagnostic approach to polyuria.

Mr George's management should consist of the following:

1) **Adequate fluid intake**. This may be enough if his condition is mild. However, patients should be wary of dehydration.

2) **Investigation of the underlying cause**. Where no obvious cause is present (e.g. intracranial surgery), a magnetic resonance imaging (MRI) scan of the head should be performed to look for a pituitary lesion (about 25% of cases are due to intracranial tumours). Mr George should also be referred to an endocrinology unit.

3) **Replacement ADH**. If no reversible cause for the cranial diabetes insipidus is found (e.g. a pituitary tumour), patients will have to take replacement ADH for life.

Other medications are sometimes used in nephrogenic diabetes insipidus (e.g. chlorpropamide, carbamazepine) but not in cranial diabetes insipidus.

Short cases

Jane is a 17-year-old who presents to her GP complaining of increasing urinary frequency and thirst over the last month. She believes that over this month she has been passing a greater volume of urine every day. She has had no dysuria and there has been no change in the smell or colour of her urine. She has been drinking copious amounts of water in keeping with her thirst. The polydipsia has been going on since she started passing more urine, which makes sense to her. She hasn't felt particularly tired but has been losing weight – about 5 kg in the last 6 months. She has had two chest infections and a UTI in the last year, which she feels is unusual as she had always considered herself very healthy.

She has had eczema and childhood asthma in the past but is currently well and takes no medications other than the oral contraceptive pill. Her parents are alive and well with no medical history of note, but her older sister was diagnosed with diabetes mellitus 3 years ago.

What is the most likely diagnosis? Which investigation(s) will you order, and what are the diagnostic criteria?

Jane presents with polyuria, polydipsia, weight loss, and recurrent infections. With her young age and family history, the most likely diagnosis is **type 1 diabetes mellitus**. Type 1 diabetes mellitus is caused by a reduction in pancreatic β cells and lack of insulin synthesis, making the patient insulin dependent. It is thought to be an autoimmune condition: antiglutamic acid decarboxylase (GAD) autoantibodies are found in a large number of patients who are diagnosed early. There is some evidence that autoimmune destruction of islet cells may follow one or more environmental triggers such as a virus. There is also a genetic susceptibility (10 times increased risk if a first-degree family member is affected with type 1 diabetes mellitus).

A urinalysis and capillary glucose can be performed as a screening test in the GP's surgery. However, the diagnosis of diabetes mellitus is based on measures of serum glucose. The **World Health Organization (WHO) criteria** for the diagnosis of diabetes mellitus are either:

- Fasting plasma glucose ≥7.0 mM
- Plasma glucose ≥11.1 mM when taken 2 hours after ingesting 75 g of glucose ('oral glucose tolerance test')

The criteria above must be met on two separate occasions or on one occasion in the presence of symptoms suggesting diabetes mellitus.

Jane's diagnosis is confirmed and she is started on insulin replacement therapy. Six months later she is brought in to A&E in a drowsy state. Her mother tells you that earlier in the evening she was complaining of abdominal pain and had been sick. Her mother insists that she has been compliant with her insulin therapy and new diet but concedes that they have not been very good about measuring her capillary glucose regularly as she doesn't like needles. Everything else has been unremarkable, although the mother mentions that Jane came down with a cold a couple of days ago and has been off school. During this time she has been unusually irritable.

On examination, Jane is indeed drowsy with a Glasgow Coma Scale (GCS) score of 11 (Eyes = 3, Verbal = 4, Motor = 4). Her heart rate is 105 bpm, blood pressure 102/64 mmHg, temperature 37.6°C, respiratory rate 22/min, and saturations of 100% on air. She looks flushed but her tongue is dry. Respiratory and abdominal examinations are unremarkable. There are no other positive examination findings.

What has happened to Jane, and why? Why is she hyperventilating?

23

Jane has most likely suffered one of the complications of type 1 diabetes mellitus, **diabetic ketoacidosis** (note: type 2 diabetics do *not* suffer this complication as ketogenesis is inhibited with even a tiny amount of insulin). Common causes include previously undiagnosed type 1 diabetes mellitus, non-compliance (sometimes deliberate, but often forgetfulness), and illness, the latter being the most likely in Jane's case. During an illness, the body makes more corticosteroid in response to the physiological stress. Cortisol acts to antagonize the action of insulin, thus the normal insulin requirements go up during illness. Type 1 diabetics should therefore increase their insulin doses when they are unwell, and should monitor their capillary glucose to ensure they get the balance right. When you speak to Jane's mother, she tells you that they have been giving the same dose throughout and hadn't realized she needed more because of 'her cold'. With more regular capillary glucose measurement this may have been evident.

Jane's breathing pattern is what is described as **Kussmaul breathing**: rapid, deep inspiration ('air hunger' to observers). It is caused by the ketoacidosis. The decrease in pH stimulates the respiratory centre. This then goes into overdrive to try to correct the acidosis (remember that by hyperventilating, you 'blow off' CO_2 and generate a respiratory alkalosis).

23

Mrs Jeffrey is a 73-year-old woman who presents to her GP with thirst and polyuria which has been present for 6 weeks. On further questioning, it emerges that she has also had constipation, for which she has been taking two sachets of Movicol a day. Throughout this period, she has felt nauseated and fatigued.

Her past medical history is notable for several months of low back pain and atrial fibrillation, for which she takes diclofenac, atenolol, and aspirin; and vaginal prolapse, which the gynaecologists manage with pessaries. On examination, she is afebrile but appears dehydrated, with a dry tongue. There are no other positive findings.

The GP orders blood tests, which show:

RBC	4.7×10^{12} cells/L
WCC	8×10^9 cells/L
Hb	9.4 g/dL
MCV	92 fL
Platelets	210×10^9 cells/L
Blood glucose	4.8 mM
Na	138 mM
K	4.1 mM
Cl	99 mM
Urea	9.1 mM
Creatinine	202 µM

(RBC, red blood cell [count]; WCC, white cell count; Hb, haemoglobin; MCV, mean corpuscular volume) Urinalysis is negative for glucose, ketones, leucocytes, or nitrites.

What do the blood tests show? What is the most likely diagnosis? How does this explain her symptoms and blood results? What other blood tests would you like to request?

This lady has presented with polyuria, constipation, fatigue, and back pain. She has a **normocytic anaemia** (low Hb with normal MCV) and **renal impairment** (raised urea and creatinine). The other results shown (WCC, platelets, glucose, and electrolytes) are within the normal ranges. **Hypercalcaemia due to bone malignancy** could explain this constellation of symptoms and blood results. High calcium levels reduce activation of voltage-gated sodium channels, thus reducing neuromuscular excitation and causing constipation. The high calcium also causes a nephrogenic diabetes insipidus (mechanism unknown), hence the polyuria. The anaemia (due to chronic malignancy or bone marrow infiltration) would explain the fatigue, and the bone malignancy (metastasis or multiple myeloma) would explain the bone pain.

The blood tests not shown above that you should request include **serum calcium**, to confirm the hypercalcaemia. If this is high, the GP should then arrange:

* **Alkaline phosphatase (ALP).** This will be raised in bone metastasis (which activates ALP producing osteoblasts) but not in multiple myeloma (which activates only osteoclasts).

* **Serum and urine electrophoresis**, looking for paraprotein (an oligoclonal band) found in multiple myeloma.

* **Lumbar radiograph**, looking for lytic lesions where she has the pain.

The above tests were performed and suggested multiple myeloma, which was confirmed with a bone marrow biopsy.

23

Mr Salvatore is a 23-year-old fisherman who lives at home with his parents and has schizophrenia. For the past 4 weeks his parents note that he has been drinking and passing large quantities of water. They are worried that this may be related to his medications, as they know there can be many different side-effects. Mr Salvatore himself is not bothered by his symptoms although he agrees that he has been drinking and peeing a lot. There is nothing of note on examination (and notably, no signs of dehydration), although he displays disordered thought in conversation. He takes olanzapine for his schizophrenia and his parents say he has been compliant with this, although they add he's been a bit more muddled than usual over the past few days.

The results of his initial blood tests are as follows:

RBC	4.4×10^{12} cells/L
WCC	5×10^9 cells/L
Hb	13.7 g/dL
MCV	89 fL
Platelets	265×10^9 cells/L
Blood glucose	4.0 mM
Na	121 mM
K	3.2 mM
Cl	93 mM
Urea	4.1 mM
Creatinine	52 μM

Urinalysis is negative for glucose, ketones, leucocytes, or nitrites, and urine osmolality is 201 mOsm/L.

What do the blood results show? What is the most likely diagnosis? What test should you order next?

The patient has normal blood glucose, ruling out diabetes mellitus. He also has both a dilute serum (low electrolytes including hyponatraemia) and a dilute urine (201 mOsm/L), but no signs of dehydration. The patient is basically overhydrated – a sign of **primary polydipsia**. This patient should undergo a **water deprivation test** to confirm the diagnosis (his urine osmolality will increase as his body is deprived of water), and be referred for specialist management by psychiatry.

The diagnosis of primary polydipsia is most commonly seen in schizophrenics, although the reason for this is unknown. The management involves fluid restriction, and in some people certain antipsychotics can be helpful (e.g. clozapine).

Viva questions

What are the long-term complications of diabetes mellitus?

Diabetes mellitus affects the vascular system, thus the common complications can be divided into macrovascular and microvascular:

- Macrovascular (affecting any of the three major vascular beds)
  - Ischaemic heart disease
  - Cerebrovascular disease
  - Peripheral vascular disease
- Microvascular
  - Retinopathy
  - Neuropathy (e.g. 'glove-and-stocking' paraesthesia, autonomic dysfunction, mononeuritis multiplex)
  - Nephropathy (nephrotic syndrome)

In addition, diabetics can get lipohypertrophy around injection sites, and a variety of other skin complications have been described.

What is the pathology of hyperosmotic non-ketotic acidosis (HONK)?

HONK is a life-threatening complication of type 2 diabetes mellitus. It is characterized by severe hyperglycaemia in the absence of any ketosis. The hyperglycaemia may be precipitated by any number of factors, including illness, dehydration, and/or non-compliance with diabetic medications. As the patient is a type 2 diabetic, they still produce insulin – but the amount produced is insufficient to control the hyperglycaemia. However, because only a small amount of insulin is needed to inhibit ketogenesis, this is sufficient to prevent ketosis.

The hyperglycaemia has two deleterious complications:

1) Fluid shifts under osmosis from the extravascular (including interstitial) compartment to the intravascular compartment. Thus, there is cellular dehydration.
2) There is an osmotic diuresis, with subsequent water loss in the urine. This can result in hypovolaemia.

If the hypovolaemia becomes severe, patients become vulnerable to shock, thrombosis, and neurological impairment.

Where is ADH produced, where does it act, and what does it do?

ADH is produced in the posterior pituitary in response to even slight increases in serum Na concentration. It acts in the collecting duct of the nephron in the kidney, where it causes an increase in the number of aquaporin channels. Normally the membrane of the collecting duct is relatively impermeable to water, preventing the water in the dilute 'urine' from passing down the osmotic gradient into the 'plasma'. By causing the insertion of aquaporin channels in the membrane, ADH makes it more permeable to water, which then diffuses across, leaving more concentrated urine. Thus, ADH is crucial for retaining fluid, e.g. when dehydrated or overnight (when we drink less).

What is the mechanism of action of the following diabetic drugs: biguanides (e.g. metformin); glitazones (or thiazolidinediones, e.g. rosiglitazone); sulphonylureas (e.g. glibenclamide); meglitinides (e.g. nateglinide); α-glucosidase inhibitors (e.g. acarbose)?

- **Biguanides** (metformin) decrease hepatic glucose production and increase peripheral glucose uptake by an unknown mechanism(s)

- **Glitazones** (or thiazolidinediones) activate peroxisome proliferator-activated receptor gamma (PPAR-γ), a nuclear transcription factor that increases lipoprotein lipase (LPL), and fatty acid transporter protein 1 (FATP1) transcription, amongst other genes involved in lipid metabolism, to increase peripheral insulin sensitivity (and hence glucose uptake by peripheral tissues, e.g. muscle and adipose tissue)

- **Sulphonylureas** and **meglitinides** increase insulin secretion by blocking the K_{ATP} channel in pancreatic β cells, causing depolarization and calcium entry, stimulating insulin secretion

- **α-Glucosidase inhibitors** decrease glucose absorption in the intestine

For a range of Single Best Answer questions related to the topic of this chapter go to www.oxfordtextbooks.co.uk/orc/ocms/

Groin lump

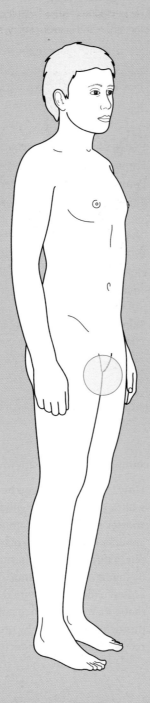

Core case

Mr Harcourt is a 36-year-old firefighter who is referred to the general surgical outpatient clinic by his general practitioner (GP) because he has a groin lump.

What is your differential diagnosis for a groin lump? Try to think of the anatomical structures in the groin region, and any pathology that may arise from those structures.

Considering the anatomy and associated pathology in a systematic fashion, the lump may represent:

> **Psoas sheath** → psoas abscess or psoas bursa
> **Femoral nerve** → neuroma
> **Femoral artery** → femoral aneurysm or pseudo-aneurysm
> **Femoral vein/long saphenous vein** → saphena varix (dilated saphenous vein due to incompetence at the sapheno-femoral junction)
> **Lymph nodes** → lymphadenopathy (infectious or malignant)
> **Hernial orifices** → inguinal hernia, femoral hernia
> **Testicular apparatus** → ectopic testis, undescended testis, hydrocele of cord
> **Skin/subcutis** → lipoma, infected abscess (e.g. from intravenous (IV) drug use), sebaceous cyst

What questions should you ask about the lump itself that might help you characterize it?

In common with lumps anywhere on the body, you will need to establish:

- **How long has the lump been there?** Many of the diagnoses mentioned above will develop rather insidiously, but there are some that may have a rather shorter history. For example, a patient may develop a femoral artery pseudo-aneurysm (a collection of blood outside the vessel lumen) following angiography, a direct inguinal hernia may be precipitated by a period of heavy lifting, or inguinal lymphadenopathy may follow a lower limb infection. Ectopic or undescended testes would be present from birth, but it is extremely unlikely that a man would reach adulthood in the Western world without having had this defect corrected by orchidopexy (orchid = testis, -pexy = fixation in correct position) or orchidectomy (orchid = testis, -ectomy = removal).

- **Is the lump always there? Does it reduce when the patient lies down?** This question relates to hernias and saphena varix. Increases in intra-abdominal pressure, for example during coughing or straining at stool, may cause hernias to increase in size. A saphena varix may increase in size if the patient stands for long periods of time as retrograde flow through incompetent venous valves will allow blood to pool. A saphena varix will disappear completely when the patient lies down.

- **Has the lump got bigger, smaller, or stayed the same size?** Almost all of the pathologies on our differential (with the possible exception of ectopic/undescended testes) may change in size over time. Rapid changes in size may hint at an infective process such as a psoas abscess or lymphadenopathy.

- **Is the lump painful?** Reducible and incarcerated hernias may or may not be painful (they are more often mildly uncomfortable), whereas a strangulated hernia will be acutely painful. A groin abscess or infected pseudo-aneurysm may also be painful.

- **Are there any other lumps?** There may be another lump in the other groin (about 20% of inguinal hernias are bilateral). Equally, inguinal lymphadenopathy may occur in conjunction with more widespread lymphadenopathy.

What questions should you ask if you suspect a hernia?

If the history is suggestive of a hernia, you should ask:

- **Has there been any abdominal pain?** The main risks of hernia formation are bowel obstruction (when the flow of bowel contents is interrupted) and bowel strangulation (when the blood supply to a section of bowel is compromised and thus ischaemia ensues). Hernias may present as an emergency due to either of the above, but even with an elective presentation (following the discovery of a groin lump) it is possible to have a history of intermittent episodes of obstruction as bowel moves in and out of a hernial orifice. Such episodes of obstruction would result in colicky abdominal pain, together with abdominal distension, vomiting, and absolute constipation if the obstruction was prolonged.

- **Has the patient been straining at stool, struggling to pass urine, or suffering from a chronic cough? Do either their job or pastimes involve heavy lifting?** All of these factors will increase intra-abdominal pressure and increase the likelihood of hernias.

- **Has the patient had any prior operations in the groin?** Previous surgery can of course predispose to incisional hernias. More importantly, a history of inguinal or femoral hernias may raise such diagnoses to the top of the differential list, and may dictate a different approach to repair (for example, laparoscopic hernia repair may be indicated for recurrent hernias).

24

What questions should you ask if you suspect an infective process or malignancy?

Questions that are more relevant to lymphadenopathy include:

- **Has there been any trauma or infection in the lower limbs or groin?**
- **Have there been any anal/scrotal/skin symptoms (e.g. rectal bleeding)?** Inguinal lymphadenopathy may represent metastatic spread from anal cancer, scrotal cancer, or melanoma.
- **Does he have a fever?** Febrile symptoms make an infective pathology such as a psoas abscess or lymphadenopathy more likely. Note that fever is also one of the 'B symptoms' of lymphoma along with weight loss, night sweats, and anorexia – one of the important differential diagnoses for lymphadenopathy.
- **Has there been any weight loss, night sweats, or pruritus?** The former two are general features of malignancy while pruritus is another symptom of lymphoma.

Mr Harcourt explains that the lump has probably been in his right groin for a couple of months. He can't remember exactly when or why he first noticed it, but says that he was first aware of a rather dull ache in his groin. The lump appeared relatively insidiously. On further questioning he explains that the lump isn't always there. It will invariably be present if he's had an active day at work, but may not make an appearance if he's just lounging around at home. When the lump appears it is always the same size. It has never extended into his scrotum. He says that it is never truly painful, but will ache at the end of the day.

He has no previous surgical history, and is otherwise fit and well. He takes no medications.

The next stage is to examine Mr Harcourt.

How would you approach the examination of a groin lump?

The first step is to ensure that the patient is *adequately exposed* – and this means being able to fully inspect both groins and the abdomen. You will also need to examine the external genitalia, but to preserve the patient's dignity it is best to leave the genitalia covered until you need to examine them.

It is fine to start with the patient lying down, but you will also need to repeat the examination with the patient *standing up*.

Look at *both sides* of the groin for any masses or scars from previous surgery.

What particular features of the lump should you characterize during palpation?

There are a number of key features that you will need to establish during palpation:

Site

- **Where is the lump?** It is crucially important that you are familiar with the anatomy of the inguinal region, as knowing the normal surface landmarks for structures will enable you to establish the origin of a lump (see Fig. 24.1). A saphena varix will lie over the sapheno-femoral junction.[†] As far as hernias are concerned, try to establish whether the **neck of the swelling** is:
  - Superior and medial to the pubic tubercle (inguinal hernia)
  - Inferior and lateral to the pubic tubercle (femoral hernia)

(Note that the anatomical relations refer to the neck of the hernia and not the swelling itself.)

[†] The site of the saphena varix corresponds with the sapheno-femoral junction, 2–3 cm inferolateral to the pubic tubercle. Another way of thinking about this is to remember that the femoral vein (hence sapheno-femoral junction) lies just medial to the femoral artery – which is itself located at the mid-inguinal point.

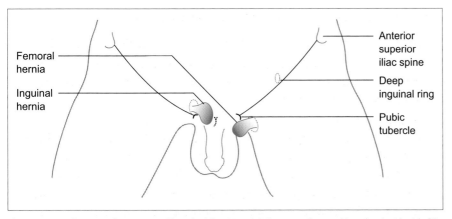

Figure 24.1 Diagram of anatomy of inguinal (patient right) versus femoral hernias (patient left).

- **Which tissue layer does the lump lie within?** Is it cutaneous, subcutaneous (lipoma), or associated with the deeper tissues?
- **Does the lump extend into the scrotum?** If so, this is almost certainly an indirect inguinal hernia (rarely a direct inguinal hernia).

Size

How big is the lump? Whilst this might not affect the management, it is part of a complete characterization of any lump and surgeons will always ask for this information.

Is the lump tender and/or warm?

- The skin overlying a strangulated hernia is likely to be red and inflamed, and there may be signs of toxicity (if there is bowel necrosis) and signs of bowel obstruction.
- Reducible hernias may be tender to palpation.
- Groin abscesses, reactive lymph nodes, or infected pseudo-aneurysms may also be warm and tender to palpation, and associated with overlying erythema.

Is the lump solid or fluctuant?

Swollen lymph nodes are solid. A hernia, saphena varix, femoral aneurysm, psoas bursa, or hydrocele of the cord will be softer and may be fluctuant.

Is the lump pulsatile?

A truly pulsatile lump can only be a femoral aneurysm (either a true aneurysm or pseudo-aneurysm). Remember, however, that you may detect a transmitted pulse if, for example, a swollen lymph node overlies the femoral artery.

Does the lump have a cough impulse?

This means that the lump expands and increases in tension during coughing – and is thus diagnostic of hernias as these will expand in response to increased intra-abdominal pressure, pushing more of the contents through the abdominal wall defect, unless incarcerated. It does not mean that the lump moves in response to coughing. To detect this you should put your hands over the lump (or where the patient says the lump appears) and ask the patient to cough. Direct inguinal

24

hernias will typically expand outwards (through the defect in the posterior wall of the inguinal canal) whereas indirect inguinal hernias will tend to expand along the path of the inguinal canal.

Is the lump reducible? If so, in which direction does it reduce?

- The only reducible groin lumps are hernias or a saphena varix. Saphena varix is rare – it is a soft, bluish swelling that is only seen when the patient stands. It will empty with minimal palpation and fill upon release of the pressure.

- The direction of reducibility is most useful for distinguishing between direct and indirect inguinal hernias. The former tend to reduce superiorly and posteriorly whereas the latter reduce superolaterally and posteriorly (indirect hernias tend to reduce along the length of the inguinal canal).

- Remember that not all hernias are reducible.

What further information will percussion and auscultation of the lump add?

Percussion and auscultation may give further clues as to the identification of the contents of the hernial sac, but are not performed by all clinicians. If the sac contains omentum it may be dull to percussion and there may be no bowel sounds audible over the lump. By contrast, if the hernia contains bowel it is likely to be resonant to percussion and bowel sounds may be audible.

Mr Harcourt is initially examined lying on the bed. No groin swellings are visible on general inspection but a mass with a cough impulse is felt in the right groin when Mr Harcourt is asked to cough. The lump does not reduce spontaneously. It is oval shaped, 4 cm long, and fluctuant. The neck of the lump is medial and superior to the pubic tubercle. The lump is resonant to percussion and bowel sounds are audible when auscultating the lump.

His abdomen is palpated while he is lying down, and nothing abnormal is noted. The external genitalia are normal.

Mr Harcourt is asked to stand and the examination is repeated. The lump does not appear until Mr Harcourt is asked to cough. He is able to comfortably reduce the swelling when he is lying down.

Why was the rest of Mr Harcourt's abdomen examined?

Which diagnosis do you think is most likely?

24

The rest of Mr Harcourt's abdomen was examined to check for any abdominal masses (such as ascites, a tumour, or constipation) which would increase intra-abdominal pressure and predispose to hernia formation.

The history and examination findings are highly suggestive of a **reducible inguinal hernia** – a fluctuant mass, with a cough impulse, that has its origin superior and medial to the pubic tubercle.

Is there a simple bedside test that will help you to distinguish between a direct or indirect hernia?

The key lies in appreciating the origins of direct versus indirect inguinal hernias (Fig. 24.2).

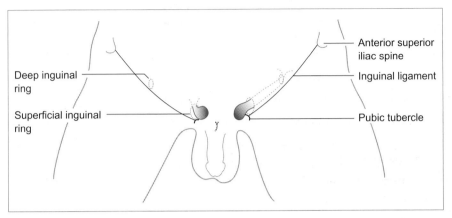

Figure 24.2 Anatomy of direct (patient right) versus indirect (patient left) inguinal hernias.

With direct inguinal hernias, the hernial sac protrudes through a defect in the transversalis fascia which forms the posterior wall of the inguinal canal. By contrast, the sac of an indirect inguinal hernia protrudes through the deep inguinal ring at the lateral end of the inguinal canal. As such, it should be possible to control an indirect inguinal hernia by applying pressure to the deep inguinal ring. To do this you will need to reduce the hernia and then place a finger over the deep ring (at the midpoint of the inguinal ligament). Now ask the patient to cough. If the hernia reappears while your finger is still occluding the deep ring then the hernia must be direct (or you have your finger in the wrong place!). An indirect hernia will reappear only when pressure over the deep ring is released.

About 75% of adult hernias are indirect and about 25% are direct. Note that it is possible for direct and indirect hernias to coexist as a 'pantaloon hernia'.

In truth, the correct diagnosis of direct versus indirect inguinal hernia is often only made in the operating theatre as clinical examination is only correct about 50% of the time! Indirect inguinal hernias have their origin lateral to the inferior epigastric artery (which lies medial to the deep inguinal ring) while direct hernias have their origin medial to the inferior epigastric artery.

Once Mr Harcourt has reduced the groin swelling, the examiner places his hand over the right deep inguinal ring and asks Mr Harcourt to cough. The lump does not reappear. The examiner then removes his hand, asks the patient to cough again, and observes that the lump appears.

What is the diagnosis and how should Mr Harcourt be managed?

24

The examination evidence is consistent with a **right reducible indirect inguinal hernia**.

Indirect hernias have a higher risk of strangulation than direct hernias as the hernial sac passes through a smaller defect (compared with the hole in the transversalis fascia that direct hernias pass through) – this also explains why direct hernias have a greater tendency to spontaneously reduce when patients lie down.

Appropriate management would be an elective surgical repair.

Short cases

Mr Guscott is a 78-year-old retired headmaster who presents to his local accident and emergency (A&E) at 8 p.m. with sudden-onset crushing chest pain that radiates to his left arm. He had a myocardial infarction aged 60, and two-vessel coronary artery bypass graft when he was 63, and has been admitted to hospital twice over the last year with acute coronary syndrome. He takes aspirin, carvedilol, ramipril, atorvastatin, and nicorandil. He smokes 30 cigarettes a day, and says that his exercise tolerance is 'nil'.

A medical student clerks Mr Guscott once his condition has stabilized. As part of a thorough examination the student notes that he has a prominent swelling in his right groin. The swelling is fluctuant, has a cough impulse, and points towards the pubic tubercle. The neck of the swelling is superior and medial to the pubic tubercle. The swelling does not extend into the scrotum. It is not tender and the overlying skin is normal. It reduces with ease and reappears as soon as Mr Guscott is asked to stand up. He is encouraged to reduce the swelling, and does so, but pressure applied by the student over the deep inguinal ring fails to control the hernia, which reappears as soon as Mr Guscott is asked to cough. The lump is dull to percussion and bowel sounds are not audible over it. The rest of the abdominal examination is unremarkable and the external genitalia are normal. Mr Guscott says that he has had the lump for years, and that it hasn't given him any trouble.

The student presents his clerking on the ward round the following morning. He describes the lump and suggests that Mr Guscott is referred to the general surgeons.

What is the most likely diagnosis for the groin lump? How should it be managed?

The examination suggests that this is a **direct inguinal hernia**. The location of the neck of the hernia medial and superior to the pubic tubercle distinguishes this from a femoral hernia. The fact that the swelling appears as soon as the patient stands, coupled with the fact that pressure over the deep inguinal ring fails to control the lump, is highly suggestive of a direct hernia.

Although indirect hernias are still more common than direct hernias in the elderly, direct hernias are more common than they are in the younger population. As direct hernias have a wider neck than indirect hernias they are at less risk of strangulation. This affords a more conservative approach to their management. Options include:

* **Doing nothing** – and reassuring the patient that this is a common and relatively benign condition. If the patient is overweight you may advise them to lose some weight as this will help to reduce intra-abdominal pressure.

* Recommending that the patient **wears a truss** to prevent bowel obstruction. There is limited evidence that they work, perhaps because of compliance issues, but they remain very popular with patients. Note that you should never put a truss over an irreducible hernia.

* **Surgical repair.**

The significance of Mr Guscott's past medical history is that he is a very poor candidate for general anaesthesia. Some surgeons advocate the use of local anaesthesia for surgical repair in such patients, but many would favour conservative management (particularly in this case, given that Mr Guscott is asymptomatic from his hernia).

Mrs Taylor is a 72-year-old lady who presents to her GP with a lump in her groin. She first noticed the lump a week ago. The lump has been present for the whole of the last week – it has never disappeared and does not appear to have changed in size. Mrs Taylor reports that it is slightly tender. She is not aware of any other lumps and says that she is otherwise fit and well.

She takes a thiazide for hypertension and a bisphosphonate for osteoporosis. She has got three children, one of whom was born by Caesarean section. She had a cholecystectomy in her 40s.

On examination, Mrs Taylor has a fluctuant lump of diameter 2 cm in her left groin, the neck of which is inferior and lateral to the pubic tubercle. There is a non-convincing cough impulse. It is not possible to reduce the lump with gentle traction. The lump is not tender to gentle palpation, and there is no overlying erythema.

The right groin and abdominal examination are unremarkable.

What is the most likely diagnosis?

How urgently would you refer Mrs Taylor to the surgeons?

Mrs Taylor's history and examination are consistent with the diagnosis of a **femoral hernia** as she has a fluctuant mass, the neck of which sits inferior and lateral to the pubic tubercle. Femoral hernias are more common in women than in men. However, inguinal hernias are still more common than femoral hernias in women.

Femoral hernias have a higher risk of strangulation than inguinal hernias (as they have a narrower neck). She should be **referred to the surgeons without delay**. A truss should never be used for femoral hernias.

Mrs Taylor is referred to the surgeons. Three days after her original GP consultation she returns to the surgery. She says that for the past 6 hours the lump in her groin has been far more painful. The overlying skin is also warm and red. Following further questioning by her GP she says that she has had colicky abdominal pain for the past 4 hours. She hasn't been to the toilet but is unsure whether she has passed any flatus. She has not vomited.

On examination, there is a tender red swelling in her left groin. She is febrile (38.2°C), her pulse is 106 bpm regular, and her blood pressure is 137/86 mmHg.

What has happened to Mrs Taylor?

What is the next course of action?

It is likely that Mrs Taylor's **hernia has strangulated**. There are local signs of inflammation (a red and tender lump), together with systemic signs (tachycardia and fever). Additionally, the colicky abdominal pain hints that she is developing small bowel obstruction. The other features that we expect to see with intestinal obstruction – namely vomiting, absolute constipation, and abdominal distension – may not have developed yet as the history is still quite short and she has a *distal* obstruction.

Mrs Taylor must now be **seen by the surgeons as an emergency** as there is a risk of bowel necrosis and perforation. The operative mortality for strangulated hernia repairs is almost 10 times higher than that for elective hernia repairs.

24

Mr Johnson is a 52-year-old publican who presents to his GP with a lump in his right groin. He says that the lump has been there 'for ages', but that he has not been concerned about it as it gives him no pain and hasn't changed in size or location. His wife thinks that it is a hernia and wants him to get it checked. Her brother has recently had an inguinal hernia repair and she wonders whether the same may be suitable for her husband as she worries about his ability to cope with lifting beer barrels around the pub. Mr Johnson explains that he only ever notices the lump when he is standing up. Following further questioning he states that he has had no abdominal pain and is not aware of any other lumps.

His past medical history is significant for a right-sided hip replacement 2 years ago. His stay in hospital was complicated by a deep vein thrombosis in his right thigh that was treated with 6 months of warfarin therapy. He says that he is otherwise fit and well. He takes seretide and salbutamol inhalers for asthma, allopurinol for gout, and sildenafil for Mrs Johnson.

Mr Johnson is asked to remove his trousers and pants and is examined standing up. On inspection, Mr Johnson is noted to have marked varicosities over the inferomedial aspect of his right thigh. Examination reveals a fluctuant swelling in his right groin, approximately 2 cm inferior and lateral to the pubic tubercle. The lump points down the leg, is approximately 1.5 cm × 1 cm, and has a bluish tinge. It is non-tender to palpation and there is an expansile cough impulse. The lump easily reduces with light palpation, and reappears as soon as the examiner's finger is removed. No bowel sounds are audible over the lump, and it is non-pulsatile. Mr Johnson is asked to lie down and the lump disappears within seconds. Examination of the rest of the abdomen and external genitalia is unremarkable.

Which diagnosis is most likely?

The differential diagnosis for a non-tender, fluctuant groin lump with a cough impulse is a hernia or saphena varix. The position of the swelling inferior and lateral to the pubic tubercle narrows the differential to a femoral hernia or saphena varix. The fact that this swelling has a bluish tinge, is easily reduced, and disappears as soon as the patient lies flat, makes **saphena varix** more likely. The history of a deep vein thrombosis (DVT) and examination findings of other venous varicosities in the right leg add further support to this diagnosis.

Short case

Mr Pemberton is a 26-year-old artist. He first noticed a firm lump in his left groin 1 week ago, and now presents to his GP. He is certain it wasn't there before. The lump is non-tender, and has not changed in size or location. He has been checking his groin several times a day, and also while in bed at night, and reports that the lump is always there. He says that he feels otherwise well. He has no significant past medical history and is taking no medications.

Examination reveals a firm rubbery lump, 1.5 cm in diameter, in the left groin crease. The lump is relatively mobile and does not appear to be tethered to underlying structures. It is not possible to reduce the lump. Examination of the right groin, abdomen, and external genitalia is unremarkable.

What is the most likely diagnosis? What can cause such a lump? How would you proceed to investigate the possible underlying cause?

This lump is consistent with **inguinal lymphadenopathy**.

When considering the causes of inguinal lymphadenopathy it is usual to divide our differential into local versus systemic, and infective versus neoplastic causes (Table 24.1).

Table 24.1 Causes of inguinal lymphadenopathy

	Systemic	Local
Infective	Tuberculosis/HIV	Non-specific lymphadenopathy from groin/lower limb infection
		Others, e.g. lymphogranuloma venereum (very rare in the West)
Neoplastic	Lymphoma	Metastases: from primary in lower limb, external genitalia,[†] or perianal region
	Leukaemia	Melanoma

[†] Remember that the testes drain to para-aortic and not inguinal lymph nodes.

The first step in investigating the potential cause of inguinal lymphadenopathy is to take a more detailed history. You may have to specifically enquire about:

- Any recent lower limb trauma or infection
- Potential exposure to specific pathogens such as tuberculosis/HIV
- Any preceding ulcers? – the painful lymph nodes seen with lymphogranuloma venereum are preceded by an ulcer
- Symptoms of anal cancer such as bleeding
- Symptoms of systemic malignancy – night sweats, fever, weight loss, pruritus.

The majority of cases of inguinal lymphadenopathy will be a response to non-specific groin or lower limb infection. It is thus very important that you also examine the leg for signs of an infective or malignant (e.g. melanoma) source. If the history

24

and examination findings raise any other suspicions, there are a number of further investigations that can be carried out:

- Full blood count and film: looking for features of leukaemia.
- Fine needle aspirate: sending samples for cytology (lymphoma) and microbiology (infection). Note that it is often very difficult to diagnose low-grade lymphoma by fine needle aspiration, and core biopsy may be required.
- An excisional biopsy may be required if a diagnosis has still not been made.

Viva questions

Define a 'hernia', 'fistula', 'sinus', and 'stoma'

- A **hernia** is the abnormal protrusion of the contents of a cavity through the wall that normally contains it.
- A **fistula** is an abnormal communication between two epithelial surfaces, such as two hollow organs or between a hollow organ and the exterior.
- A **sinus** is a blind-ended tract between an epithelial surface and a cavity lined with granulation tissue.
- A **stoma** is the artificial opening of an internal tube (e.g. gastrointestinal (GI) tract, ureter) that has been brought to the surface.

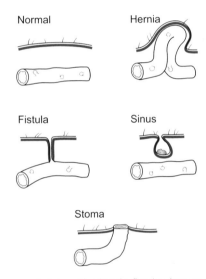

Figure 24.3 Diagram comparing the normal state with a hernia, fistula, sinus, and stoma.

What is the most common type of hernia in women?

Indirect inguinal hernias are the most common hernias in men and women. Don't fall into the trap of saying femoral hernias – while it is true that femoral hernias are the only hernia that is more common in women than in men, indirect inguinal hernias are still more common.

What is the difference between reducible, irreducible, incarcerated, obstructed, and strangulated hernias?

- A **reducible hernia.** can be pushed back into the right place.
- An **irreducible hernia** cannot be pushed back into the right place. This is not a problem for the patient *per se* but is at risk of causing problems. A hernia may be irreducible because it is:
  - **Incarcerated**: stuck in the abnormal position because either there are adhesions between the hernial sac and surrounding structures, or there are adhesions between structures within the sac such that the sac is now wider than its neck and no longer able to pass through the wall defect.
  - **Obstructed**: the neck of the hernial sac provides an obstruction to the passage of flow through the bowel (but the blood supply of the bowel is intact).
  - **Strangulated**: if the bowel becomes so constricted by the neck of the hernial sac that the blood supply is compromised it is referred to as a strangulated hernia. This is a major problem for the patient as their bowel will necrose rapidly from ischaemia.

What are the contents of the inguinal canal?

If you watch a hernia operation it is almost guaranteed that somebody will ask you to name the contents of the inguinal canal. The male canal contains the ilio-inguinal nerve and spermatic cord, while the female canal contains the ilio-inguinal nerve and round ligament Perhaps the easiest way to remember the contents of the spermatic cord is to think of structures arising in sets of three. Hence there are:

- Three layers of fascia:
  - external spermatic fascia (from the external oblique aponeurosis)
  - cremasteric fascia (from the internal oblique aponeurosis)
  - internal spermatic fascia (from the transversalis fascia)
- Three arteries:
  - the gonadal artery (arising directly from the aorta)
  - the cremasteric artery (arising from the inferior epigastric artery)
  - the artery of the vas (arising from the inferior vesical artery)
- Three veins, which mirror the arteries:
  - testicular vein/pampiniform plexus
  - cremasteric vein
  - vein of the vas
- Three nerves:
  - ilioinguinal nerve (which lies outside the spermatic cord)
  - sympathetic supply from T10 and T11
  - genital branch of the genitofemoral nerve
- Three other things:
  - vas deferens
  - lymphatics
  - patent processus vaginalis (if present)

24

What are the boundaries of Hesselbach's triangle and what is its significance?

Whether an inguinal hernia is direct or indirect is defined according to its relationship to Hesselbach's triangle (Fig. 24.4). The borders of the triangle are as follows: medially, rectus sheath; inferiorly, inguinal ligament; superiorly, inferior epigastric artery. An inguinal hernia that arises within Hesselbach's triangle is direct, whereas indirect hernias arise lateral to the inferior epigastric artery and thus lateral to the triangle.

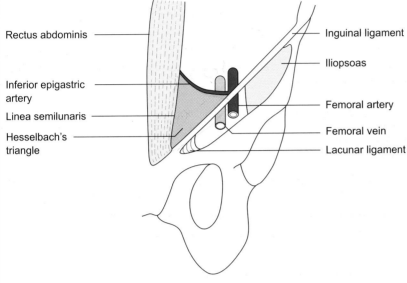

Rectus abdominis

Inferior epigastric artery

Linea semilunaris

Hesselbach's triangle

Inguinal ligament

Iliopsoas

Femoral artery

Femoral vein

Lacunar ligament

Figure 24.4 Hesselbach's triangle.

What are the boundaries of the inguinal canal?

- **Anterior:** skin, superficial fascia, external oblique aponeurosis, and internal oblique for lateral third.
- **Posterior:** conjoint tendon medially and transversalis fascia laterally.
- **Roof:** arching fibres of internal oblique and transversus abdominis.
- **Floor:** inguinal ligament.

Figure 24.5 shows a cross-section of the inguinal canal at its medial end.

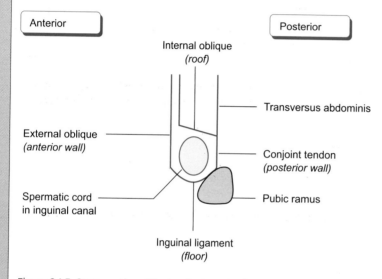

Figure 24.5 Cross-section of the inguinal canal at its medial end.

What are the boundaries of the femoral canal?

- **Anterior:** inguinal ligament.
- **Posterior:** pectineal ligament and pectineus.
- **Medial:** lacunar ligament.
- **Lateral:** femoral vein.

What is the difference between herniotomy, herniorraphy, and hernioplasty?

A **herniotomy** refers to the surgical excision of a hernial sac. **Herniorrhaphy** involves the repair of a hernia using locally available tissues (for example, a sutured repair such as the Bassini). **Hernioplasty** involves the repair of a hernia using synthetic material such as a mesh.

The inguinal hernias which typically occur in childhood are due to a patent processus vaginalis and thus the repair is usually a herniotomy as there is rarely a weakness in the inguinal canal which needs repairing. By contrast, adult hernias are due to a defect in the boundaries of the inguinal canal and are thus usually repaired by herniotomy in conjunction with herniorrhaphy/hernioplasty.

What are the potential complications of a surgical hernia repair?

When asked to list complications for any procedure you should take a systematic approach. Thus you may recognize complications of surgery in general, including anaesthetic complications, and complications peculiar to the particular procedure:

1) Potential **complications of surgery in general**:
   - Haemorrhage[†]
   - Infection[†]
   - Thromboembolism (DVT or pulmonary embolism (PE))
   - Anaesthetic complications (e.g. inadequate analgesia, respiratory depression, urinary retention, cardiac depression)
   - Death

2) Potential **complications of hernia repair**:
   - Hernia recurrence
   - Ischaemic orchitis/testicular atrophy
   - Bruising of scrotum and penis
   - Cutaneous anaesthesia or hyperaethesia (but note that is considerable overlap in the cutaneous areas supplied by the iliohypogastric, ilioinguinal, and genitofemoral nerves).

Note that it is important to be familiar with complications so as to be able to explain the risks to patients in the process of soliciting their consent.

[†] Haemorrhage following hernia repair may be seen as scrotal haematoma. Infection is more likely if a mesh repair is performed.

24

> **What is the difference between the *mid-inguinal point* and the *midpoint of the inguinal ligament*?**

- The **mid-inguinal point** is half-way between the anterior superior iliac spine (ASIS) and the symphysis pubis. It represents the surface landmark of the *femoral artery*.

- The **midpoint of inguinal ligament** is half-way between the ASIS and the pubic tubercle. It represents the surface landmark of the *deep inguinal ring*.

Figure 24.6 summarizes these differences.

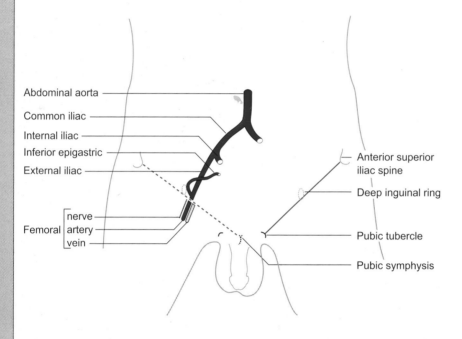

Figure 24.6 The mid-inguinal point versus the midpoint of the inguinal ligament.

 For a range of Single Best Answer questions related to the topic of this chapter go to www.oxfordtextbooks.co.uk/orc/farne/

24

Scrotal mass

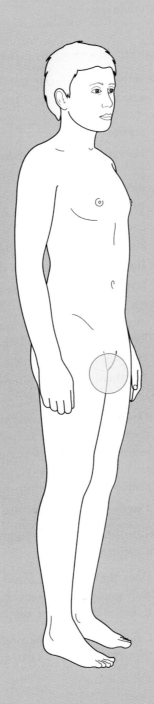

Core case

! *Read through the sections in red, covering up the sections in white that follow so that you don't see the answer. At the end of each red section, try to answer the question before reading on.*

Core case

Mr Collons is a 36-year-old Pilates instructor who presents to his general practitioner (GP) because he has noticed a lump in his scrotum.

Before you examine Mr Collons it would be prudent to establish a few more details about this 'lump'. What else what you like to know?

In common with lumps anywhere on the body, you will need to establish:

* **Is the lump painful?** This is an absolutely critical question. An acutely swollen and tender scrotum is testicular torsion until proven otherwise, and should thus be regarded as a surgical emergency. Most cases of testicular malignancy are not painful.

* **How long has the lump been there?** A testicular torsion will only have been present for hours/days whereas a testicular tumour may have been present for weeks/months.

* **What made the patient first notice the lump?** It may be that Mr Collons checks his testes regularly, but it is equally likely that this may be a chance finding – perhaps following some minor trauma to his scrotum.

* **Has the lump got bigger, smaller, or stayed the same size?**

* **Is the lump always there?** This is not such a strange question as it may sound. An inguinal hernia may extend into the scrotum in response to increases in intra-abdominal pressure, such as during periods of exertion or after prolonged periods of standing. Varicoceles can vary in size throughout the day, and will typically disappear when the patient lies flat.

* **Are there any other lumps?** The pathology may not be confined just to the testicles.

* **Does he have any other symptoms?** You should ask about symptoms of urinary tract infection (dysuria, polyuria, suprapubic pain, offensive-smelling urine, urgency, strangury, haematuria) and symptoms suggestive of sexually transmitted infections (such as purulent urethral discharge) in order to identify possible sources of infection which may have ascended into the testis and/or epididymis.

* **Has there been any trauma to the testes?**

There is one further question that can be particularly informative regarding scrotal swellings:

* **Does the testis feel heavy?** While there are no symptoms that are truly pathognomonic for testicular cancer, this symptom should raise suspicions... if clinical examination supports the diagnosis.

* **Can you get above the swelling/lump?** Meaning, is the swelling confined to the scrotum or does it extend proximally into the groin?

On further questioning you establish that Mr Collons' partner first noticed the swelling in his scrotum 2 weeks ago. He doesn't usually check himself for lumps, but following this discovery he has been checking his scrotum daily whilst having his morning shower. The lump is always there and hasn't changed size. Like many men, he didn't want to rush to the doctor to have his testicles examined, but says that his partner kept urging him to get it checked out. Furthermore, he admits that he has become progressively more anxious that something isn't quite right.

When quizzed about pain, he says that he hasn't had any true pain, but his left testicle has a bit of a dull ache and just doesn't feel right. He has otherwise felt well and has had no urethral discharge or features of urinary tract infection.

You will need to examine Mr Collons. Other than tenderness, what are the four key characteristics of a scrotal mass that will enable you to narrow your differential diagnosis?

- **Is it possible to palpate the testis separately from the swelling/lump?** Whilst examining the scrotal contents you should make every effort to ensure that you can clearly identify the spermatic cord, epididymis, and testis. If you can't distinguish these separate structures due to the presence of a lump or swelling, you should aim to establish which of the remaining structures you can palpate.

- **Does it transilluminate?** When you shine a torchlight into the mass it will glow if full of fluid, but will be opaque if it is a solid structure.

- **Is the mass tender or not?**

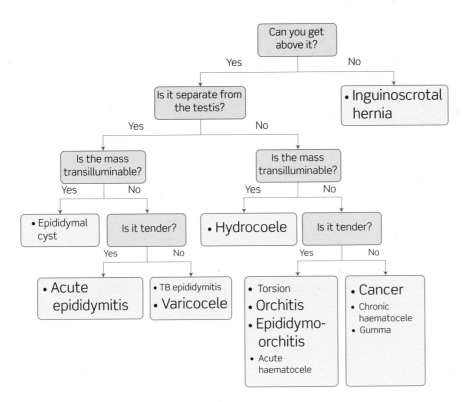

Figure 25.1 Diagnostic approach to a scrotal mass.

25

> What is your differential diagnosis of scrotal masses? Can you organize the above four questions into a flow chart that helps you sort out your differential diagnosis?

Figure 25.1 shows a flow chart for differential diagnosis of scrotal masses. Diagnoses listed in a smaller font are rare.

A cautious but wise maxim is to consider any acutely swollen and tender scrotum as testicular torsion until proven otherwise. As this condition rapidly progresses to irreversible testicular ischaemia it must be treated as an emergency (see Chapter 16).

> Upon examination of Mr Collons' scrotum, you can discern a mass in the left hemiscrotum. It is possible to palpate the testis, and the mass is within the testis and confined to it (i.e. you can get above it). More precisely, the mass is on the lower pole of the testis – it is approximately 1 cm in diameter, protrudes beyond the natural curvature of the testis, but has a smooth surface. The mass is not fluctuant and does not transilluminate. The epididymis and spermatic cord can be palpated as distinct from the mass. The testes are not tender to palpation. The overlying scrotum appears normal and there is no erythema.
>
> What is the most likely pathology?

The history and examination findings are highly suggestive of a **testicular tumour** – a non-tender solid mass within the testis, associated with abnormal testicular sensation. Tumours may present as a 'nodule' within the testis, or as an ill-defined circumferential swelling.

If the swelling had been circumferential, rather than projecting beyond the natural curvature of the testis, then the differential would also include a chronic haematocele or a gumma (syphilitic infection of the testis). A chronic haematocele may develop following an acute bleed that is noticed but ignored, or following a bleed that the patient is oblivious to. The clotted blood within the tunica vaginalis contracts and hardens around the testis, producing a mass that is clinically indistinguishable from a tumour. To be certain of the diagnosis it is necessary to surgically explore the scrotum. Figure 25.2 shows the different types of scrotal mass.

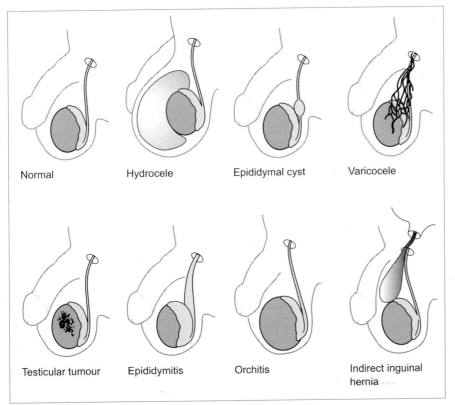

Figure 25.2 Line drawing showing different types of scrotal mass.
Reproduced from Judge RD, Zuidema GD, Fitzgerald FT (1989). *Clinical Diagnosis: a Physiologic Approach*, 5th edn. Little Brown & Co, Boston.

> Are you aware of any risk factors for this disease?

The single biggest risk factor is a history of undescended or maldescended testes. As many as 10% of patients will give a history of orchidopexy (surgical placement of the testis within the scrotum).

> Bearing in mind the maxim that solid testicular lumps are tumours until proven otherwise, the GP prepares to refer Mr Collons for urgent urological review. Prior to doing so he will wish to assess whether there is any evidence for metastatic spread.
>
> Which lymph nodes should the GP palpate?

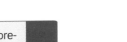

Remember that the testes themselves drain to para-aortic nodes whereas the scrotal skin drains to inguinal nodes. There was no evidence of scrotal skin involvement and so the GP should focus his examination on the para-aortic nodes (palpating for a mass in the centre of the abdomen, above the umbilicus) and the supraclavicular nodes. Note that most patients' body habitus is such that para-aortic nodes are impalpable.

> **What are the systemic symptoms of malignancy?**

The systemic symptoms that you should enquire about in anyone with suspected malignancy are weight loss, fatigue, and night sweats. You could ask more specific questions relating to particular sites of metastases – including respiratory symptoms, back pain, or neurological symptoms.

> Mr Collons is urgently referred to a urologist.
>
> **Which investigations are likely to be ordered?**

In the first instance, the most appropriate investigation is an **ultrasound scan** of both testes. In experienced hands this test has a sensitivity of almost 100%.

If the ultrasound scan is highly suggestive of a tumour, the next stage is to request **tumour markers**. The role of tumour markers is three-fold: aiding diagnosis (in conjunction with histology), monitoring response to treatment, and monitoring for relapse. α-Fetoprotein (AFP) is expressed by 50–70% of teratomas but is not usually expressed by seminomas. β-Human chorionic gonadotropin (β-HCG) is expressed by 40–60% of teratomas and about 30% of seminomas. Lactate dehydrogenase (LDH) is a less specific marker but is more common in seminomas. Blood samples are taken prior to, during, and following treatment.

Staging scans will also be requested – the most suitable being a plain chest radiograph and computed tomography (CT) scan of chest/abdomen/pelvis.

> Shortly after his appointment with the urologist Mr Collons underwent a radical left orchidectomy. Sperm was collected for storage prior to the procedure, as a safeguard against any reduction in fertility following surgery and subsequent radiotherapy. Histology showed the tumour to be a seminoma with no evidence of metastatic spread. Fortunately, seminomas are highly radiosensitive and Mr Collons is expected to have very good survival prospects following his post-operative radiotherapy.

25

Short cases

Dr Barlow is a 43-year-old engineering lecturer who presents with a mass in his scrotum. He says that he has been checking his testicles regularly over the past year and has been prompted to do so by media coverage of testicular cancer, but is slightly unsure what is normal. He reports that he has felt some sort of lump in his right scrotum for much of the past year, but as it was small and painless he had not presented to his GP. However, he now feels that the lump may have grown slightly and it is becoming mildly painful. He is otherwise fit and well, with no significant past medical history.

Examination reveals an irregularly shaped fluctuant mass superior and posterior to the right testis. It is possible to get above the mass. The mass transilluminates and is tender to palpation. It is approximately 15 mm in diameter and feels multilocular. The right testis is palpable and feels normal, as does the left testis. The overlying scrotal skin is normal.

What is the most likely diagnosis?

The examination findings are consistent with the diagnosis of an **epididymal cyst**. These are fluid-filled swellings, derived from the epididymal collecting tubules, and are relatively common in middle-aged and elderly men. The characteristic features are that the swelling is:

- Distinct from the testis (strictly superior and posterior to it).
- It is possible to get above the swelling, thus differentiating it from an inguino-scrotal hernia.
- The swelling is cystic and is thus fluctuant and transilluminable.

Epididymal cysts are frequently multiple or multilocular, and may be bilateral. Although epididymal cysts are usually painless they may sometimes be tender. It is possible for the cysts to reach quite impressive sizes – sometimes >5 cm in diameter. Epididymal cysts are often confirmed by ultrasound and are not usually removed unless they are symptomatic (e.g. they may chafe the legs or cause unsightly bulges in the trousers).

It is worth noting that spermatoceles are a subtype of epididymal cyst that contains milky fluid rather than the usual clear fluid. As it is only possible to make this distinction following removal or aspiration of the cyst it is best to avoid using the term spermatocele.

25

Mike is a 22-year-old rower who presents with a lump in his scrotum. The lump has got progressively larger over the past 6 months and is starting to cause him some discomfort. He complains of a dull ache in his scrotum following training sessions – particularly after lifting heavy weights. He is otherwise fit and well, with no significant past medical history.

Mike is examined whilst standing up. The lump feels like 'a bag of worms', and sits below and behind his left testis. It is possible to get above the lump.

What is the most likely diagnosis? Why was Mike examined whilst standing up? What treatment would you offer him?

The 'bag of worms' is a classic description of the dilated tortuous veins that comprise a **varicocele**. In common with varicose veins elsewhere in the body, these varicosities of the pampiniform plexus are responsive to changes in venous pressure and may thus increase in size at the end of the day (due to venous pooling) or following strenuous exercise.

The veins should empty when the patient lies down and thus a varicocele will only be palpable if the patient is standing up.

As many as 10–25% of men will have a varicocele, and this figure may be as high as 40% in infertile men, although it is controversial as to whether there is any causative link. The first step when offering Mike treatment is to **reassure him** that varicoceles are incredibly common. **Scrotal support**, by means of a jockstrap or tighter pants may relieve him of some of the discomfort. If his varicocele becomes painful he may wish to consider treatment. Options include **embolization**, **surgical ligation**, or **sclerotherapy** of the veins draining the testis.

Mr Hoff is a 53-year-old pub singer who presents because he is concerned that his testicle is growing in size. He has no pain or discomfort, and was initially rather proud of his large appendage but is now concerned that it might not stop growing. He has no history of testicular cancer, trauma, or infection. He is otherwise fit and well.

Examination reveals a large fluctuant mass of 7 cm diameter in his right hemiscrotum. It is possible to feel the spermatic cord above the lump, but it is not possible to clearly distinguish the right testis as it is within the swelling. The mass transilluminates brightly and is non-tender.

What is the most likely diagnosis? What is the significance of a negative history of testicular cancer, trauma, and infection?

This is a **hydrocele** – a collection of fluid within the tunica vaginalis. The key features in the examination are that there is fluid (hence the lump is fluctuant) surrounding the testis and thus it is not possible to palpate the testis itself. If this were an epididymal cyst, the testis would still be palpable. It is possible to feel the spermatic cord above the swelling – thus distinguishing this from an inguinoscrotal hernia (the situation is rather more complicated with childhood hydroceles). Hydroceles may reach impressive sizes and contain as much as 500 mL of fluid.

The significance of a negative history of trauma, infection, or testicular cancer is that there are two sorts of hydrocele: primary (idiopathic), and secondary to the aforementioned testicular insults. Secondary hydroceles usually present in men in their 20s to 40s, as this age group is most susceptible to the initiating pathologies. Treatment options differ according to whether the hydrocele is primary or secondary. With secondary hydroceles, treatment is of the underlying condition. With primary hydroceles, options are to do nothing, aspirate the fluid collection (most will recur), or undergo surgery.

25

Mr Blofelt is a 32-year-old club rep who has just returned from a season in Ibiza. He presents with a 10-hour history of pain and swelling in his scrotum. He has had a headache and rigors, and believes that he has a temperature. On direct questioning he admits to having had some penile discharge and painful micturition over the previous 3 days. He says that he was 'very' sexually active whilst on his recent travels.

Examination reveals a swollen, red, tender, warm right hemi-scrotum. The right epididymis and right testis are very tender to palpation. Prehn's sign (relief of pain upon elevating the scrotum) is positive, and the cremasteric reflex (elevation of the testes upon stroking the inner thigh) is present (although neither sign is pathognomonic). There is no visible urethral discharge. His temperature is 38.3°C, pulse 105 bpm regular, and blood pressure 147/82 mmHg.

What is your differential diagnosis? Which diagnosis is most likely? What investigations would you like to order?

Remember that an acutely painful testis in a young man should always make you suspect testicular torsion. Although we must consider torsion in this instance the history and examination are more suggestive of **epididymo-orchitis**. Mr Blofelt has had systemic symptoms, is febrile, and provides a history that is suggestive of a sexually transmitted infection. Acute infections of the testis and epididymis usually ascend via the vas, having arisen in the urinary tract or as sexually transmitted infections.

It would be wise to request the following tests:

- Bloods: **full blood count** (looking for a leucocytosis) and **blood culture**.
- Urine: **dipstick** (looking for positive leucocytes and nitrites), **microscopy, culture, and sensitivities (MC&S)** – looking for culprits of the infection.
- You should advise a **urethral swab** and **genitourinary medicine (GUM) screen**.

Treatment is likely to involve bed rest, scrotal elevation, and appropriate antibiotics for at least a month. Contact tracing may be considered if this proves to be a *Chlamydia* or *Gonococcus* infection.

Your threshold for investigating a possible testicular torsion should be low and some surgeons advocate surgical exploration of any acutely painful testis (particularly in children). Surgical investigation provides an immediate and certain answer and avoids missing torsion, which has grave consequences – although this advantage must be balanced with the risks of surgery (bleeding, infection, anaesthetic risk). Sometimes, with a low pre-test probability of torsion, duplex ultrasound can be helpful in avoiding unnecessary surgical exploration.

Viva questions

Why is a radical orchidectomy performed via an inguinal incision rather than a scrotal incision?

Removing a malignant testis via a scrotal incision would potentially risk seeding malignant cells into the scrotum during the procedure. The significance of this lies in the lymphatic drainage of the testes and scrotum – the former drain to para-aortic nodes whereas the scrotum drains to inguinal nodes.

Does orchidopexy reduce the cancer risk of previously undescended testes?

Orchidopexy does not reduce the cancer risk of undescended or maldescended testes *per se*. It does, however, mean that the testes (which are abnormal and hence have an inherently higher cancer risk) can now be checked easily and hence cancer can theoretically be detected at an earlier stage.

What are the most common types of testicular tumour?

The two most important types to know about are seminomas and teratomas as these combined represent 90% of testicular tumours. Teratomas typically affect men aged 20–30 whereas seminomas classically affect men in their 30s to 50s.

Are varicoceles more common on the right or left? Why is this?

Almost 98% of idiopathic varicoceles present on the left. Various theories have been put forward, but the most consistent explanation relates to the anatomy of the venous drainage of the testes. The right gonadal vein drains directly into the inferior vena cava, and does so at an oblique angle. By contrast, the left gonadal vein drains into the left renal vein at a 90° angle. It is believed that this draining arrangement contributes to the development of varicosities.

What might you consider if a left-sided varicocele appears suddenly in a previously normal scrotum?

The sudden appearance of a left-sided varicocele is a rare, but important, presentation of renal tumours (clear cell adenocarcinoma in adults and nephroblastoma in children) as both of these tumours may invade the left renal vein and hence compromise drainage of the left gonadal vein.

Which pathogens are most likely to cause epididymo-orchitis in patients <35 years and >35 years?

In men <35 years of age sexually transmitted infections are the most likely source of ascending infection, thus consider *Chlamydia trachomatis* and *Neisseria gonorrhoea*. In men >35 years of age, urinary tract pathogens such as *Escherichia coli* are most likely.

Which pathogen might you consider in a boy who presented to his GP with a swelling adjacent to the angle of his jaw 8 days ago, and now presents with a swollen testis?

You should consider the mumps virus. Mumps orchitis is a blood-borne infection and may present without any previous history of parotid swelling.

What is idiopathic scrotal oedema?

This is a condition that primarily affects pre-pubescent boys, peaking around 6–7 years. The boy presents with acute-onset erythematous, oedematous scrotal swelling, which is often bilateral and may extend into the groin. A key feature which helps distinguish idiopathic scrotal oedema from other causes of the 'acute testis/scrotum' is that the child is often unconcerned about the swelling (they may be slightly tender to palpation) and will often be running around A&E completely bemused by the amount of attention being paid to their nether regions. This is in stark contrast to a boy with testicular torsion, hydatid torsion, or epididymo-orchitis – all three of which would result in pain.

Idiopathic scrotal oedema will resolve over 48–72 hours and needs no further management other than reassurance (of parents and child) and analgesia.

 For a range of Single Best Answer questions related to the topic of this chapter go to
www.oxfordtextbooks.co.uk/orc/ocms/

Limb weakness

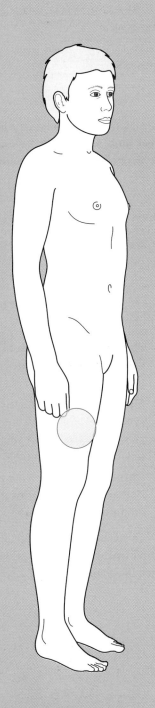

Approach

Approach

Limb weakness is a complex presentation to unravel. As with any other clinical situation, the broad approach involves resuscitation where appropriate, followed by history, examination, and suitable investigations as dictated by the history and examination findings. However, it helps to have a diagnostic approach in mind before you approach the patient with limb weakness.

Limb weakness is a symptom and therefore subjective. Thus, it is important to establish what exactly the patient means by limb weakness.

What could be confused for weakness?

The definition of weakness is important, because many patients who self-describe a 'weak limb' will actually have a clumsy limb (**ataxia**), a numb limb (**reduced sensation**), or a limb that is too **painful** to move.

One of the most important elements in a history of limb weakness is the time course.

How does the time course help with your diagnosis?

The time course of the onset of the symptoms in general reflects the time course of the underlying pathology:

- **Sudden onset** (seconds to minutes) usually implies either trauma or certain vascular insults, e.g. stroke, transient ischaemic attack (TIA), subarachnoid haemorrhage.

- **Subacute onset** (hours to days) is seen in pathologies such as Guillain–Barré syndrome (progressive autoimmune demyelination), venous thrombosis (progressive blockage of a vein), or a subdural haematoma (progressive enlargement of the haematoma).

- **Chronic onset** (weeks to months), is consistent with pathologies such as a slow-growing tumour or motor neuron disease (progressive degeneration of motor neurons).

As only acute and subacute limb weakness will present acutely to generalists in hospital (chronic onset cases will most likely be referred to neurology), we have limited the chapter to these cases.

26

A full neurological examination will enable you to fully define the deficit(s) – both the motor symptoms (including the pattern of limb weakness) and any other signs (e.g. language).

Having defined the deficit(s), you should think about where the lesion could be. The lesion should be localized clinically rather than by using imaging, as there is a risk of misattributing the pathological symptoms to an incidental finding (i.e. imaging should be used to confirm your clinical impression).

Three pieces of information that will help you localize the lesion clinically are:

1. What is the pattern of weakness?
2. Are there signs of a lower or upper motor neuron lesion (LMN or UMN)?
3. Are there other (non-motor) localizing signs, e.g. involvement of language, attention, or eye signs?

Let's take each in turn.

1. What are the potential different patterns of weakness (e.g. hemiparesis)? For each, where could the lesion(s) be?

The pattern of weakness is described using a combination of the terms as follows:

The prefix mono- implies one limb

The prefix hemi- implies half of the body

The prefix para- implies the lower limbs

The prefixes tetra- or quadra- imply all four limbs

The suffix -paresis implies weakness (can still move)

The suffix -plegia implies complete paralysis

So, for example, a patient with a weak left arm and leg (with or without a weak left face) would be described as having a left hemiparesis, whereas a patient with paralysed legs has a paraplegia.

Limb movement requires an intact pathway from the cerebral cortex, down the corona radiata, internal capsule, and pons, along the corticospinal tract of the spinal cord, out along a nerve root, and down a peripheral nerve to the neuromuscular junction and muscle itself (see Fig. 26.1). If a patient has limb weakness, there must be a lesion somewhere in this pathway.

Different patterns of weakness suggest the different possibilities for the site of the lesion (Table 26.1).

26

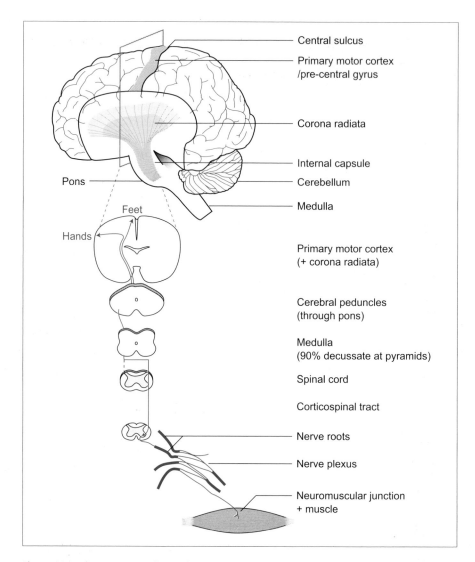

Figure 26.1 The motor tract from primary motor cortex to muscle.

Table 26.1 Different patterns of weakness and possible lesion sites

Pattern of weakness	Site of lesion
Full body hemiparesis	Contralateral cerebral motor cortex (e.g. widespread stroke)
	Contralateral corona radiata, internal capsule, or pons (e.g. stroke)
Limb hemiparesis	Contralateral cerebral motor cortex (e.g. stroke)
	Contralateral corona radiata, internal capsule, or pons (e.g. stroke)
	Ipsilateral spinal lateral motor tract (e.g. cervical disc prolapse)
Isolated limb weakness (arm or leg)	Contralateral cerebral motor cortex (e.g. localized stroke)
	Contralateral corona radiata, internal capsule, or pons (e.g. stroke)
	Ipsilateral peripheral nerve root (e.g. osteophyte)
	Ipsilateral peripheral nerve plexus (e.g. trauma to brachial plexus)
	Ipsilateral peripheral nerve *per se* (e.g. angiogram sheath injury to the femoral nerve)
Paraparesis	Bilateral cerebral motor cortex (e.g. parasagittal meningioma)
	Bilateral motor spinal tracts (e.g. cord compression)
	Cauda equina (e.g. lumbar intervertebral disc prolapse)
	Bilateral lumbosacral plexus (e.g. Guillain–Barré syndrome)
Tetraplegia	Bilateral motor tracts of cervical spinal cord (e.g. traumatic spinal cord transection at C5)
	Peripheral nerves (demyelinating disease, i.e. Guillain–Barré syndrome)
Proximal muscle weakness	Neuromuscular junction (e.g. myasthenia gravis, Eaton–Lambert syndrome)
	Muscle (e.g. polymyositis, dermatomyositis) or secondary to other conditions (e.g. hyperparathyroidism) or drugs (e.g. statins)
Several episodes separated in time and space	Various sites in central nervous system (e.g. multiple sclerosis)

26

In an UMN lesion, the pathology causing the muscle weakness lies within the central nervous system (CNS; spinal cord and brain). In a LMN lesion, the pathology is peripheral, i.e. between the spinal cord and the muscle.

The signs that distinguish between UMN and LMN lesions are shown in Table 26.2.

Table 26.2 Differences between UMN and LMN signs

UMN signs	LMN signs
↑ Tone	↓ Tone
↑ Reflexes	↓ Reflexes
↑ Plantars (Babinski reflex)	Fasciculations (sometimes)
Clonus (sometimes)	Wasting

Pathology in the neuromuscular junction and muscle most commonly causes proximal muscle weakness with *normal* tone and reflexes.

If you get confused about these signs, it may help to remember that in *lower* motor neuron lesions tone and reflexes are *lowered* or reduced, with the converse applying to UMN lesions. Also, it is worth noting that UMN lesions may paradoxically present with normal or reduced tone and reflexes in the initial phase, because of spinal shock.

Weakness accompanied by UMN signs may be termed 'pyramidal' and the increased tone 'spasticity', whereas if the signs are of a LMN lesion it may be called 'flaccid'. The term pyramidal relates to the fact that the descending motor neurons pass through the medullary pyramids (and on to the corticospinal tract). In a **pyramidal pattern of weakness**, extensors are disproportionately weaker than flexors in the upper limb and vice versa in the lower limb. This gives rise to the classic stroke posture: flexed upper limb and extended lower limb.

26

Language defects

These suggest pathology in the **cortex of the dominant hemisphere** (usually the left, even if the patient is left-handed). Look specifically for:

- **Receptive dysphasia.** The patient speaks fluently (although often with jumbled words and phrases) but cannot comprehend language. This suggests a lesion to Wernicke's area (in the temporal lobe) of the dominant hemisphere.

- **Expressive dysphasia.** The patient can comprehend language and follow instructions, but cannot find words or speak fluently (classically with correct phrases but like a telegram with missing 'link words'). This suggests a lesion to Broca's area (in the frontal lobe) of the dominant hemisphere. Indeed, Broca's original patient could only say the word 'tan'!

Attention defects

These suggest a lesion to the **parietal cortex**.

- **Neglect.** The patient ignores half of their sensory world. This can be distinguished from hemianaesthesia or hemianopia by asking the patient to draw a clock; the patient with neglect will only draw half of the clock face.
- **Extinction.** This is subtly different from neglect in that the patient ignores half of their sensory world *only* when presented with simultaneous stimuli to both sides.

Eye signs

Depending on the specific defect, these suggest a lesion at different points of the visual pathway. There are many potential lesions and defects, but those that arise most commonly in the context of limb weakness include:

- **Complete blindness** in one eye. The lesion is likely to be in the optic nerve (e.g. optic neuritis) or globe itself.
- **Homonymous hemianopia,** or loss of the same half of the field of vision in both eyes. It suggests a lesion (ischaemia, mass) at some point between the optic chiasm and the visual cortex, on the contralateral side ... but beware that visual neglect due to lesions to the parietal cortex can mimic homonymous hemianopia.
- **Eye deviation.** If the eyes deviate away from the weak side, this suggests a cortical lesion. If the eyes deviate towards the weak side, this suggests a brainstem lesion.

There are other higher cortical functions you can test for (e.g. graphaesthesia, astereognosis, apraxia, acalculia), to see if the lesion is cortical rather than lying in deeper brain structures (e.g. the internal capsule), but it is unusual to do so in the acute setting.

Sensory symptoms

For example paraesthesia or loss of one or all of the sensory modalities. In a weak limb with LMN signs, sensory signs can help distinguish between a nerve root or peripheral nerve lesion (sensory signs present) and a neuromuscular or muscular lesion (absent). In limb weakness with UMN signs, sensory loss can indicate damage to specific tracts in the spinal cord: spinothalamic (pain and temperature), dorsal columns (light touch, vibration, position sense or proprioception), as well as corticospinal (motor). This helps distinguish types of spinal cord pathology (e.g. an anterior spinal artery infarct spares dorsal columns).

26

Once you have decided clinically where the lesion causing the limb weakness is likely to be, you should start thinking about what *type of lesion* it could be. This will guide your investigations (e.g. computed tomography (CT) is good for showing brain haemorrhages but magnetic resonance imaging (MRI) is better for showing demyelinating diseases).

What diseases can cause limb weakness? Think about it in terms of pathologies that could affect each part of the motor pathway (see Fig. 26.1).

Table 26.3 Possible types of lesions

Site of lesion (clinically)	Possible type of lesion
Cerebral cortex, corona radiata, internal capsule, pons	Infarct
	Haemorrhage
	Central demyelinating disease (i.e. multiple sclerosis)
	Abscess
	Rapidly growing tumour (e.g. meningioma during pregnancy)
Corticospinal tract in the spinal cord	Compression (e.g. due to disc prolapse)
	Demyelination
	Transection
	Infarct (rare given blood supply of spinal cord)
Nerve root (radiculopathy)	Impingement by osteophytes, spondylosis, or bulging disc
Nerve plexus, peripheral motor nerve	Transection/trauma
	Peripheral demyelinating disease (e.g. Guillain–Barré syndrome)
	Compression by a mass (e.g. haematoma)
	Other (e.g. vasculitis, diabetes mellitus, alcohol)
Neuromuscular junction	Autoantibodies interfering with synaptic transmission (e.g. myasthenia gravis, Lambert–Eaton syndrome)
Muscle	Myositis

In addition, motor neuron disease and subacute combined degeneration of the cord (SACD, due to vitamin B_{12} deficiency) can cause UMN and/or LMN signs in any anatomical pattern although both of these diseases usually present as a *chronic* limb weakness rather than an *acute* limb weakness.

26

Finally, you should look for an underlying cause where this isn't already defined by the answer to the question above (e.g. multiple sclerosis, motor neuron disease). Thus an infarct may be due to emboli coming from atherosclerosis of the carotid arteries, or from the heart if it is in atrial fibrillation or has suffered a recent infarct with mural thrombosis.

What clues will you look for on examination for an underlying cause of limb weakness?

Cardiovascular examination

- Any signs suggesting a source of embolus that could have caused a stroke or TIA
    - Signs of endocarditis (e.g. splinter haemorrhages, cardiac murmurs)?
    - Atrial fibrillation?
    - Carotid bruits?
- Hypertension? Hypertension is a risk factor for both ischaemic and haemorrhagic strokes, but remember that strokes can themselves cause secondary hypertension.
- Signs of widespread atherosclerosis, i.e. peripheral vascular or ischaemic heart disease. Either makes atherosclerosis in the cerebral vasculature more likely.

Fundoscopy

- Hypertensive retinopathy, specifically arteriovenous nipping, flame haemorrhages, and silver or copper wiring of arterioles. Hypertension is a likely contributory cause in any stroke.
- Diabetic retinopathy, specifically cotton wool spots, dot-blot haemorrhages, hard exudates, macular oedema, proliferative retinopathy (new vessels around the disc).
- Raised intracranial pressure (which may suggest an intracranial mass), i.e. papilloedema.

The overall approach outlined above is summarized in the flow chart in Fig. 26.2.

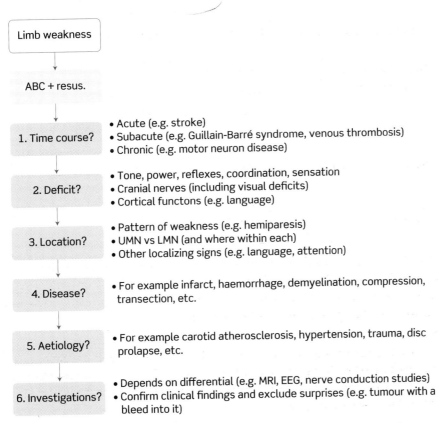

Figure 26.2 A suggested diagnostic approach for acute limb weakness. ABC + resus., airways, breathing, and circulation + resuscitation; UMN, upper motor neuron; LMN, lower motor neuron.

26

Core case

Mr Walker is a 62-year-old right-handed farmer who has been brought into the Medical Admissions Unit with acute-onset limb weakness. The emergency team have already assessed his airways, breathing, and circulation (ABC) and he is stable. Mr Walker tells you that he was walking at a cattle market when he suddenly developed a weakness in his left leg that made him go 'wobbly'. He tried to hold on to a fence but found that he couldn't move his left arm. An ambulance was called and he came to hospital. He isn't aware of his weakness getting worse or of any other symptoms, and denies previous episodes.

His past medical history is remarkable only for the lack of a distal phalanx on the little finger of his right hand due to an accident on the farm. When asked, he admits he occasionally gets some chest pain if he over-exerts himself. He has smoked two packs of cigarettes a day since he was 16. He drinks a single pint of ale every evening at his local pub. He lives with his wife and one of his two sons at a local farm. His family history is unremarkable, with both of his parents dying of 'old age' in their late 70s; his only sister is alive and well. He takes no medications and has no allergies.

Based on the history, how would you describe Mr Walker's deficit?

On examination, what should you be looking for?

Mr Walker has presented with **acute left-sided hemiparesis** (from the description it is unclear whether the face is affected or not).

You should use the clinical examination to confirm the pattern of weakness from the history, to determine whether the lesion is UMN or LMN, and to elicit any additional (non-motor) localizing signs. At the same time you should be thinking of the possible underlying causes and looking for clues as to which of these is the culprit.

You examine Mr Walker. On inspection you note that the left corner of his mouth is drooping and his left arm is lying completely still, although he is moving his right arm normally.

Examination of his left arm reveals decreased tone, power 0/5 on the MRC scale (for definition of the MRC scale see the Viva questions), decreased reflexes, and decreased (but still present) sensation to both pin-prick and vibration. The left lower limb shows decreased tone, power 3/5 on the MRC scale, present patellar reflex, and upgoing plantar reflex and normal pin-prick and vibration sensation. There are no abnormalities on examination of the right upper and lower limbs.

Examination of his cranial nerves reveals several positive findings. Visual field testing reveals a loss of the left field of vision in both eyes. On examination of his facial movements, the patient is unable to blow out his cheek or grin on the left side. However, he is still able to wrinkle both sides of his forehead and blink normally. His tongue deviates towards the side of the limb weakness (left). His speech is spontaneous and fluent but slurred.

Cardiovascular examination reveals a regular heart rate of 80 bpm, blood pressure 170/100 mmHg, and a bruit in his right carotid. Peripheral pulses are all present. Respiratory examination is unremarkable except for tar stains on his fingers.

What has the examination told you about: the pattern of weakness; whether there are UMN or LMN signs; the presence of other localizing signs; and consequently, the most likely site(s) of the lesion?

From the examination you can deduce the following about the location of the lesion:

- **Pattern of weakness:** Mr Walker is unable to blow out his cheek or grin on the left, but note that forehead wrinkling and blinking is present bilaterally (we will come to this shortly). Therefore he has a left-sided facial weakness. This confirms that he has a **full-body, left-sided hemiparesis**. Note that the arm and face weakness is greater than the leg weakness, where there is some residual movement (3/5 on the MRC scale).

- **UMN versus LMN:** the decreased tone in his limbs is consistent with either a LMN lesion or the acute phase of an UMN lesion. But the intact knee reflex and upgoing plantar reflexes and the ability to wrinkle his forehead on both sides confirm that it is an **UMN lesion**. Sparing of forehead wrinkling and blink distinguishes UMN facial weakness from LMN facial nerve palsy: in a LMN lesion the final common pathway to the frontalis and orbicularis muscle is destroyed, but these muscles have bilateral UMN representation and are therefore spared in a unilateral UMN lesion.

- **Other localizing signs:** Mr Walker has **homonymous hemianopia** (loss of the left half of his visual field in both eyes). This suggests a lesion in the **right cortex** affecting the optic radiation as well as the motor pathway. There are no language impairments other than dysarthria, which is most likely due to acute tongue and facial muscle weakness.

- **Likely location of lesion:** clinically, Mr Walker has got signs of an UMN lesion, suggesting the lesion is somewhere in the CNS. He also has a homonymous hemianopia, suggesting the lesion is in the cerebral cortex (rather than the spinal cord) and is affecting the optic tract (between the optic chiasm and lateral geniculate nucleus), both optic radiations (between the lateral geniculate nucleus and occipital visual cortex), or the occipital visual cortex. The left-sided hemiparesis and left-sided homonymous hemianopia suggest the lesion is on the right side. Thus, Mr Walker has a lesion in his **right cerebral cortex**.

> What is the differential for the type of lesion? Are there any clues to the aetiology from the examination above?

The possibilities include:

> Stroke (infarct or haemorrhage)
> Cerebral mass (e.g. tumour, abscess – potentially with a bleed into it)
> Todd's palsy (post-seizure paralysis)
> Migraine
> Hypoglycaemia (can present with localized signs although it is unclear how)

26

The weakness is greater in the arm and face than the leg. From neuroanatomy we know that the most medial part of the primary motor cortex maps to the lower limb, whereas the more lateral areas map to the upper limb and face (see Fig. 26.3). Moreover, we know that the medial primary motor cortex is primarily supplied by the anterior cerebral artery (ACA), whereas the rest of the primary motor cortex is supplied by the middle cerebral artery (MCA; see figure). The MCA also supplies the right posterior parietal cortex, where damage can cause a contralateral hemineglect.

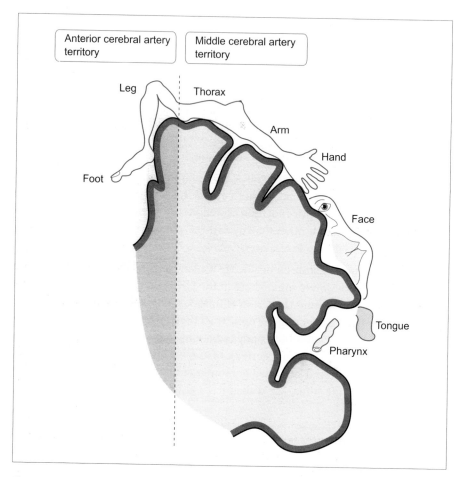

Figure 26.3 The primary motor cortex and its blood supply.

Thus, Mr Walker's pattern of weakness and the acute time course is suggestive of a right MCA stroke, either resulting from an infarct or mimicked by haemorrhage. On examination, there was a right carotid bruit, which could represent the source of emboli causing an infarct.

Having decided that a right-sided MCA stroke is the most likely diagnosis, what first-line investigations will you arrange?

26

Bloods

- **Full blood count:** this may reveal a cause for arterial occlusion (e.g. polycythaemia, thrombocytosis) or haemorrhage (e.g. thrombocytopenia).

- **Blood glucose:** although you have made a diagnosis of stroke, you must rule out hypoglycaemia as a cause for the limb weakness – it is possible the patient has both had a stroke and is hypoglycaemic.
- **Blood clotting:** particularly important if the patient is on warfarin and also to exclude a haemophilia or coagulopathy.

Imaging

- **CT head scan.** Although stroke is a clinical diagnosis, you must determine whether this is an ischaemic stroke or a haemorrhagic stroke. A CT head scan should be performed as soon as possible (certainly within 24 hours, but immediately if possible) on all patients with suspected stroke. Also, a CT will help rule out alternative diagnoses such as a space-occupying lesion in the right hemisphere. Although MRI is more sensitive at picking up the initial stages of ischaemia, CT is better at viewing haemorrhages (fresh blood is bright white), and is quicker and more readily available than MRI. Note that while CT can pick up fresh blood straight away, it can take up to 24 hours for infarction to become apparent on a CT scan.
- **Electrocardiogram (ECG):** looking for atrial fibrillation, a potential cause of emboli.

Second-line investigations

Note that patients can have 'dual pathology', e.g. both carotid stenosis and atrial fibrillation. Finding one potential cause should not preclude a search for another. If the head CT or MRI confirm an ischaemic stroke or the patient has a TIA (i.e. the neurological deficit has resolved in <24 hours), a patient should have both of the following investigations:

- **Carotid Doppler ultrasonography:** an ultrasound of the carotid arteries will identify or exclude carotid artery atheromas that could be the source of emboli causing the stroke. Clinical examination for carotid bruits is not a sensitive way of detecting carotid artery stenosis.
- **Echocardiogram:** an echocardiogram will help identify a cardiac source of emboli (e.g. indicated by atrial fibrillation, a recent myocardial infarction, an abnormal ECG, a heart murmur, ischaemic events affecting more than one cerebral artery territory).

Mr Walker's blood glucose is 5.3 mM and his clotting is normal (international normalized ratio (INR) 1.1). His ECG is normal. The CT head scan excludes a haemorrhage, suggesting that the stroke is likely to be ischaemic.

Why is it important to find out if the stroke was ischaemic or haemorrhagic?

26

Ischaemic strokes (about 80% of strokes) are usually caused by embolism or *in situ* thrombosis occluding a cerebral artery and are therefore potentially treatable by thrombolysis (e.g. with tissue plasminogen activator, tPA), provided this is started within 3 hours of onset of symptoms, as well as antiplatelet therapy.

However, antiplatelet treatment and particularly thrombolysis are likely to make a haemorrhagic stroke worse!

There is little in the way of acute management for the approximately 20% of strokes that are haemorrhagic other than supportive measures.

> Your Consultant agrees with the diagnosis of right-sided MCA ischaemic stroke.
>
> **How should Mr Walker be managed acutely?**

Strokes are a medical emergency, to be treated with the same sense of urgency as a myocardial infarction. After checking his need for resuscitation (ABC), Mr Walker will need:

- **Thrombolysis.** Mr Walker has had an ischaemic stroke less than 3 hours ago and is therefore a candidate for thrombolytic therapy. You must first check for contraindications to this therapy. Provided these are absent and he is in a centre that has the necessary resources, he is a candidate for thrombolysis using tPA.

- **Antiplatelet drugs.** Antiplatelet drugs (typically aspirin) have been shown to improve outcomes in ischaemic stroke, probably from early secondary prevention. They are given as soon as a haemorrhagic stroke has been excluded by imaging but are delayed 24 hours if the patient receives thrombolysis.

- **Venous thromboembolism (VTE) prophylaxis:** stroke patients are largely immobile and therefore at increased risk of thromboembolic events (deep vein thrombosis and/or pulmonary embolus) due to blood stasis. This can be prevented by using compression stockings on the legs and, for ischaemic stroke patients, subcutaneous heparin. Note that subcutaneous heparin is sometimes also given to patients with a haemorrhagic stroke but only some time after the event, once cerebral bleeding has stopped.

- **Stroke unit/specialist ward.** Mr Walker needs transferring to a specialist stroke unit where he can be looked after by a **multidisciplinary team** consisting of specialist nurses (e.g. who will manoeuvre the patient regularly to avoid bedsores), specialist speech and language therapists (SALT) who are experts at assessing, for example, whether a patient is safe to swallow food and liquids without choking, specialist occupational therapists (e.g. who will assess how a patient can start to mobilize and gain independence again), and social workers (e.g. who will consider the financial and community care needs of the patients upon their discharge).

There is still not enough evidence that any **neuroprotective agent** is safe or beneficial to patients, despite the fact that they have attracted much media attention.

> Thinking beyond the acute setting, what medical complications of stroke should you be worried about? What actions can you take to minimize the likelihood of these occurring?

26

- **Pressure ulcers:** patients who are immobile are at risk of developing bedsores (very quickly), which can then become infected. Bedsores can be prevented by regularly moving the patient and/or having them on a special inflatable mattress which periodically varies the area of the body that is resting most heavily on the mattress.

* **Aspiration pneumonia:** stroke patients often have difficulty swallowing and are therefore at risk of aspirating food, fluids, or gastric secretions, leading to pneumonia. This can be prevented by carrying out a swallowing assessment and, if necessary, feeding the patient via a nasogastric (NG) tube.

* **VTE** and **recurrent ischaemic stroke:** as discussed above under acute management.

In patients with a suspected stroke you should always assess disability, as this is critical in establishing the level of care and support they need on the ward.

Which elements should form part of your disability screen? Why is each important?

You should assess the patient in terms of the following:

* **Glasgow Coma Scale (GCS) score:** the GCS will have been recorded as part of the initial survey (under D for Disability, after ABC). Remember that the GCS score reflects the patient's best response. Thus, because this patient can move his right side normally he scores 15/15, indicating no impairment of consciousness. The GCS is used to monitor progress and/or inform a decision to intervene (e.g. intubating). The GCS score on admission also gives an indication of prognosis.

* **Swallow:** an assessment is required to see if the patient is safe to swallow solids and/or fluids. If not, they are at risk of aspiration and may need a secure airway and/or NG tube. It will also determine how they are given fluids and nutrition.

* **Speech and language:** you will have assessed this as part of your neurological examination, but a speech and language therapist may be additionally involved to aid communication between the patient, staff, and family.

* **Visual fields:** a patient with severely impaired visual fields will need care to avoid tripping over, to avoid food or water being placed outside their field of vision, etc.

* **Gait:** it is vital to determine whether a patient is safe to walk or not. If they cannot walk, they will need prophylaxis for deep vein thrombosis and pressure sores secondary to immobility.

A week after his admission, Mr Walker is recovering. He is in good spirits and determined to 'get back to normal'. His left facial palsy is still present, but improving. His left arm has developed a spastic weakness but power is now 3/5 and he can grab objects albeit clumsily. The tone in his left leg is almost normal and although power is still only 4/5, the occupational therapist is keen to attempt walking soon.

How should Mr Walker be managed now that the acute phase is over?

26

* **Risk factor reduction:** Mr Walker has two modifiable risk factors that should be addressed before discharge:
    - **Carotid artery disease:** Mr Walker's right carotid bruit suggests carotid artery stenosis due to atherosclerotic disease. It is quite probably the source of the

embolus responsible for his right-sided MCA stroke. Mr Walker should have a Doppler ultrasound of his carotid arteries within a week of the onset of his stroke. If this shows a stenosis of >70%, Mr Walker may benefit (before discharge) from either a carotid endarterectomy or a carotid artery stenting within 2 weeks of the onset of his stroke (the evidence for this comes from the NASCET and ECST trials[1-3]). There is still considerable debate about the risk–benefit ratio of these procedures and which of the two procedures is preferable.

- **Smoking:** Mr Walker should be advised to stop smoking, as this is a significant risk factor for all atherosclerotic disease, including strokes.

• **Drug prophylaxis:** patients who have suffered an ischaemic stroke benefit from three lifelong medications:
  - Daily antiplatelet prophylaxis (e.g. aspirin ± dipyridamole) to reduce the chances of further thrombotic events. This should also be started before discharge.[4]
  - Daily statin, even if cholesterol levels are normal.[5]
  - Daily angiotensin-converting enzyme (ACE) inhibitor and/or thiazide diuretic, aiming for a blood pressure of <130/85 mmHg (or <120/80 mmHg if diabetic).[6]

• **Discharge with community care:** Mr Walker is now probably fit enough for discharge to an intermediate community hospital nearer his home. This will allow him to continue to recover and adapt to his new circumstances in an environment that is still supportive (with nurses, occupational therapists, physiotherapists, and access to physicians) but hopefully closer to his home. In time, pending a full assessment from the individuals in his multidisciplinary team (e.g. occupational therapist, physiotherapist) and in the context of his social circumstances (e.g. is there anyone who could help care for him or will he need carers?), Mr Walker will hopefully return home.

Follow-up: it is important that his GP monitors him for any of the stroke risk factors picked up in hospital and continue to manage these as relevant.

Acute management of stroke is summarized in Fig. 26.4.

[1] North American Symptomatic Carotid Endarterectomy Trial Collaborators (1991). Beneficial effect of carotid endarterectomy in symptomatic patients with high-grade carotid stenosis. *New Engl J Med*, **325**: 445–453.

[2] European Carotid Surgery Trialists' Collaborative Group (1998). Randomised trial of endarterectomy for recently symptomatic carotid stenosis: final results of the MRC European Carotid Surgery Trial (ECST). *Lancet*, **351**: 1379–1387.

[3] Barnett HJ, Taylor DW, Eliasziw M *et al.* (1998). Benefit of carotid endarterectomy in patients with symptomatic moderate or severe stenosis. North American Symptomatic Carotid Endarterectomy Trial Collaborators. *New Engl J Med*, **339**: 1415–1425.

[4] Diener HC, Cunha L, Forbes C, Sivenius J, Smets P, Lowenthal A (1996). European Stroke Prevention Study. 2. Dipyridamole and acetylsalicylic acid in the secondary prevention of stroke. *J Neurol Sci*, **143**: 1–13.

[5] Collins R, Armitage J, Parish S, Sleight P, Peto R (2004). Effects of cholesterol-lowering with simvastatin on stroke and other major vascular events in 20536 people with cerebrovascular disease or other high-risk conditions. *Lancet*, **363**: 757–767.

[6] Hankey GJ (2003). Angiotensin-converting enzyme inhibitors for stroke prevention: is there HOPE for PROGRESS after LIFE? *Stroke*, **34**: 354–356.

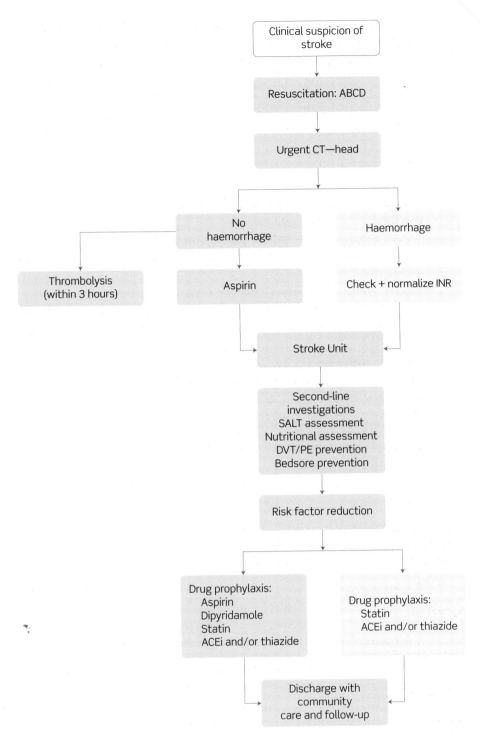

Figure 26.4 Flow chart for acute management of stroke. ABCD, airways, breathing, circulation, and disability; INR, international normalized ratio; SALT, speech and language therapists; DVT, deep vein thrombosis; PE, pulmonary embolism; ACEi, angiotensin-converting enzyme inhibitor.

26

Short cases

Mr P Browne is a 57-year-old investment banker who has been attending a ball to celebrate his daughter's engagement. At the ball, Mr Browne remembers feeling unusually short of breath dancing the Charleston and took a break to have a cocktail. He suddenly dropped the cocktail he was holding and found himself unable to move his right arm. His daughter noticed that his speech was slurred. They called for an ambulance but by the time Mr Browne arrived in hospital, his speech was back to normal. On examination, his right arm was still weak (4/5 on the MRC scale) but much improved from before, when he said he was unable to move it at all. The remainder of the neurological examination was unremarkable. His heart rate was irregularly irregular and his blood pressure 154/95 mmHg. An ECG showed no P-waves, confirming his heart was in atrial fibrillation.

Mr Browne's past medical history includes an appendicectomy and hypertension, for which he takes an ACE inhibitor (ramipril). He admitted feeling unusually short of breath playing cricket over the past few weeks. He has never smoked and drinks only socially (he insists this is less than 10 units a week). He lives at home with his second wife and although he still works, they are both hoping to retire to the south of France soon.

How would you assess Mr Browne in terms of the framework above (i.e. time course, deficit, location, disease, aetiology)? What is the most likely diagnosis? How should he be managed? How would you decide if warfarin is indicated?

1) Time course: acute onset, short-lived, and self-resolving.
2) Deficit: right hemiparesis and dysarthria on history (but no UMN/LMN signs on examination).
3) Location: ?left primary motor cortex.
4) Disease: reversible vascular insult, i.e. **TIA**.
5) Aetiology: emboli from either the left atrium, as he is in **atrial fibrillation**, or the carotids. His **uncontrolled hypertension** is additionally a risk factor for atherosclerosis, which may be a source of emboli, and small vessel haemorrhages.

TIAs are usually caused by small emboli lodging in cerebral arteries and causing cerebral ischaemia. Unlike in stroke, the clots in TIAs dissolve naturally under the action of the plasmin system before any lasting neurological defect can develop. Hence TIAs resolve spontaneously (80% within an hour, 100% within 24 hours) and leave no long-term deficit.

Management

Although TIAs self-resolve, the management is as for stroke: you need to establish the likely source of the emboli. If you don't and the cause is left untreated, about 25% will have a further TIA, a stroke, or a fatal cerebrovascular event within 90 days. The risk is highest early on (especially the first 24 hours), then decays. Having dealt with the cause, you should also look for and manage any other risk factors. In Mr Browne's case, you will need to address his atrial fibrillation, which increases the risk of TIA/stroke fivefold, and uncontrolled hypertension, as well as looking for other risk factors.

Warfarin

You should first exclude the carotids as a source of emboli by carotid Doppler ultra-sound. If this is clear, a cardiac source is most likely, particularly given Mr Browne's atrial fibrillation. Provided there are no contraindications, he is then suitable for anticoagulant therapy with either warfarin or aspirin. Although warfarin decreases the risk of embolic stroke, it increases the risk of haemorrhage, thus a scoring system (CHADS2) has been devised to determine when the benefits outweigh the risks. The CHADS2 score is calculated as follows:

Cardiac failure (1 point)

Hypertension (1 point)

Age >75 years (1 point)

Diabetes mellitus (1 point)

Stroke or TIA history (2 points)

A CHADS2 score of ≥2 warrants warfarin, as the benefits outweigh the risks. Patients with a CHADS2 score of 0 should instead be given aspirin, and those with a score of 1 may be given either (equivocal evidence) depending on your assessment of the patient. There is no benefit of adding aspirin to warfarin in terms of stroke prophylaxis, but it may be indicated for other reasons (e.g. risk of cardiovascular disease). Mr Browne has a CHADS2 score of 3 (hypertension and he has just had a TIA) so (but delay this until after surgery if he is to have a carotid endarterectomy during the same admission), he should be started on lifelong anticoagulation with warfarin.

26

Short case

Mr Bell is a 62-year-old gentleman who is referred to his local hospital because of a recent onset of leg weakness. He first noticed his legs becoming weak about a fortnight ago, when he found himself struggling to get out of the armchair or his car. The weakness progressed to the point where he had to use his wife's walking frame to get around the house, but since 2 days ago he has been unable to walk at all.

A year ago Mr Bell had a right coronary artery stent after a myocardial infarction, but has no other past medical history of note. He currently takes aspirin and simvastatin. His family history is remarkable for three of his five siblings developing colorectal cancer in their early 60s. He is a retired police officer who lives with his wife in a bungalow. He smoked two packs of cigarettes a day for most of his adult life, giving up only 2 years ago at the insistence of his daughter. He has not had any alcohol for some years.

On examination, both of Mr Bell's legs have increased tone and clonus, reduced power (2/5 on hip flexion and knee flexion), brisk patellar reflexes and ankle reflexes, upgoing plantar reflexes, and coordination which is difficult to test accurately due to the weakness. He has lost vibration sensation below the hips and pin-prick (pain) sensation below the umbilicus. His anal sphincter tone and perianal sensation are normal on digital rectal examination. Examination of his upper limbs, cranial nerves, cardiovascular, and respiratory systems is unremarkable and he is apyrexial.

How would you assess Mr Bell in terms of the framework above? What is the most likely diagnosis? What investigation(s) should be arranged in light of his history and examination?

1) Time course: gradual onset (weeks).

2) Deficit: spastic (UMN) paraparesis (bilateral leg weakness) + bilateral sensory loss in the lower limbs.

3) Location: ?spinal cord lesion around T10 in the cord (corresponds to a vertebral level around T6). There are UMN signs, thus it must be in the spinal cord or brain. The weakness is bilateral, and two cortical lesions are less likely than a single spinal lesion. The loss of pain sensation below the umbilicus, a landmark for the T10 dermatome, suggests a lesion around T10. Because the spinal cord is shorter than the spinal column, the vertebral level will be around T6.

4) Disease: the most likely cause is **cord compression**.

5) Aetiology: cord compression may be due to disc herniation, spondylolisthesis, or any other space-occupying lesion, i.e. a tumour, abscess, cyst, or haematoma. The subacute onset argues against e.g. haematoma.

Investigations

You should order an investigation to confirm your clinical suspicion, which in this case would be a **spinal MRI**. This will provide more information about the type of lesion (e.g. spondylolisthesis, tumour, etc.).

Mrs Bean is a 26-year-old post-doctoral laboratory researcher who presents to her GP complaining of a weak left leg. She describes that she first noticed an odd tingling sensation spreading up her leg about a week ago, which is still present. A few days after the tingling, she found herself tripping over several times in a single day. By this morning, she was limping and could not manage the stairs at home alone.

Nothing like this has ever happened before and she does not recall any trauma. She has never been admitted to hospital before but says that about a year ago she had some eye problems whilst travelling in Africa. She recalls that her right eye became painful and that she had blurred vision for almost a week, before it gradually resolved. She did not seek medical help at the time as she was 'in the middle of nowhere' and put it down to 'some weird infection'. She currently takes the combined oral contraceptive pill and sumatriptan for her occasional migraines. Her family history is unremarkable. She does not smoke and drinks only very occasionally. She lives with her husband and their 2-year-old child.

There are a number of notable features on neurological examination: when you get Mrs Bean to *rapidly* move her eyes from extreme right gaze to extreme left gaze, you notice that the right eye is slow to adduct relative to the left and abnormal nystagmus of the left eye. Adduction on convergence is normal. In addition, there is a relative afferent pupillary defect (Marcus Gunn pupil) on the right. On examination of her limbs you find that despite the tingling in her left leg, sensation in both legs is objectively intact. However, her left leg has increased tone, decreased power (3/5 on hip flexion and knee flexion), brisk patellar reflex, an upgoing plantar reflex, but normal coordination. Although she has not noticed anything in her right leg, this too has decreased power considering the patient's young age (4/5 on hip flexion and knee flexion), although tone, reflexes, and coordination are normal on the right.

How would you assess Mrs Bean in terms of the framework above? What is the most likely diagnosis? What investigations should you order to support this diagnosis?

1) Time course: gradual (1 week), ?previous episode.

2) Deficit: spastic (UMN) paraparesis (bilateral leg weakness) with a relative afferent papillary defect (RAPD) and internuclear ophthalmoplegia (INO; slow adduction of her right eye during saccadic movements and leading eye nystagmus with preserved adduction on convergent gaze).

3) Location: ?spinal cord lesion. The UMN signs mean it must be in the spinal cord or brain, and the bilateral nature makes the spinal cord more likely. However, INO indicates an additional lesion in her right medial longitudinal fasciculus. The previous episode of loss of vision suggests a further lesion in the optic nerve (at an earlier time).

4) Disease: multiple lesions at different times over a period of months or years are consistent with a demyelinating disorder. The UMN signs and involvement of vision indicate central (rather than peripheral) demyelination, i.e. **multiple sclerosis**. Stroke is unlikely given her age, the gradual onset, and the bilateral pattern of weakness with additional lesion(s).

5) Aetiology: the underlying cause of multiple sclerosis is unknown.

Multiple sclerosis characteristically causes central nervous lesions that are disseminated in space and time, and is strongly associated with both optic neuritis and INO. The earlier acute episode of a painful eye with blurred vision that spontaneously resolved after a week is highly suggestive of inflammation of her right optic nerve (optic neuritis). The right RAPD adds further weight to a diagnosis of a previous right optic nerve lesion.

26

Multiple sclerosis is, at least in part, an autoimmune disease in which Tc cells destroy the myelin sheath around neurons in the CNS at unpredictable locations and times, with some demyelination being reversible but some being permanent.

Investigations

Various paraclinical investigations can help confirm a clinical diagnosis of multiple sclerosis, but should only be made by an experienced neurologist because of the great fear and misunderstanding that it causes in many patients:

- **Lumbar puncture,** looking for oligoclonal bands. In multiple sclerosis, it is characteristic to find elevated levels of multiple IgG antibodies in the cerebrospinal fluid (CSF) compared with the blood serum. These are known as oligoclonal bands because the various different antibodies arise from multiple B-cell clones (oligoclonal) and appear as dark 'bands' on a protein gel used to visualize the proteins found in the CSF or the serum. These antibodies should be matched with a serum sample in order to elucidate whether they originate in the CSF or are features of a systemic immune response. Note that oligoclonal bands are a non-specific sign of multiple sclerosis.

- **MRI of the brain and spinal cord,** looking for plaques. As its name implies, multiple sclerosis causes many sclerotic (demyelinated) plaques to appear throughout the CNS. These can be visualized using MRI and help confirm a diagnosis of multiple sclerosis.

- **Visually evoked potentials:** optic neuritis leads to demyelination of the optic nerve and therefore slower electrical conduction along this nerve. It is possible to measure the activation of both visual cortices (occipital areas of both brain hemispheres) in response to visual stimulation. Delayed response indicates slow electrical conduction and a lesion along the optic pathway that may not be apparent clinically.

Viva questions

A young man is rushed into his local A&E after crashing his motorbike at high speed. Advanced trauma life support (ATLS) protocols are promptly followed by the trauma team, and the patient is found to be suffering from no life-threatening injuries. The trauma surgeon proceeds to examine the patient's limbs.

The patient has sustained a complex, closed, supracondylar fracture of the distal metaphysis of his right humerus. The patient has lost sensation over the medial aspect of his right hand on both the dorsal and palmar side and has weakness in finger adduction and abduction. The patient can still extend and flex his wrist, and has strong thumb abduction. However, abduction in his other fingers is weak.

What lesion has this patient most likely sustained during his accident that can explain the pattern of weakness?

The complex, distal fracture of his right humerus has probably injured his **ulnar nerve**. This would explain the weakness of the *intrinsic interossei* muscles of his right hand (responsible for abduction and adduction of the fingers) and the loss of sensation over the medial third of this hand (Fig. 26.5).

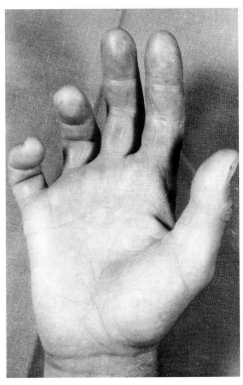

Figure 26.5 A hand with ulnar palsy.
From *Oxford Textbook of Medicine*, 4th edn, Vol. 3, Fig. 2, p.1185

Brown–Sequard syndrome is a rare neurological condition most commonly due to intrinsic cord lesions, e.g. multiple sclerosis, but classically seen in penetrating trauma to the spine or spinal fractures during road traffic accidents. Whilst rare, it is a favourite topic of examiners because it illustrates the neuroanatomy of the spinal cord. **Can you explain the features of Brown–Sequard syndrome anatomically?**

Each half of the spinal cord contains (amongst many others):

- Upper motor neurons innervating the *ipsilateral* side of the body.
- Dorsal column neurons (vibration, proprioception, fine touch) innervating the *ipsilateral* side of the body.
- Spinothalamic neurons (pain, temperature, light touch) innervating the *contralateral* side of the body.

Thus, section of half of the spinal cord results in loss of power (paralysis) and loss of vibration, proprioception, and fine touch on the same side of the body below the lesion, but loss of pain and temperature on the opposite side of the body (usually a few vertebral levels below the lesion, as spinothalamic neurons do not cross immediately upon entering the spinal cord).

What is the ABCD2 scoring system for prognosis in TIAs?

The ABCD2 score is used to identify individuals at high early risk of stroke after TIA. Its parameters are:

Age: 1 point for age >60 years

Blood pressure: 1 point for >140/90 mmHg

Clinical features: 1 point for speech disturbance without weakness, 2 points for unilateral weakness

Duration of symptoms: 1 point for 10–59 minutes, 2 points for >60 minutes

Diabetes: 1 point

Stroke risk up to 90 days after the event with a score of:
   0–3: low
   4–5: moderate
   6–7: high

What scale is used to grade limb weakness?

Power (and therefore weakness) in muscles is graded using the MRC scale for power:

Grade 5: normal power

Grade 4: can move limb against gravity and some resistance exerted by examiner

Grade 3: can move limb against gravity

Grade 2: movement only if gravity is eliminated

Grade 1: flicker is perceptible in the muscle

Grade 0: no movement

For a range of Single Best Answer questions related to the topic of this chapter go to
www.oxfordtextbooks.co.uk/orc/ocms/

Acute joint pain

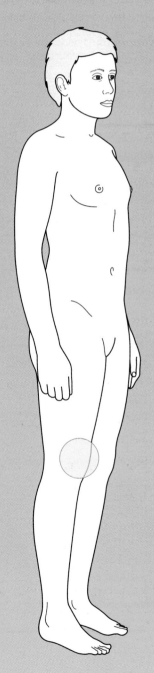

Core case

Read through the sections in red, covering up the sections in white that follow so that you don't see the answer. At the end of each red section, try to answer the question before reading on.

Core case

Mr Sullivan, a 54-year-old magazine editor, presents to accident and emergency (A&E) with knee pain that has been present since he woke up. He denies any recent trauma to the joint.

What diagnosis must you exclude in a patient with acute joint pain and why?

The 'must exclude' diagnosis is **septic arthritis**. Not only can it destroy articular cartilage within days if not treated (hence permanently reducing joint function), but it is also associated with a mortality of about 10% due to underlying bacteraemia.

Joint pain can be due to pathology in the joint or from structures outside the joint (i.e. not a true arthritis).

What are the articular causes of a single, acutely painful joint (i.e. monoarthritis)? What periarticular and non-articular pathologies can cause an acute arthropathy?

Remember that pain may be referred from elsewhere. For example, hip pathology may present as knee pain, and lumbar spine pathology may present as hip pain. The causes of a single, acutely painful joint include those shown in Table 27.1.

Table 27.1 Causes of a single, acutely painful joint

Articular	Periarticular	Non-articular
• **Trauma** (resulting in, e.g., fracture, meniscal tear, haemarthrosis)	• **Ligament injury**	• Nerve entrapment
• **Gout**	• **Tendonitis**	• **Radiculopathy**
• **Pseudogout**	• Bursitis	• Bone malignancy
• **Septic arthritis**	• Fasciitis	• Osteomyelitis
• Seronegative spondyloarthropathy	• Epicondylitis	• Neuroma
• Transient synovitis	• Periostitis	
• First presentation of chronic mono- or polyarthritis (e.g. rheumatoid arthritis)		
• Sarcoidosis		
• Amyloidosis		
• Vasculitis		
• SLE		
• Rheumatic fever		

27

What questions in the history will help you narrow down the differential?	

- **Pain.** You should characterize the pain as for any other pain along the lines of SOCRATES (see Chapter 1). Pain that worsens with movement and improves with rest is likely to be non-inflammatory. An acute onset (hours) is consistent with septic arthritis, gout/pseudogout, and trauma. A more insidious onset is more common in conditions like bursitis and tendonitis, where> the relevant anatomical structure becomes inflamed with overuse. Chronic onset suggests osteoarthritis (note that some rheumatologists prefer the term osteoarthrosis to reflect the fact that the inflammation is not the primary pathology). The severity of pain can usefully be assessed by asking about joint function – for example, can the patient weight bear?

- **Trauma.** Mr Sullivan has already said he remembers there being no trauma, but you must always ask and make sure. Even the slightest of knocks can cause significant pain. However, this does not exclude other diagnoses – trauma can precipitate infection or gout, for example.

- **Common risk factors for gout.** There are many potential causes of gout, but the more common ones that you should ask about include use of thiazide diuretics, recent heavy alcohol intake, chronic renal failure, and chemotherapy (high cell apoptosis, leading to degradation of DNA and excess urate). A history of renal stones or previous episodes of gout also makes gout more likely.

- **Common risk factors for septic arthritis.** Again there are many possible risk factors, but the key ones are immunosuppression (e.g. diabetes, HIV, steroid use) and any prosthetic joints.

- **Risk factors for haemarthrosis.** Typically due to a coagulopathy (e.g. classically haemophilia), although anticoagulant use is also a risk factor.

- **Past medical history**
  - **Recent gastrointestinal (GI) or urethral infection?** Reactive arthritis can develop after either of these types of infection. You should take a sexual history as a gonococcal infection may be asymptomatic, and can lead to septic (rather than reactive) arthritis (via haematogenous spread).
  - **Previous episodes?** Think first of recurrent conditions like crystal arthropathies and overuse injuries.
  - **Rheumatological disease?** This is as relevant for joint pathology as a past surgical history is for abdominal pathology.

- **Other joints.** The involvement of several joints *sequentially* is characteristic of gonococcus or rheumatic fever. The involvement of several joints *simultaneously* suggests a first presentation of a chronic polyarthritis such as rheumatoid or psoriatic arthritis. If you suspect the latter, you should ask about psoriasis.

- **Drug history.** A variety of drugs (e.g. thiazides, low-dose aspirin, or ciclosporin) can predispose to gout. Steroids predispose to osteoporosis, with subsequent pathological fractures, although pathological fractures are usually in the spine and very rarely in the knee.

27

Mr Sullivan tells you the pain in his left knee is a sharp pain and is severe. It was there when he woke up this morning and is still present when you clerk him mid-afternoon. He's tried paracetamol and ibuprofen but they have had no effect. He does not think he has had a fever.[†] He says his knee is red, hot, slightly swollen, and tender. There are no breaks in the skin.

Mr Sullivan is partial to wine and drinks half a bottle to a bottle with meals most nights. He has eczema and hayfever but no other ailments currently or previously. He uses a steroid cream, steroid nasal spray, and cetirizine tablets. He is married and has not had sex with another partner for over 5 years. No other joints are involved.

Any monoarticular pain requires examination of the relevant joint.

Describe how you would approach your examination of Mr Sullivan's knee. What features would help you distinguish articular from periarticular pain?

[†] Note that fever is not a very useful symptom, as it is neither specific nor sensitive enough to diagnose or exclude septic arthritis.

You should examine the relevant joint *and* one joint above and below, as pain may be referred from these joints. In Mr Sullivan's case, this means the knee, hip, and ankle – and the other knee for comparison.

Your joint examination should be based around 'look, feel, move':

- **Look:** inspect the joint for erythema, scars, swelling, muscle wasting, bony deformities. Make the most of symmetry and compare left with right, as in some individuals it may be difficult to tell if a joint is swollen or in some other way abnormal!

- **Feel** for any **effusions**; for **tenderness** on the bones, ligaments, tendons, or along the joint line; for **temperature** (in case of infection or inflammation); and for **neurovascular status**. Checking neurovascular status is crucial, as a neuropathy or vasculopathy (either causing the pain or secondary to joint damage) may rapidly lead to irreversible damage and loss of function.

- **Move:** being careful and gentle with the painful joint, test the **full range** of passive and active movement. There are additionally numerous special tests for each joint (many of them eponymous!) for which the reader is referred to a suitable orthopaedics resource.

Articular conditions are more likely to present with a diffusely inflamed joint (red, hot, painful) and pain on passive as well as active motion.

Periarticular conditions tend to have a focal point of tenderness on palpation (in bursitis this would be over the bursa; in tendonitis, over the tendon) and pain is usually much worse on active movement than on passive movement.

Many conditions causing acute monoarticular pain may have signs beyond the joint.

What would you look for on examination beyond the joint(s)?

You should keep an eye out for the following:

- **Skin:**
  - **Tophi:** deposits of urate crystals that can be found anywhere on the body usually around joints and bones. They are hard lumps that sometimes

break through the skin with a chalky appearance (Fig. 27.1). If present, they suggest chronic gout.

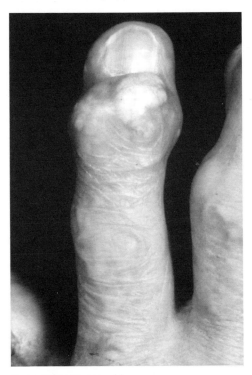

Figure 27.1 Gouty tophi.
Reproduced from Warrell et al., (2005), *Oxford Textbook of Medicine* vol 3, 4th Edition, p71, Fig 4. Oxford University Press.

- **Rheumatoid nodules:** subcutaneous nodules, classically found on elbows and ears, which are pathognomonic of rheumatoid arthritis.
- A variety of **rashes** are seen in conditions that can also cause arthritis e.g. psoriasis, systemic lupus erythematosus (SLE).

- **Nails:** look for pitting, subungual hyperkeratosis, and onycholysis – all signs of psoriasis, associated with psoriatic arthritis.
- **Uveitis** (inflammation of the middle layer of the eye), evidenced by a painful red eye with diminished vision, and sometimes an irregularly shaped pupil. This is often associated with HLA-B27-positive inflammatory arthropathies.
- **Mouth ulcers** which may be evidence of inflammatory bowel disease (particularly Crohn's disease), itself associated with arthropathy.
- Lung signs suggestive of **fibrosis** (e.g. clubbing, late inspiratory crackles), as pulmonary fibrosis is a complication sometimes seen in various inflammatory arthropathies.

Do not overly focus on these, as beyond the skin and nail signs these are relatively rare in someone presenting with acute joint pain (and indeed, outside of a rheumatology clinic!).

27

You examine Mr Sullivan. He has patches of eczema on his forearms and knees. He does not appear systemically unwell and is afebrile. His left knee is swollen and red compared with his right. On palpation it is warm and there is no effusion. You find he is diffusely tender to palpation around the joint, but not especially along the joint line, the patellar ligament, or patella. His dorsalis pedis and posterior tibial pulses are present, and sensation is normal throughout his lower leg. Active and passive knee flexion are markedly reduced due to pain (as a result you cannot test for strength). His right hip and ankle are not tender and have a normal range of movement.

Taking this information into account, what is the differential and how will you proceed?

The diagnosis is still not clear despite the history and examination – both septic arthritis and crystal arthropathies remain equally likely. In such cases you *must* perform **arthrocentesis** to exclude septic arthritis, given the seriousness of this condition. Arthrocentesis is the most useful diagnostic tool for discriminating between septic arthritis and other causes of acute monoarticular pain. It has the added benefit of offering symptomatic relief. Unfortunately the signs and symptoms of septic arthritis – fever, joint pain, and swelling – are non-specific and do not help distinguish it from some of the other causes of monoarticular pain

What are the possible findings and what do they mean?

You will want to perform microscopy (cell count and crystals), Gram stain, and culture on the joint fluid aspirate. There are several possible findings:

1) **Crystals.** Present in gout (urate crystals – negatively birefringent and needle shaped) and pseudogout (calcium pyrophosphate crystals – positively birefringent and rhomboid shaped). Detected by microscopy (Fig. 27.2).

2) **Infection.** Cloudy aspirate with elevated white blood cell count, a high neutrophil component, and bacteria visible on microscopy, with positive cultures a few days later, indicate septic arthritis. Note, however, that the white cell count may also be elevated in crystal arthropathies. Also note there is a false negative rate of about 20–25% in gonococcal septic arthritis. If you suspect gonococcus, you should request additional tests (below).

3) **Blood.** Haemarthrosis is seen in trauma with or without a fracture. If fat globules are present, it strongly suggests a fracture (the fat comes from the bone marrow).

4) **White cells.** In the absence of crystals, blood, and infection (all of which cause inflammation as well), inflammation as evidenced by white cells could be due to reactive arthritis (Reiter's syndrome), enteric arthropathy (due to inflammatory bowel disease), rheumatoid arthritis, psoriatic arthritis, and rheumatic fever. Non-inflammatory aspirate (clear and with a normal white cell count) usually suggests trauma or osteoarthritis.

27

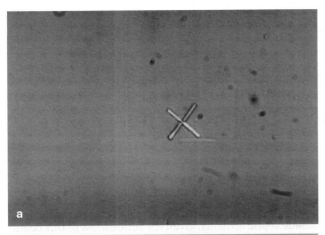

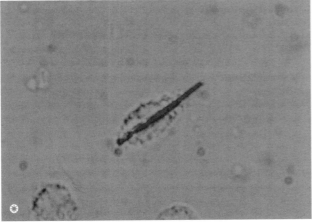

Figure 27.2 Negatively birefringent crystals, typical of gout.

Reproduced from Isenberg et al., (2004), *Oxford Textbook of Rheumatology*, 3rd Edition, plate 189. Oxford University Press.

Arthrocentesis is usually the only first-line investigation indicated. However, there are a number of other investigations that you may consider depending on the history and findings from arthrocentesis:

- **Cultures:** take swabs of skin lesions, or of throat, urethra, cervix, and rectum if gonococcal arthritis is a possibility. Blood cultures should be requested if there is a clinical suspicion of sepsis, although results may be negative in early infection.

- **Bloods**
  - **Full blood count (FBC), C-reactive protein (CRP), and erythrocyte sedimentation rate (ESR):** these will reveal any widespread inflammatory and/ or infectious process. Osteomyelitis will also result in deranged inflammatory markers (e.g. ESR and CRP) but not always a raised white cell count.
  - **Prothrombin time (PT) and activated partial thromboplastin time (APTT):** if arthrocentesis reveals a haemarthrosis in the absence of trauma sufficient to explain the injury, these should be requested to screen for a coagulopathy.

27

- **Rheumatological investigations:** if you suspect rheumatological disease, you may want to request rheumatoid factor, anticyclic citrullinated peptide (anti-CCP) antibodies, antinuclear antibody (ANA), and other autoantibodies.
- **Serum urate?** Patients who develop gout have often had hyperuricaemia for years, although during acute gout their serum urate is often normal or low. For this reason it should *not* be ordered in the acute setting. Also note that asymptomatic hyperuricaemia is fairly common in the population and thus a finding of elevated urate is not very helpful in diagnosis.

- **Imaging:** imaging rarely contributes anything to the diagnosis of non-traumatic, acute monoarthritis. As with serum urate, it may occasionally be misleading as pathology unrelated to the acute monoarthritis may be picked up, e.g. osteoarthritis. However:
  - **Radiographs** are useful if there has been trauma as they identify fractures and, depending on the site, some effusions (e.g. elbow).
  - **Magnetic resonance imaging (MRI)** is the imaging of choice for soft tissue injuries and other extra-articular pathology, e.g. osteomyelitis. If you have excluded intra-articular pathology, MRI can be very helpful.

As with all presentations, resist the temptation to request a 'standard' panel of investigations as they may misdirect you. This is particularly the case with investigations such as ANA, which are relatively non-specific.

> You perform arthrocentesis on Mr Sullivan and send the aspirate to the lab. The microbiology report notes the presence of 'negatively birefringent crystals' and a negative Gram stain; cultures are pending.
>
> **What is the diagnosis? Why is the Gram stain result important?**

Urate crystals are negatively birefringent, needle-shaped crystals and therefore Mr Sullivan has **gout**. Gout most commonly affects the big toe (podagra), but the knee is the second most common joint affected and thus Mr Sullivan's presentation is not atypical. Calcium pyrophosphate crystals seen in pseudogout are positively birefringent, rhomboid-shaped crystals.

Even in the presence of crystals, it is crucial to exclude septic arthritis, which may coexist with a crystal arthropathy. Hence Gram staining, and cultures, remain crucial to the diagnosis.

> **What are the options for managing Mr Sullivan? What contraindications might drive your management?**

Treatment of gout can be divided into **acute** and **chronic.**

Acute management

During the acute episode of gout, the following medications can be helpful:

- **Non-steroidal anti-inflammatory drugs (NSAIDs),** which are contra-indicated in patients with peptic ulcer disease, acute or chronic renal failure, heart failure, asthma, or pregnancy.

27

- **Colchicine,** if administered within 24 hours, can provide dramatic relief. However, it is contraindicated in patients with renal or hepatic impairment and causes severe GI side-effects unless used in low doses.

- **Corticosteroid injections** either injected into the joint, or given systemically, are useful in patients who cannot take NSAIDs or colchicine.

Interestingly, aspirin is contraindicated in gout because low doses can cause hyperuricaemia by impairing urate excretion. However, this effect appears to be dose dependent, such that daily, low-dose aspirin used for preventing cardiovascular events increases urate levels far less than full-dose aspirin. For this reason, many patients with gout and significant cardiovascular risk factors continue to be prescribed low-dose aspirin, as a single acute cardiovascular event is arguably a worse outcome than occasional episodes of gout, which may (or may not) be caused by the low-dose aspirin in any case.

Chronic management

In the longer term, you will want to investigate Mr Sullivan for hyperuricaemia. If present, this can be treated using three strategies, although none of these will work in the acute setting:

- **Decrease urate production: allopurinol** is an inhibitor of xanthine oxidase and limits the production of urate during the degradation of nucleic acids. The dose of allopurinol is titrated to the serum or urinary levels of urate until these are reduced to normal levels. The dose must be reduced in patients with renal or hepatic impairment and must be stopped if it causes a rash, as this tends to pre-empt more serious side-effects. *Colchicine must always be co-prescribed with allopurinol for the first 6 weeks because the initial doses of allopurinol can paradoxically result in acute gout.*

- **Increase urate excretion: sulfinpyrazone** and **probenecid** are drugs that inhibit the reuptake of urate at the proximal convoluted tubules in the kidneys, thereby increasing urate excretion. They are useful for patients who cannot tolerate allopurinol.

- **Increase degradation of urate: rasburicase** is a uricase enzyme that can be administered to patients with severe hyperuricaemia due to chemotherapy.

27

Short cases

Mrs Hanbury is a 32-year-old school teacher who presents with an acutely tender left elbow that she knocked whilst gardening at the weekend. She took ibuprofen and paracetamol at night to alleviate the pain but was unable to sleep and has come in to A&E because it is getting worse. She says it hurts 'no matter what I do' and is tearful. She drinks the occasional glass of white wine, has had no recent medical problems, and is on the combined oral contraceptive pill but nothing else.

You examine Mrs Hanbury's left elbow. It appears swollen compared with the right elbow and is red and tender. You also note the presence of lots of scratches on the skin over her elbow, which she explains are from her gardening. Sensation and capillary refill are normal in her left hand. However, she finds active and passive motion exquisitely painful. Her pulse is 88 bpm, blood pressure 110/58 mmHg, temperature 38.4°C, respiratory rate 14/min, and saturations 99% on room air.

The radiologist performs arthrocentesis of the affected elbow under ultrasound guidance. The aspirate, which is yellow and turbid, is sent off to the laboratories for appropriate analysis.

What diagnosis should you be worried about? How should Mrs Hanbury be managed whilst you wait for the results of the arthrocentesis?

Mrs Hanbury has a very painful joint that developed acutely, with evidence of trauma to the skin (possible route of entry for infection, although most septic arthritis is due to haematogenous spread). The joint is clinically inflamed (red, hot, swollen, tender) and painful to both active *and* passive motion. She is also pyrexic, and has a yellow, turbid aspirate that would be consistent with pus. The diagnosis you should be worried about is **septic arthritis**.

If you suspect septic arthritis you should immediately start **analgesia,** take **blood cultures** to help identify the responsible pathogen, and start **broad-spectrum empirical antibiotics** (in accordance with local guidelines, to be adjusted when sensitivities are known). If the diagnosis is confirmed, she will need **joint aspiration and lavage**, either arthroscopically or as an open surgical procedure.

Mrs Jones is a 48-year-old shop assistant at a supermarket who presents to the Minor Injuries Department with pain in her right shoulder that has been ongoing for some days but is getting worse and is limiting her activities. She gets the pain around the front of the shoulder, and it occurs when she tries to move the joint. She is a keen tennis player and has been playing a lot recently, so thought it might be a strain. As a result she has tried 'RICE' – rest, ice, compression, elevation (she has some first aid training) – with some relief. There has been no trauma and no redness or swelling although her shoulder is tender. Her past medical history is notable for anxiety, for which she takes citalopram, and asthma, which is managed using a salbutamol inhaler as required. She dislocated the same shoulder when she was 22 and although she hasn't dislocated it since, she feels 'it isn't right' and that it 'pops out a bit' at times. Her job involves shifts of stacking shelves, which is very repetitive. She has not had a cold and is not sexually active. She does not drink and is a vegetarian.

She is apyrexial and comfortable at rest, and is wearing a self-fashioned sling. You expose both her arms, and on inspection her right and left shoulders look the same. However, her right shoulder is tender over the bicipital groove, unlike her left. Shoulder flexion reproduces the pain, although abduction, adduction, and internal and external rotation are normal. Special tests of the rotator cuff muscles are also normal. On examination of the elbow, you find elbow flexion and forearm supination cause pain.

What is the most likely diagnosis? What investigation would you consider for this lady? How might you manage her?

Mrs Jones has **bicipital tendonitis**, an overuse injury particularly common in those performing repetitive lifting activities (such as stacking shelves). It usually coexists with other shoulder pathology including rotator cuff damage and shoulder instability. Mrs Jones probably has the latter, having dislocated her shoulder and reporting it feels like it 'pops out a bit' at times. Tenderness over the bicipital groove suggests inflammation of the long head of the biceps tendon that passes through that groove. Pain on shoulder flexion, elbow flexion, and supination is classic in this condition.

She should be managed with **analgesia** (regular paracetamol and cautious use of anti-inflammatories such as NSAIDs because of her asthma) and **rest**. If the pain is severe or persists, it is sometimes helpful to administer a **corticosteroid injection** into the affected space (e.g. the bicipital groove) but *never* into the tendon itself, as this can cause it to rupture.

If her symptoms do not resolve, the investigation of choice would be **MRI** given that this is a soft tissue injury. This is particularly the case given her history of shoulder problems, as you will want to check the rotator cuff and other structures for damage as well.

27

Mrs Sermon is an 81-year-old living in a nursing home who is referred for a painful, immobile right leg. You ask where the pain is and she tells you it is primarily in her right thigh but her right knee and hip are also sore. It came on over the past 2 days and was not associated with any trauma. The pain has not worsened over the last 2 days. She has an indwelling catheter for incontinence control, which she has had for the last 2 months as her dementia appears to have deteriorated. She takes a thiazide for hypertension and simvastatin for her cholesterol. She does not drink. Her past medical history is remarkable for a right hip replacement 7 years ago, with which she has had no problems to date. There is no other medical history of note. However, the nursing staff tell you that Mrs Sermon's urine has been dark and smelly for the last day, and was positive for leucocytes and nitrites on urinalysis that morning.

She has a temperature of 38.1°C but is haemodynamically stable. She is a thin lady and you can see that her right thigh is swollen relative to the left, and red. The knees look the same. You notice the scar from her hip replacement. On palpation, her right thigh is warm and extremely tender. Passive flexion of the knee or hip brings on pain in her right thigh, not the joints themselves. Distal pulses are present and sensation is intact throughout her right leg.

You decide to admit Mrs Sermon for further investigation and, potentially, treatment. There is no significant effusion around the knee and, given the clinical picture, you decide not to perform arthrocentesis, at least for the time being. Bloods are taken, which show a white cell count of 14.1×10^9 cells/L and a CRP of 28.8 mg/dL. Blood cultures are also taken and a urine sample is sent off for microscopy, culture, and sensitivities. Radiographs are also requested and show no bony abnormality.

What is the most likely diagnosis? How might you confirm this? How should she be treated in the acute setting?

Mrs Sermon has a 2-day history of an acutely painful limb. The pain, inflammation, and tenderness are primarily in the right thigh, arguing in favour of a non-articular cause. Of note in the history is the indwelling catheter, the fever and elevated inflammatory markers, and the urinalysis suggesting a urinary tract infection. The combined information suggests a *possible diagnosis* of **osteomyelitis**, the most likely cause being haematogenous spread from the urinary tract infection.

MRI has a high sensitivity for osteomyelitis early in the disease process. Radionuclide bone scanning and computed tomography (CT) imaging are alternatives for confirming your diagnosis.

Mrs Sermon will need a long course of suitable intravenous (IV) antibiotics (follow local guidelines and consult your local microbiology department, as prior to cultures empirical therapy is often based on age and presentation). She should be referred to the orthopaedic surgeons. Cultures will be required to check for sensitivities.

Mr Taylor is a 27-year-old fitness instructor who presents with a 3-day history of a painful, stiff left knee and difficulty walking. The pain is always there and has not improved despite rest and analgesia. There has been no trauma to his knee. He says he has had some trouble recently with a sore eye and blurred vision. He also suffers from mouth ulcers, and has a couple at present. On direct questioning, he tells you that he has developed a rash on his glans penis and has had urethral discharge for the past 2 weeks with dysuria. He has had a number of male sexual partners over the last couple of months and has not yet been to the sexual health clinic, which he insists he was planning to do. There is no history of gout or other illness, and he takes no medications. He enjoys wine but does not drink heavily.

On examination, he has a temperature of 37.6°C and a hot, red, swollen, and very tender knee. All active and passive movements of his left knee are painful. In addition, you note his eye is red.

Arthrocentesis reveals a clear fluid with no blood or crystals. Gram stain and cultures are pending, as are urethral, rectal, and pharyngeal swabs and bloods.

Based on the history and examination findings, what is the most likely diagnosis? If you are correct, what is the management?

Mr Taylor's history of urethral and eye symptoms, and the clinical finding of a red eye in addition to an inflamed joint, are highly suggestive of **reactive arthritis (Reiter's syndrome)**.

Reiter's syndrome is an inflammatory arthropathy that typically affects patients with the HLA-B27 genetic allele and follows an episode of either gastroenteritis (*Salmonella* spp., *Campylobacter* spp., *Shigella* spp.) or sexually transmitted urethritis (*Chlamydia trachomatis*). The syndrome classically causes a triad of uveitis, urethritis, and arthritis (remembered as *'can't see, can't pee, can't climb a tree'*).

You should consider all of the following in your management plan:

1) Analgesia (NSAIDs or, if necessary, corticosteroid injection)

2) Rest

3) IV antibiotics until cultures are back to exclude a septic arthritis

4) If you suspect *Chlamydia* (or gonorrhoea, although this typically causes a septic arthritis), treat as per local antibiotic guidelines

5) Ophthalmology referral (as an inpatient)

6) Referral to a sexual health clinic (for contact tracing, advice, and screening for sexually transmitted diseases)

7) Rheumatology follow-up in outpatients (as there is a risk of chronic arthritis)

27

Viva questions

Describe the pathophysiological circumstances in which serum urate might be elevated.

Remember that urate is the major end product of the degradation of purine (a component of nucleic acids). Thus there are a number of causes of hyperuricaemia:

1) Primary (90%)
   – Enzyme defects resulting in overproduction of urate ± underexcretion of urate
2) Secondary (10%)
   – Increased nucleic acid turnover, e.g. leukaemia, polycythaemia, cytotoxic drugs
   – Underexcretion, e.g. chronic renal disease, drugs (diuretics, low-dose aspirin, excess alcohol which competitively inhibits urate excretion), starvation

When is a rheumatological referral warranted for patients with painful joints?

You should consider referring patients with:

- suspected inflammatory polyarthritis; *or*
- recurrent monoarthritis unresponsive to treatment.

What are the most likely infective organisms in a native joint compared with a prosthetic joint?

- **Native joint infection:** *Staphylococcus aureus* is the most common infective organism of joints in all patients. In immunosuppressed patients one might find *Mycobacterium tuberculosis*. In patients with a possible or proven sexually transmitted disease one might find *Neisseria gonorrhoeae*. In patients with sickle cell disease one might find *Salmonella* spp.
- **Prosthetic joint:** *Staphylococcus epidermidis* is commonly implicated in infection of prosthetic joints. This probably reflects its ability to attach itself to artificial surfaces and its abundance (it is a major component of everyone's skin flora).

What are the features of osteoarthritis on a plain radiograph?

An osteoarthritic joint has a characteristic radiograph (Fig. 27.3) that may include some or all of the following features. These can be easily remembered using the mnemonic LOSS:

- Loss of joint space
- Osteophyte formation
- Subchondral sclerosis
- Subchondral cysts

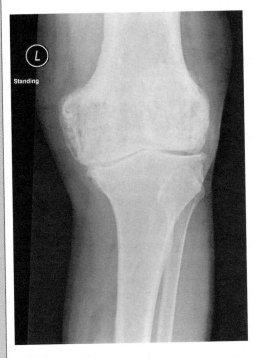

Figure 27.3 Radiograph of knee with osteoarthritic changes.

For a range of Single Best Answer questions related to the topic of this chapter go to
www.oxfordtextbooks.co.uk/orc/ocms/

27

Swollen calf

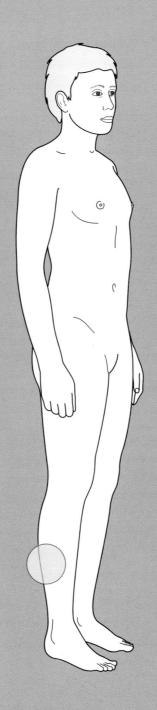

Core case

> Mrs McDonald is a 48-year-old cleaning lady who presents to a local hospital complaining of a swollen right calf that has appeared over that last few hours.
>
> **What is your differential diagnosis for an acutely swollen limb?**

Core case

The main causes of an acutely swollen limb are:

> ## Deep vein thrombosis (DVT)
> ## Cellulitis
> ## Ruptured Baker's cyst
> ### Muscular strain
> Septic arthritis
> Lymphoedema
> Pelvic tumour (e.g. ovarian) compressing iliac vein
> Allergic response to insect bite
> Compartment syndrome

Note that it is possible for different pathologies to coexist: a patient may present with a DVT and ruptured Baker's cyst, for example. Also, many patients will get a swollen leg following surgery to that leg, but this shouldn't present much of a diagnostic challenge and therefore is not included in the list above.

> **Would your differential diagnosis be different if *both* of her legs were swollen?**

Yes, because most of the diseases listed above are local diseases and it would be highly unlikely for the patient to have two similar events in both legs. Instead, it would be more likely that the patient has either a systemic problem or a problem affecting central vessels. However, it is worth remembering that a DVT can arise in a patient with pre-existing bilateral leg oedema, so don't rule out a DVT just because both legs are swollen.

Causes for bilaterally swollen legs are:

> Right heart failure (in isolation or together with left heart failure)
>
> Pregnancy
>
> Vasodilators (e.g. calcium-channel blockers)
>
> Hypoalbuminaemia: from renal failure (nephrotic syndrome), liver failure, or malabsorption/ malnutrition
>
> Pelvic tumour (e.g. ovarian) compressing the inferior vena cava
>
> Venous insufficiency

What specific questions would you ask Mrs McDonald during your history-taking? Think of questions that will provide key clues to help rule in or rule out particular diagnoses.

- Are there any risk factors for venous thrombosis?
  - **Hypercoagulable blood?** Trauma, surgery within the last month, pregnancy, active cancer, obesity (body mass index (BMI) $>30 \text{ kg/m}^2$), combined oral contraceptive pill or hormone replacement therapy, family history or past medical history of DVTs
  - **Stasis?** Bed rest (>3 days) or long-haul flight (>12 hours)
  - **Vessel injury?** Trauma, surgery.
- **Has she felt breathless, had any chest pain, or coughed up any blood?** If DVT is high on your differential list, it would be wise to enquire about symptoms of a possible pulmonary embolism (PE).
- **Has she had any cuts, insect bites, or other wounds to her right leg?** If the patient has recently had a wound in her right leg, infective diseases such as cellulitis and septic arthritis become much more likely.
- **Is the swelling getting bigger?** Cellulitis can spread fairly rapidly along the affected limb, whereas the other pathologies are more likely to remain confined in the short term.
- **Has she had any abdominal pain? Has she noticed any blood in her faeces? Has she had any unusual vaginal bleeding? Has she noticed any weight loss, fever, or malaise?** If you are considering a pelvic malignancy as the cause of the limb swelling, you can ask for symptoms that are suggestive of colon, ovarian, or uterine malignancies.
- **Has she recently had radiotherapy or surgery to her right leg or abdomen?** Radiotherapy or surgery may have damaged the lymphatic drainage from her affected limb, causing the accumulation of lymph (lymphoedema).
- **Does moving the joints in her leg elicit the pain?** Patients with septic arthritis will tell you that movement of the affected joint brings on *excruciating* pain in the joint. Patients with compartment syndrome in their calf will tell you that moving the ankles and toes brings on pain in their calf (as this causes the flexors of the foot to move within the compressed compartment of the calf).

28

Mrs McDonald is in town visiting her daughter, who is getting married next week. She arrived yesterday after a 10-hour overnight bus journey and noticed that her right calf started swelling within a few hours of arriving. She can still walk on her affected limb, which is only slightly painful but 'feels very hot'. She thinks the swelling has been the same for the past few hours. She has not noticed any cuts, bites, or wounds in her right leg. She has not had any recent surgery, but started taking hormone replacement therapy last month to help with the unbearable hot flushes that she was getting from her menopause – her last period was 5 months ago and she has had no vaginal bleeding since. She has never had any cancer or radiotherapy, but did have her appendix removed when she was a teenager. Her past medical history is otherwise unremarkable. She has been trying to lose weight recently in preparation for her daughter's wedding but admits to limited success in her efforts as her BMI is still >30 kg/m².

Can you identify risk factors for any of your differential diagnoses in the history?

- **Long-distance travel:** several studies have shown an increased risk of venous thrombosis in people who are immobilized through travelling for more than 8 hours non-stop. It is important to realize that what matters is the prolonged immobility, and not the type of transport used. Thus, most lay people will (wrongly) associate DVTs with all forms of flying (irrespective of duration) whilst few people will consider long-haul bus, train, or car journeys as a risk for DVT. Also, it is important to note that most studies suggest that the increased risk of DVT associated with long-distance journeys applies only to people with other predisposing risk factors for DVT, although patients may not be aware of these at the time of travelling.

- **Oestrogen- and progesterone-based therapies:** several studies have shown that medications involving oestrogen and/or progesterone analogues (e.g. contraceptive pills in fertile women, hormone replacement therapy for menopausal women, tamoxifen in breast cancer patients) increase the risk of venous thrombosis. However, it is important to note that most people taking oestrogen/progesterone-based medications will have a low baseline risk of venous thrombosis, and so increasing that risk only moderately will still result in a risk that is low overall.

- **Obesity:** obesity also increases the risk of thrombotic disease.

Having taken a history, you examine Mrs McDonald.

Is there anything in particular you will look for on examination that might help you sort out your differential diagnoses?

- **Cuts, bites, wounds, or superficial infections:** patients often haven't noticed small cuts, puncture wounds, or insect bites so look carefully for these all over the affected limb. Also check between the toes for fungal infection as a portal of entry.

- **Location of the swelling:** septic arthritis is likely to produce inflammation that is principally over a joint (e.g. the ankle, the knee). Compartment syndrome is likely to produce inflammation which is confined to the calf or thigh muscle compartments but spares the joints. A ruptured synovial sac in the knee ('Baker's cyst') would emerge from the popliteal fossa and track down into the calf.

28

- **Extent of swelling:** measure the extent of swelling using a tape measure to compare the circumference of both limbs at the same point (e.g. 10 cm below the tibial tuberosity). Also, mark the area of swelling with a pen so that you can monitor a progressing cellulitis.

- **Lymphadenopathy:** check for swollen lymph nodes along the affected leg and in the inguinal fold, as lymphadenopathy would be highly suggestive of an infection in the limb.

- **Abdominal masses:** an abdominal mass in the right lower quadrant would suggest a tumour that could be compressing the right iliac vein.

- **Neurovascular status of the limb:** it is imperative that you check and document the sensation, motor function, and pulses of the affected limb distal to the swelling. These can be affected by compartment syndrome, and compromise of neurovascular status is a surgical emergency.

- **Pain on gentle passive movement:** septic arthritis will elicit pain in the affected joint whereas pain in the calf is suggestive of compartment syndrome. Note that the joint should be moved gently and slowly to avoid dislodging any DVTs into the circulation.

Mrs McDonald looks systemically well but her right calf is indeed swollen (pitting oedema), red, warm, and tender from just below the knee to just above her ankle. Her right calf is 4.5 cm greater in circumference than her left calf. There are no wounds visible on her leg and no lymph nodes palpable in her right leg or right groin. Palpation of the popliteal fossa reveals no swelling. Slow, passive movement of the ankle and toes does not elicit any pain, only mild discomfort in her right calf. Her sensation to light touch is preserved throughout her right limb. Her posterior tibial pulses are present. Dorsalis pedis is not palpable on either leg, but capillary refill time in the toes of both feet is <2 seconds. Power on dorsiflexion, plantar flexion, and big toe dorsiflexion (extensor hallucis longus) is 5/5 on the MRC scale for both feet. There are no abdominal masses palpable.

The history, examination, and risk factors mentioned by Mrs McDonald should have narrowed your differential diagnosis down to just three 'most likely' diagnoses. Which are they?

DVT, ruptured Baker's cyst, or cellulitis.

Do you know of any scoring systems to help you decide how this lady should be investigated?

The pre-test probability of a patient having a DVT can be estimated using the Wells' scoring system for DVT (Table 28.1).

28

Table 28.1 The Wells' scoring system for DVT

Criteria	Points
Entire leg swollen	1
Calf swollen >3 cm (circumference) compared with the other leg	1
Pitting oedema confined to the leg (affected side)	1
Paralysed or immobilized leg	1
Bed rest for >3 days or surgery within the last 4 weeks	1
Tenderness along the course of deep veins of the leg	1
Collateral superficial veins visible on leg (non-varicose)	1
Active cancer (treatment within last 6 months or palliative)	1
Previous DVT	1
Alternative diagnosis more likely than DVT[†]	−2

Score 0 = low (3%) probability of DVT
Score 1–2 = moderate (17%) probability of DVT
Score >2 = high (75%) probability of DVT

[†] This refers to patients in whom the clinical history and examination strongly point towards a particular diagnosis for a swollen limb that is not a DVT. Thus, a patient with a rapidly spreading, shiny, red swelling over the calf and an obviously purulent puncture wound over the sole of the foot is quite likely to have cellulitis.

Mrs McDonald has a Wells' score of 2 (pitting oedema, calf swollen >3 cm).

Given Mrs McDonald's Wells' score, what investigations will you arrange?

The flow chart in Fig. 28.1 is useful for deciding the investigations in suspected DVT using the Wells' score. Note that D-dimer is used to exclude DVT only if the Wells, score is low (0); ultrasound is used to exclude DVT if the Wells' score is moderate (1 or 2), whilst both D-dimer and ultrasound are used to exclude DVT if the Wells' score is high (3 or more).

• **Doppler ultrasound of the right calf:** this is the most sensitive, rapid, and non-invasive way of visualizing a DVT in the lower leg (it does not detect isolated thrombi in the femoral or iliac veins). Ultrasound will also enable a ruptured Baker's cyst to be diagnosed.

• **Serum D-dimer levels:** D-dimers (fibrin degradation products) can be elevated by DVTs and PE, but also in various other situations such as acute coronary syndromes, atrial fibrillation, pneumonia, vasculitis, sickle cell crises, superficial phlebitis, malignancies, and disseminated intravascular coagulation. Elevated D-dimers have >90% sensitivity for DVT, but only 30–40% specificity. An elevated D-dimer is therefore not useful in positively diagnosing a DVT. However, a normal D-dimer level is useful because it rules out a DVT in someone with a low Wells' score without the need for an ultrasound. Also,

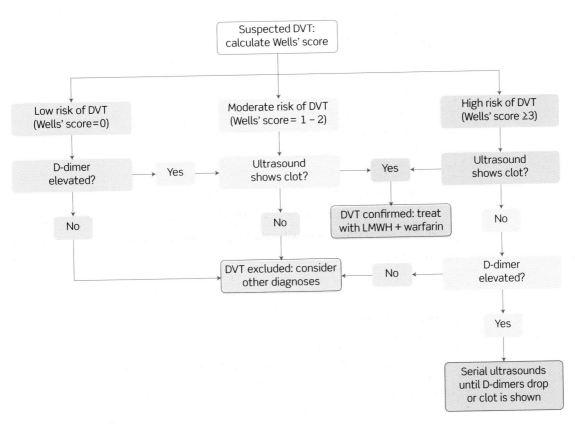

Figure 28.1 Diagnostic approach for a suspected deep vein thrombosis (DVT).

an elevated D-dimer in someone with a high Wells' score is an indication for doing serial ultrasounds (rather than a single investigation – if the first ultrasound scan is negative). Ultimately, however, it is the ultrasound that will positively diagnose the DVT.

♦ **Full blood count (FBC) and clotting studies:** a FBC may reveal a high white cell count (WCC; you still haven't ruled out cellulitis) or a high red blood cell count (RBC; polycythaemia – a rare cause of DVT) and clotting studies may reveal deranged coagulation.

> The Doppler ultrasound of Mrs McDonald's right calf showed an occlusion in one of her deep veins consistent with a DVT. Her serum D-dimer was not requested and her FBC was normal.
>
> **How will you manage Mrs McDonald?**

Mrs McDonald has had a diagnosis of **DVT** confirmed by Doppler ultrasound. Her management should include:

♦ **Anticoagulation.** This is to prevent clot extension, PE, and recurrence. Acutely, patients should be given low-molecular weight heparin (LMWH). LMWH is administered via a subcutaneous (SC) injection and is dosed according to the patient's weight. In addition they should be started on warfarin and have their international normalized ratio (INR) measured until it is stable in the

28

target range (2–3) at which point the LMWH can be stopped. The optimal duration of anticoagulation therapy is debated and varies with a number of factors such as location (above/below knee), previous DVTs, and the presence of risk factors. Mrs McDonald will require 3 months on warfarin.

• **Compression stockings.** To prevent acute recurrence. Mrs McDonald should also be advised to wear compression stockings on long-haul travel (or at other times of prolonged stasis).

• **Lifestyle advice.** Lifestyle advice, e.g. cessation of hormone replacement therapy (HRT) or the combined oral contraceptive pill, weight loss. These are risk factors for DVT that you should address.

Short cases

> Mr Bullen is a 34-year-old gardener who is on the trauma unit of his local hospital because he has broken his right tibia. He presented yesterday morning having been hit by a car while attempting to cross the road. He was diagnosed with a closed, transverse, minimally displaced fracture of the right tibial shaft which required internal fixation.
>
> You have been bleeped by the nurse on the Trauma Unit. Mr Bullen is complaining that his leg is 'excruciatingly painful' and that he cannot feel his toes. You attend and confirm that he cannot feel you touching his cold toes, which protrude from the cast. You immediately cut and remove the cast to reveal a right calf that is red, tender, swollen, and with skin that looks tense and shiny. There is no pitting oedema. Passive movement of his right toes or ankle causes severe pain. Sensation to light touch is diminished over the distal portion of his right calf, over the dorsum of his right foot, and over his toes. His right posterior tibial pulse is palpable but his dorsalis pedis is not, although it is palpable on the left leg.
>
> **What is the diagnosis? How will you manage this patient?**

Mr Bullen has features that are strongly suggestive of **compartment syndrome**: a tense, shiny, swollen limb that is painful to passive movement and has neurovascular compromise. Inflammation due to trauma (accidental or iatrogenic) is the most common cause of compartment syndrome. Limbs have muscle groups surrounded by tight inelastic fascia. The inflammation in a confined compartment can occlude the deep veins, impeding venous drainage of the limb, which therefore starts to swell – further occluding the deep veins. Pressures in the affected limb can become high enough to cause ischaemia and necrosis of all the tissues in the limb, leading to an irreversible atrophy of the limb known as **Volkmann's contracture**.

Compartment syndrome is a **surgical emergency** requiring urgent decompression via a **fasciotomy**. The skin, subcutaneous tissue, and tight fascia surrounding the affected limb are all divided and left open for a few days so that the pressure is relieved and the inflammation can resolve. Two longitudinal incisions are made in the leg in order to decompress all four compartments (anterior and lateral compartments via an anterolateral incision, and superficial and deep posterior compartments via a medial incision).

28

Miss Patel is a 21-year-old student who has just returned from celebrating the end of her university studies with her friends at a Mediterranean coastal resort in Catalunya. A few days after her return, her left ankle started to swell. She has presented because the swelling has been spreading up her leg and into her foot. She does not use the contraceptive pill. She has never had a 'blood clot in her legs or lungs' before, and has not had any recent surgery. Her past medical history is unremarkable. Her flight back from Catalunya lasted only 2.5 hours.

Inspection reveals a red, swollen distal calf, ankle, and dorsum of the foot; although a tape measure reveals that the swelling is actually only 1 cm more than her right limb. The swelling is warm, soft, and tender to touch but has no pitting oedema nor visible superficial veins. A small punctum is visible just next to her lateral malleolus, and she explains that it is a mosquito bite that was particularly itchy. Passive movement of her ankle and toes does not elicit any pain, although it is uncomfortable because of the swelling. No other lumps or bumps are palpable in the leg or abdomen. The patient is apyrexial.

What is the most likely working diagnosis and how will you manage this patient?

It is likely that Miss Patel has either **cellulitis** or an **inflammatory response to the mosquito bite** over her left ankle. Her Wells' score is 0 and therefore a DVT is unlikely (and can be ruled out if her serum D-dimer is negative). She has no signs of septic arthritis or compartment syndrome and is young for a pelvic malignancy.

Management of Miss Patel should include:

- **FBC:** looking for signs of bacterial infection (a neutrophilia).

- **Serum D-dimer:** given her Wells' score of 0, a negative D-dimer will rule out a DVT without need for an ultrasound. Unfortunately Miss Patel's D-dimer will be elevated in any case as she has an infection, thus the test will be of no diagnostic value in her case.

- **Doppler ultrasound:** as Miss Patel's D-dimer is unlikely to exclude a DVT, you will need to request an ultrasound of her calf to exclude the possibility of DVT.

- **Antibiotics:** an antibiotic that covers both streptococci and staphylococci should be used, such as flucloxacillin, in case this is cellulitis.

- **Topical steroids and oral antihistamines:** given the story that suggests that the mosquito bite may have triggered the episode, you should also consider that the swelling may simply be an inflammatory response to the mosquito bite (essentially an allergic response to the mosquito bite). If so, the inflammatory response will benefit from topical steroids (to dampen the immune response) and antihistamines (as histamine release by mast cells is likely to be driving the inflammation).

Mr Leroy is a 72-year-old gentleman who limps into hospital using a walking stick. He complains of a painful, swollen right calf since he woke up this morning. He has a past medical history of osteoarthrosis in his right knee and low-grade (papillary) bladder cancer for which he has received a cystoscopic resection and for which he receives ongoing, regular irrigation of his bladder with BCG (Bacille Calmette–Guérin, which is usually used for tuberculosis vaccination). On examination, his right calf is swollen (2 cm), pitting, warm, red, and tender all over (not specifically along the veins), with the inflammation extending up into the popliteal fossa. There are no other masses palpable in his leg or abdomen. His right foot has normal sensation, power, and pulses. Passive movement of his ankle and toes brings on mild pain in his calf. Suspecting a DVT because of his Wells' score (pitting oedema, active cancer = 2), a Doppler ultrasound of his leg is arranged but no occlusion of any deep veins can be seen.

What is the most likely diagnosis and how should the patient be managed?

Short case

This patient probably has a **ruptured Baker's cyst**. This is caused by rupture of a synovial sac protruding from the knee in the popliteal fossa, usually in patients with arthropathy of the knee. The fluid from the ruptured synovial sac ('Baker's cyst') can then track down into the calf, producing signs that are clinically indistinguishable from a DVT. However, the Doppler ultrasound helps to rule out a DVT, making the diagnosis of ruptured Baker's cyst the more likely one.

Treatment is by **aspiration of the fluid** and **injection of corticosteroids** into the knee, to reduce the inflammation and alleviate the pain.

28

Viva questions

A concerned patient comes to seek advice on how to prevent DVTs whilst travelling, because their brother suffered from a DVT after a long-haul flight last year. The patient explains that they will be flying from London (Heathrow) to Istanbul (Turkey), before taking a bus to the Cappadocia region of Turkey. The patient wants to know if he should take aspirin and wear compression stockings during the flight.

Several studies have shown that the risk of DVT whilst travelling is only increased if the patient is immobile for >8 hours and has other risk factors for DVT (although the patient may not be aware of these). The flight from London to Istanbul will take less than 8 hours and therefore poses little risk of DVT for this patient. However, the bus journey from Istanbul to Cappadocia is likely to take >8 hours and involve far less opportunity to mobilize than during the flight, so the patient may wish to wear compression stockings during the bus journey, rather than the flight. The Antiplatelet Trialist Collaboration[1] showed that aspirin can reduce the incidence of DVT by up to 25% in post-surgical patients, but as yet there is no evidence of aspirin being beneficial in preventing DVT in long-haul flights.

[1] Antiplatelet Trialists' Collaboration (1994). Collaborative review of randomized trials of antiplatelet therapy. III: reduction in venous thrombosis and pulmonary embolism by antiplatelet prophylaxis among surgical and medical patients. *BMJ*, **308**: 235–246.

Several congenital mutations, acquired diseases, and drugs can all make a patient's blood more likely to clot. Can you name them?

Congenital mutations

- Factor V Leiden mutation (5% of Caucasians)
- Prothrombin G20210A mutation (2% of Caucasians)
- Antithrombin III deficiency (0.4% of Caucasians)
- Protein C deficiency (0.5% of Caucasians)
- Protein S deficiency (0.5% of Caucasians)

Diseases

- Any form of malignancy
- Antiphospholipid syndrome
- Disseminated intravascular coagulation
- Polycythaemia

Drugs

- Combined oral contraceptive pill
- Hormone replacement therapy
- Heparin-induced thrombocytopaenia (HIT), which can counterintuitively cause thrombosis by an unknown mechanism but which can fortunately be prevented by using LMWH instead of full-length heparin
- Procoagulant drugs (e.g. for nosebleeds or menorrhagia), such as tranexamic acid or aprotinin

What components of the clotting cascade does warfarin interfere with? What additional drug should all patients starting on warfarin be placed on and why?

Warfarin is a competitive antagonist of vitamin K, the cofactor used by liver hepatocytes to synthesize factors II, VII, IX, X, protein C, and protein S.

Warfarin can take a few days to have an effect on clotting because it inhibits the synthesis of coagulation factors, and these have to become depleted. Also, warfarin can initially cause a paradoxical increase in clotting because of the depletion of protein C and protein S (anticoagulant) before the depletion of other clotting factors (procoagulant). For this reason, patients are started on LMWH for up to 5 days or until the INR >2 for two consecutive days.

What are the main contraindications and side-effects of warfarin therapy? What advice would you give a patient starting on warfarin?

Contraindications
- Pregnancy (warfarin is teratogenic)
- Severe hypertension (risk of haemorrhagic stroke)
- Peptic ulcer disease (risk of bleeding ulcer)

Side-effects
- Haemorrhage
- Nausea, vomiting, diarrhoea, rash (like most drugs!)
- Purple toes and skin necrosis
- Hepatic dysfunction, jaundice
- Pancreatitis

Advice for patients
- Avoid alcohol, cranberry juice, and St John's wort
- Check with GP before taking any other medication
- Consult GP if faeces or urine go dark or bloody

A patient who has been diagnosed with having a right femoral DVT is placed on LMWH and warfarin, but continues to throw off clots and suffer from small PEs. Is there any further treatment that can be offered?

You may wish to consider placing an inferior vena cava (IVC) filter using a venous catheter, to catch any clots that become dislodged.

28

A 19-year-old female who uses the oral contraceptive pill presents to A&E with a swollen left calf. She has a past medical history of non-Hodgkin's lymphoma for which she received chemotherapy until 2 months ago. A Doppler ultrasound of her leg confirms occlusion of a deep calf vein by a DVT. She is placed on LMWH and warfarin and admitted to hospital for observation. That night, she suffers a thromboembolic stroke. What may have happened?

This patient is very young for thromboembolic strokes. It is possible that her blood is in a highly coagulable state due to underlying malignancy and that this has predisposed to clot formation, but even then it would be hard to explain a clot forming in the fast-flowing arteries that supply the brain. It is more likely that the clot has formed in the slow-flowing veins and somehow reached the arteries supplying the brain without getting lodged in the lungs. The most plausible anatomical explanation is that the patient has a patent foramen ovale between her atria which has allowed for the dislodged DVT to cross into the systemic circulation and reach her brain.

This is not as far-fetched as it may sound. Echocardiographic studies show that 10% of the population have a patent foramen ovale. About 35% of embolic strokes have no identifiable source and of these, 20% of patients have a patent foramen ovale, which is presumed to have allowed for the 'paradoxical embolus' to reach the brain.

When are D-dimer levels useful in suspected DVT or PE?

D-dimer is the breakdown product of fibrin and is therefore elevated in any inflammatory process, e.g. infection, cancer, thrombosis, trauma. It is very sensitive but non-specific. In the context of suspected DVT or PE it is **only useful if the likelihood of the patient having a DVT or PE is low** (i.e. a low Wells' score). In this case, a negative D-dimer rules out a DVT or PE. This is referred as negative predictive value. Remember that if the Wells' score is not low, or there is another inflammatory process ongoing, a D-dimer is of no diagnostic value and you should not request it.

For a range of Single Best Answer questions related to the topic of this chapter go to
www.oxfordtextbooks.co.uk/orc/OCMS/

Leg ulcer

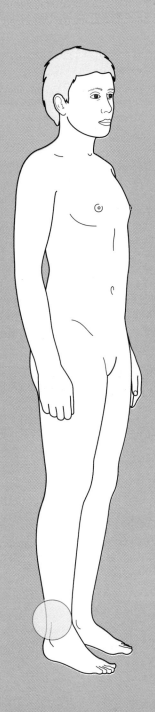

Core case

> *Read through the sections in red, covering up the sections in white that follow so that you don't see the answer. At the end of each red section, try to answer the question before reading on.*

Core case

Mrs Swanson is a 72-year-old lady admitted to hospital overnight because of increasing confusion secondary to pneumonia. On the ward round the next morning, the overnight doctor points out that Mrs Swanson also has an ulcer over her right ankle that will need investigating.

What is your differential diagnosis for a leg ulcer?

Venous ulcer
Mixed arterial/venous ulcer
Arterial (atherosclerotic) ulcer
Neuropathic ulcer
Pressure ulcer
Lymphoedema ulcer
Traumatic ulcer
Malignant ulcer (e.g. a Marjolin ulcer: a squamous cell carcinoma in a long-standing ulcer)
Vasculitic ulcer (e.g. rheumatoid arthritis, pyoderma gangrenosum)
Infective ulcer (e.g. tuberculosis, syphilis, leprosy)
Haemolytic anaemia (sickle cell, hereditary spherocytosis)

Venous ulcers account for by far the majority (about 70%), with mixed arterial/venous (about 10%) and arterial (about 10%) most of the remainder. The other causes are relatively rare with the exception of neuropathic ulcers in patients with diabetes mellitus.

Note that many leg ulcers may have a multifactorial aetiology, i.e. they may involve more than one of the pathologies above.

What do you want to know about the history of the ulcer itself, and how would each of the main types differ?

The first thing is to ask about the ulcer. You should consider:

* **Is the ulcer painful?**
  - **Venous ulcers** are caused by venous stasis in the leg and are thus *less painful when elevated* and drained of blood. However, only about 30% of venous ulcers are painful.
  - **Arterial (atherosclerotic) ulcers** are caused by ischaemia to the leg and are thus *more painful when elevated* and drained of blood. Patients often say the ulcers are painful enough to wake them up at night and that they obtain relief by lowering their leg over the side of the bed.

- **Neuropathic ulcers** are caused by loss of sensation (which predisposes to constant trauma) and are thus *not painful*.

- **How long has the ulcer been there?**
  - **Venous ulcers** are less painful and can therefore present late. They often have a long and recurring history.
  - **Arterial ulcers** tend to present relatively early because of pain. They often occur secondary to trivial trauma.
  - **Neuropathic ulcers** are associated with a loss of sensation and thus often present late.
  - A long history should arouse suspicion of a **Marjolin ulcer**, which only occurs in chronically present ulcers.

> The pathologies causing ulcers are not limited to the ulcer but will be evident in other symptoms. These will vary depending on the pathology.
>
> **What other symptoms occur in the most common pathologies causing ulcer (and therefore which symptoms should you ask about)?**

The associated symptoms you should ask about are:

- **Venous ulcers:** chronic venous insufficiency leads to **varicose veins**, stasis eczema, leading patients to complain of **itchiness**, and ankle oedema, leading to complaints of **swollen ankles** and a sensation of 'heavy feet'.

- **Arterial ulcers:** atherosclerosis is likely to be manifest systemically, thus ask about symptoms of peripheral arterial disease and coronary artery disease. These include **claudication**, **cold extremities**, and **angina** or **shortness of breath on exertion**.

- **Neuropathic ulcers:** these are associated with **sensory loss**, and patients may also have an **unsteady gait**. There is often secondary infection, and if this is by anaerobes the patient may comment on a **foul smell**.

> The probability of each type of ulcer is affected by the presence or absence of risk factors.
>
> **What risk factors should you ask about in the history?**

You should make a note of the following risk factors:

- **Venous ulcers** usually occur in patients with **varicose veins**, especially those who are **immobile** (reduced venous drainage of legs) and/or **malnourished** (reduced healing). They may also occur in patients with **recurrent deep vein thrombosis (DVT)**, an **abdominal tumour** (compressing the iliac veins), or **arteriovenous malformations** (increasing venous pressure). Major joint replacement (e.g. of a hip or knee) is also a risk factor, as up to about 25% of such operations are associated with subclinical DVTs.

- **Arterial ulcers** invariably occur in patients with risk factors for atherosclerosis (**smoking, diabetes mellitus, hypertension, hyperlipidaemia**, strong **family history** of atherosclerotic disease, **male**) and/or evidence of other

29

atherosclerotic disease: **coronary artery disease** (angina, myocardial infarction), **cerebrovascular disease** (transient ischaemic attack (TIA), stroke), **peripheral arterial disease** (claudication, impotence, abdominal aortic aneurysm (AAA)).

• **Neuropathic ulcers** mostly occur in patients with **diabetes mellitus** or **alcohol overuse**.

The key points from the history above, covering the most common ulcers, are summarized in Table 29.1.

Table 29.1 Key points in an ulcer history

	Venous	Arterial	Neuropathic
About the ulcer	Moderately painful, better on elevation. Present relatively late as not overly painful	Severe pain, worse on elevation. Present early due to pain	Painless and therefore present late
Associated symptoms	Varicose veins, stasis eczema (itchy), heavy legs, swelling around ulcer	Claudication, impotence, cold feet, angina	Loss of sensation in feet, contractures of feet
Risk factors	Varicose veins, DVT/pulmonary embolism, abdominal tumours (compressing iliac veins), arteriovenous malformations, major joint replacement	Smoking, diabetes mellitus, hypertension, hypercholesterolaemia, angina, myocardial infarction, TIA, stroke, claudication, impotence, AAA	Diabetes mellitus, poor foot care

29

Mrs Swanson is no longer confused after a night's sleep and some antibiotics for her pneumonia. She tells you that her ulcer is not really painful but that her legs often 'feel heavy' if she has been standing for a while. Her right ankle has been very itchy lately. She has not noticed any varicose veins and does not get pain in her calves when walking because of arthritis in her hip limiting her mobility. She never gets chest pain or suffers from shortness of breath. Her past medical history is remarkable for bilateral hip osteoarthritis, well-controlled hypertension, a presumed TIA 2 years ago, and chronic glaucoma in her right eye. She takes regular diclofenac with misoprostol for her hip pain, timolol and latanoprost for her glaucoma, and aspirin, simvastatin, ramipril, and bendroflumethiazide because of her hypertension and previous TIA. She smoked a packet of cigarettes every day from her 20s until her 50s. She has lived at home alone since the death of her husband 2 years ago.

What will you look for on examination? Think of what features might distinguish the most common types of leg ulcers. Also think about other signs associated with the underlying pathology that you can look for.

- **Site of the ulcer** (see Fig. 29.1)?
  - **Venous ulcers** occur where venous pressures are highest, which is the **gaiter area** of the legs (i.e. the area covered by a long sock). The most commonly affected area is just above the medial malleolus because this is the site of the medial calf perforators.
  - **Arterial ulcers** occur where arterial blood supply is worst, which tends to be the distal areas of the foot (e.g. between toes) and those that are frequently compressed (e.g. ball of foot, lateral malleolus, and bony prominences).
  - **Neuropathic ulcers** are caused by repetitive trauma in a foot that has lost sensation, and thus occur in pressure areas where the foot rubs on poorly fitting footwear (e.g. beneath the metatarsal heads).

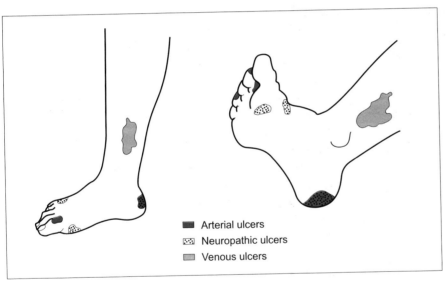

Figure 29.1 Typical locations of venous, arterial, and neuropathic ulcers.

- **Characteristics of the ulcer?**
  - **Venous ulcers: shallow, wet,** and with **irregular borders** that look white and fragile.
  - **Arterial ulcers: deep, punched out, dry,** and often elliptical.
  - **Neuropathic ulcers** often have very **thick, keratinized, raised edges** surrounding them (unlike a basal cell carcinoma, which has rolled edges that are not as thick).
  - **Pyoderma gangrenosum** (a type of ulcer associated with inflammatory bowel disease or haematological malignancies) often has a characteristic **dark blue/purple halo** around it.

29

- **Associated signs?**
  - **Venous ulcers** are due to increased hydrostatic (venous) pressure, which can also cause **oedema, extravasation,** and death of erythrocytes (**skin pigmentation**) and eventually scarring of the skin (**'atrophie blanche'**) and underlying tissue (**'lipodermatosclerosis'**). Superficial **varicose veins** or a collection of small, dark, engorged superficial veins (**'ankle flare'**) may be visible. In extreme cases, severe lipodermatosclerosis may lead to an **'inverted champagne bottle'** appearance to the leg.
  - **Arterial ulcers** are due to limb ischaemia and are therefore associated with **cold, pale limbs** with **poor capillary refill, absent or weak pulses,** and **atrophic skin changes** (dry, shiny, hairless). Buerger's test may reveal blanching of the foot on elevation to 45° and reactive hyperaemia on lowering the leg, suggesting arterial insufficiency. They usually occur in patients with widespread atherosclerotic disease. Thus, look for popliteal and AAAs, and listen for carotid, femoral, or renal artery bruits.
  - **Neuropathic ulcers** are due to loss of sensation. Typically, **vibration** and **proprioception** are lost before other modalities. **Foot deformities** may be present due to motor neuropathy or repetitive joint trauma secondary to sensory neuropathy (Charcot joints).
  - **Inguinal lymphadenopathy:** check for this if you suspect infection or malignancy as the cause of the ulcer.

Ulcer examination is summarized in Table 29.2.

Table 29.2 Summary of ulcer examination

	Venous	Arterial	Neuropathic
Site	Gaiter area (especially medial)	Ball of foot, between toes, tips of toes, lateral malleolus	Pressure areas of foot
Ulcer characteristics	Irregular, sloping, white edges	Well-defined, deep, punched out edges	Raised callous edges
Associated signs	Oedema, stasis eczema, skin pigmentation, lipodermatosclerosis, ankle flare, atrophie blanche	Cold, hairless, dry-skinned limb with weak or absent pulses. Poor capillary refill. Buerger's positive test. Carotid bruits. Abdominal aortic and/ or popliteal aneurysms	Decreased sensation (especially vibration), contractures of foot

Mrs Swanson has a single, 5 × 5 cm ulcer just above the medial malleolus of her right leg. The ulcer looks wet, has fragile looking irregular borders, and the surrounding skin is deeply pigmented. Her feet (and hands) feel slightly cold but dorsalis pedis and posterior tibial pulses are palpable in both feet. Her capillary refill time is 2 seconds in both feet. The rest of her cardiovascular exam is normal. Sensation is intact in both of her legs.

What is the most likely diagnosis? What first-line investigations will you arrange?

Mrs Swanson is an elderly lady with limited mobility who has a wet, irregular ulcer on the medial aspect of her right leg (gaiter area). Sensation is intact. There is surrounding skin pigmentation and no suggestion of arterial insufficiency on examination. The most likely diagnosis is a **venous ulcer**. Nonetheless, you should arrange the following investigations in case there is coexisting arterial disease, diabetes mellitus, or infection, as these will influence your management:

- **Bloods:** full blood count (FBC) (?infection), erythrocyte sedimentation rate (ESR), or C-reactive protein (CRP) (?vasculitis), albumin (?malnutrition), fasting lipids (?hyperlipidaemia, contributing to any atherosclerosis). In Mrs Swanson's case inflammatory markers will be unhelpful as her underlying pneumonia will cause these to be deranged. The FBC and albumin are particularly relevant because anaemia and hypoalbuminaemia are important factors that impair healing of venous ulcers but which can be addressed.

- **Capillary glucose:** a quick and reliable way of assessing whether Mrs Swanson has undiagnosed diabetes mellitus. Remember that up to 50% of type 2 diabetes mellitus is undiagnosed.

- **Urinalysis:** looking for glucose (?diabetes mellitus affecting healing) but also haematuria/proteinuria (?vasculitis).

- **Duplex ultrasound:** to assess the competence of the sapheno-femoral and sapheno-popliteal junctions, and state of the perforators and deep venous system.

- **Ankle–brachial pressure index (ABPI)**[†]: measured to exclude arterial disease as the cause. This is measured using a manual sphygmomanometer, stethoscope (for brachial pressure), and portable Doppler probe (for dorsalis pedis or posterior tibial pressure). The ABPI is the ratio of the ankle systolic pressure (either dorsalis pedis or posterior tibial) over the brachial artery systolic pressure. Even if you are clinically convinced that an ulcer is venous, it is important to measure the ABPI because if the ABPI is <0.8, the patient must *not* have a pressure bandage applied as this suggests the ulcer is actually a mixed venous/arterial ulcer and compression will make the arterial ischaemia worse. If the ABPI is <0.5, or there has been a sudden change, the patient needs urgent referral to a vascular surgeon.

- **Swabbing** an ulcer for microscopy, culture, and sensitivities (MC&S) is not routinely performed as all ulcers will have some growth. Swabbing may, however, be useful in the case of spreading cellulitis.

[†] **Beware:** patients with diabetes mellitus or chronic renal failure can have calcified (hard) arteries that give falsely high ABPI readings even in the presence of significant limb ischaemia. Oedema may also result in erroneous readings.

29

Mrs Swanson's admission blood results show leucocytosis and a raised CRP, as expected in a patient with pneumonia. Her ABPI is 0.95.

How should Mrs Swanson's ulcer be managed?

Mrs Swanson almost certainly has a **venous ulcer**. This is the result of prolonged venous stasis in her lower limb, and thus management involves:

- **Adequate nutrition,** vital for any healing process but especially relevant for venous ulcers as they tend to occur in elderly patients who may be malnourished or deficient in key vitamins and minerals (e.g. vitamin C, zinc).
- **Lifestyle modification:** encourage patients to mobilize (to encourage venous blood flow in the legs).
- **Leg elevation** whenever possible, to reduce blood pressure in the lower limb.
- **Compression bandages** applied and frequently changed by an experienced nurse, to reduce the pooling of venous blood in the lower limb. This can be done safely given that her ABPI is >0.8.
- **Graduated class I or II elastic stockings** will be helpful once the venous ulcer has healed to prevent recurrence.
- **Varicose vein surgery** may also be helpful in preventing recurrence if the ulcer was caused by obvious superficial varicosities and there is no deep vein incompetence (see viva question).

With this management, about 80% of venous ulcers will heal within 26 weeks. Those that fail to heal in this way may require skin grafting by the plastic or vascular surgeons.

Short cases

Mr Griffin is a 58-year-old gentleman who presents to his GP because of an ulcer on his left foot which has been present for 2 weeks. The ulcer causes him constant 'sharp pain' that is worse at night unless he sleeps with his foot dangling over the edge of the bed. Mr Griffin gets a stabbing pain in both calves if he walks too fast, but denies any chest pain, shortness of breath, or impotence. He also denies any itch, heaviness, or loss of sensation in his legs. He does not recall any trauma that could have caused the ulcer. His past medical history is remarkable for type 2 diabetes mellitus. He takes metformin, gliclazide, aspirin, simvastatin, and ramipril. He has smoked two packets of cigarettes a day for most of his adult life. His family history is unremarkable.

On examination, a well-demarcated, deep, dry ulcer is found over the ball of his left foot. His legs are pale, smooth, and hairless. Both feet are cold and have a capillary refill time of 5 seconds. On the right, dorsalis pedis is palpable but the posterior tibial pulse is not. On the left, neither pulse is palpable. Buerger's test is positive on both legs. The ABPI is 0.45 on the left and 0.65 on the right. Sensation in his lower limb is normal for all modalities. Examination of the rest of his cardiovascular system is unremarkable. His heart rate is 85 bpm (regular) and his blood pressure is 128/76 mmHg.

What is the diagnosis of Mr Griffin's ulcer? How should it be managed?

Mr Griffin is a gentleman with significant risk factors for atherosclerosis (lifelong smoker, diabetes mellitus) and a history of claudication on exercise. He has a well-demarcated, deep, dry ulcer on his left foot. His feet have poor capillary refill, weak or impalpable pulses, a positive Buerger's test, and an ABPI <0.8. This all suggests that Mr Griffin has an **arterial (atherosclerotic, ischaemic) ulcer** on his left lower limb. Furthermore, Mr Griffin has **critical limb ischaemia** – he has rest pain, tissue loss (the ulcer), and an ABPI <0.5 in the left leg – and therefore needs urgent referral to a vascular surgeon.

Management should involve:

- **Investigations:** remember that atherosclerosis is a systemic disease.
  - **Duplex ultrasonography of his lower limbs** (or magnetic resonance angiography) to assess the patency of the arteries and potential for revascularization or bypass surgery. Alternatively, **percutaneous angiography** can be performed to allow for assessment and treatment (angioplasty) to be done all in one
  - **Electrocardiogram (ECG)**
  - **Urinalysis** looking for proteinuria (?diabetic nephropathy) or haematuria (?vasculitis)
  - **Fasting serum lipids, fasting glucose, and HbA1c levels,** to see if Mr Griffin's lipid and glucose control are adequate
  - **FBC,** as anaemia will exacerbate any ischaemia
- **Interim management:**
  - **Dressing of the ulcer** to prevent infection, but take care to avoid the bandage being tight as this will worsen the ischaemia
  - **Analgesia**
  - **Antibiotics:** if there are any signs of infection and a swab is positive

29

- **Surgical intervention:**
  - **Angioplasty** and **stenting** can be performed if an artery is stenotic or there is a short occlusion and there is a patent artery downstream of the occlusion
  - **Bypass surgery** using a venous graft or artificial Dacron graft can be performed if angioplasty is not possible

---

Short case

Mr Griffin is admitted to hospital and has a duplex ultrasound that shows moderate stenosis of both the left and right external iliac arteries and severe stenosis (about 80%) of the left superficial femoral artery. He is placed on the waiting list for angioplasty and stenting. On the second night of Mr Griffin's admission the nursing staff bleep the duty junior doctor and ask her to come and see Mr Griffin. He states that he was awoken 2 hours ago because the pain from the ulcer in his left foot had suddenly spread to affect his entire left leg below his knee. He describes the pain as sharp and 8/10 in severity, with a tingling sensation confined to the foot. He was going to wait until the morning until he realized he was unable to move his left ankle.

On examination, Mr Griffin's left leg is significantly colder than the right. Both legs have typical Anglo-Saxon pallor but the sole of his left foot is ghostly white compared to his right. His popliteal pulse, dorsalis pedis, and posterior tibial are all impalpable on the left. On the right, dorsalis pedis is palpable but the posterior tibial pulse is not (as per his GP's findings). Sensation remains grossly intact in both legs.

What has happened to Mr Griffin? What is your next step?

Mr Griffin is a patient with known atherosclerotic disease of both lower limbs who has presented with the cardinal features of **acute limb ischaemia** which can be remembered as the **six Ps**: a painful, pale, pulseless, paralysed, perishingly cold leg with paraesthesia. This is likely to represent either thrombosis at the site of known stenosis or embolism.

Acute limb ischaemia is a **surgical emergency** that requires urgent intervention by the vascular surgeons to avoid losing the limb from irreversible ischaemic necrosis. For this reason, the next step should be to refer Mr Griffin to the vascular surgeon on call *immediately*. The vascular surgeons will then decide whether to attempt an embolectomy, percutaneous thrombolysis, revascularization angioplasty, bypass surgery, or amputation of the affected limb.

Mr Cleveland is a 52-year-old patient who has attended his local endocrinology department for a routine follow-up of his type 1 diabetes. During the consultation, Mr Cleveland points out that he has developed a painless ulcer on his right foot and his community nurse has urged him to get it checked. After removing the bandage for inspection, there is a small ulcer over the lateral aspect of the fifth metatarsophalangeal joint. The ulcer has rimmed edges and is deep. After removing some pus, it is obvious that the ulcer extends down to the bone. Mr Cleveland's feet are warm and well perfused. All pulses are palpable in Mr Cleveland's lower limbs and there is no eczema, varicose veins, or lipodermatosclerosis. However, Mr Cleveland has, for several years now, had diminished sensation to vibration in both feet. The registrar confirms that this is still the case, and that Mr Cleveland is now starting to lose his proprioception in both feet as well.

What is the likely cause of Mr Cleveland's ulcer? How should the ulcer be managed? What complication should you be concerned about?

Mr Cleveland is a patient with known diabetes mellitus who has presented with an ulcer on his foot. Diabetes mellitus increases one's risk of arterial (atherosclerotic) ulcer. However, this ulcer is directly over a pressure site (where shoes often rub), has rimmed edges, and is painless. Mr Cleveland has signs of peripheral neuropathy in both feet, whereas there are no signs of arterial disease. This is therefore a **neuropathic ulcer**.

Neuropathic ulcers in diabetics are due to repeated trauma and pressure plus a reduced ability to heal skin breaks and fight infection. For this reason, treatment involves:

- **Foot care:** avoid tight-fitting shoes until the ulcer is healed. Always wear soft, comfortable shoes thereafter and examine the feet daily.
- **Manage diabetes:** make sure diabetic control is optimized as uncontrolled hyperglycaemia will hinder ulcer repair and fighting infections.
- **Debridement:** ulcers in diabetics tend to build up necrotic tissue. This needs debriding either using special bandages (e.g. hydrogel sheets) or surgically.
- **Treat infections:** if there are clinical signs of infection.

The major complication to worry about in diabetic foot ulcers is infection. Given that Mr Cleveland's ulcer extends down to the bone you need to exclude **osteomyelitis**. Osteomyelitis should be suspected and investigated by magnetic resonance imaging (MRI) if:

- Diabetic ulcer >2 cm^2
- Visible or palpable bone in the ulcer (arguably, this represents osteomyelitis by definition)
- ESR >70 mm/hour

Mrs Glenn is an 82-year-old lady who has been referred to the surgeons at her local hospital because of a large ulcer on her right shin. Mrs Glenn lives in a nursing home because she has advanced Alzheimer's dementia. Her GP referral letter states that Mrs Glenn has had a long-standing venous ulcer (flat, wet, with irregular borders), on her right shin for the past 3 years. Management has been attempted with alginate-based compression dressings changed regularly by the nursing home staff, but the GP has noticed that the ulcer has recently changed: its central area has become raised and indurated, the ulcer smells far worse than usual, and its borders have spread and become raised.

On inspection, there is a large fungating ulcer on the right shin, surrounded by an area of lipodermato-sclerosis and skin pigmentation.

What has most likely happened to Mrs Glenn's ulcer? How should it be investigated? What is the prognosis?

Mrs Glenn has had a long-standing venous ulcer over her right pre-tibial region, as suggested by the lipodermatosclerosis, the skin pigmentation, and the GP's letter. The ulcer is now fungating, suggesting malignancy or infection. It is likely that Mrs Glenn's chronic venous ulcer has transformed into a squamous cell carcinoma – also known as a **Marjolin ulcer**.

Investigation involves a biopsy of the *peripheral* area of the ulcer (as the central area is likely to contain necrotic tissue which is hard to visualize for a histological diagnosis).

Management of a Marjolin ulcer is by wide excision and skin grafting, but the prognosis is poor and she may not be a candidate for surgery given her age and advanced, irreversible dementia.

Miss Takenawa is a 32-year-old lady who has been admitted to hospital for intravenous corticosteroid therapy for a particularly bad flare-up of her ulcerative colitis. During a teaching ward round, a medical student notices that Miss Takenawa has a small ulcer over the lateral aspect of her right leg. Miss Takenawa states that she was bitten by a midge several weeks ago whilst hiking in Scotland and assumes the ulcer has arisen because of the high-dose steroids she is currently receiving. The ulcer has a purplish halo at its border. She says it has been painful although it is now improving.

What type of ulcer has Miss Takenawa developed? How should it be managed?

Miss Takenawa is a patient with known ulcerative colitis who has developed an ulcer on her leg that has a purple halo around it. In the absence of any other obvious cause for her ulcer this is consistent with **pyoderma gangrenosum**, a complication of systemic inflammatory diseases (e.g. Crohn's disease, ulcerative colitis, rheumatoid arthritis) or haematological malignancies.

Management of pyoderma gangrenosum is with good nursing care (bandages to prevent infection and promote healing) and treatment of the underlying disease. As Miss Takenawa is already on intravenous corticosteroids, it is likely that the ulcer will improve as her ulcerative colitis settles.

29

Viva questions

What are the indications for surgery of varicose veins?

Patients with any of the following should be considered for surgery of their varicose veins under the UK National Health Service (NHS):

- Bleeding varicosity
- Unresolving or painful ulcer despite treatment
- Progressive skin changes (pigmentation, lipodermatosclerosis)
- Recurrent thrombophlebitis
- Significant impact on quality of life that has not been improved by conservative management with graded stockings.

The above criteria are based on the current National Institute for Health and Clinical Excellence (NICE) guidelines. As one can see, cosmetic reasons alone do not qualify for surgery under the NHS. Equally, there is nothing in the guidelines to suggest that a previous venous ulcer warrants surgery to prevent recurrence.

As discussed above, current NICE guidelines do not recommend prophylactic surgery of varicose veins to prevent recurrence of healed venous ulcers. Is there any evidence that surgery for varicose veins can reduce the recurrence of venous ulcers?

The **ESCHAR trial**[1] compared the long-term outcomes for patients with venous ulcers who were managed either with compression bandages alone or compression bandages plus surgery for any superficial varicose veins. The trial found that surgery did not accelerate ulcer healing times but almost halved the rate of recurrence at 4 years. The trial therefore suggests that it is better to surgically treat *superficial* varicose veins in patients who have had a venous ulcer as soon as possible, rather than waiting for a recurrent and unresolving ulcer to develop. The same benefit has not yet been found for *deep* venous disease.

[1] Gohel MS, Barwell JR, Taylor M, Chant T, Foy C, Earnshaw JJ *et al*. (2007). Long term results of compression therapy alone versus compression plus surgery in chronic venous ulceration (ESCHAR): randomised controlled trial. *BMJ*, **335**: 83.

What surgical options are there for treating varicose veins?

- **Avulsion/phlebectomy:** small incisions are made along the varicose vein and it is then pulled out with forceps.
- **Stripping:** small incisions are made at the ends of the varicose vein and an endoluminal hook and wire is used to pull the vein out.
- **Injection sclerotherapy:** this involves sealing the vein from within by injecting an irritant sclerosant. Unfortunately, the procedure is associated with skin discoloration in about 10% of patients and a 30% risk of recurrence if there is valvular incompetence, and is thus being used less often. A variant of injection sclerotherapy involves injecting a foam that blocks the vein, but there is a (small) risk of the foam embolizing into the venous system.

- **Radiofrequency ablation:** an endoluminal catheter is inserted into the long saphenous or short saphenous vein and a tip used to deliver high-energy radio waves (VNUS) that seal the vein from within. A similar procedure involves using a laser (EVLT) rather than radiowaves to achieve the same effect.

What are the risks of percutaneous angioplasty for arterial ischaemic limb disease?

Whenever you are asked about risks, try to have a structure to help you answer the question:

General risks (common to any procedure)

- Infection of puncture site
- Haemorrhage from puncture site
- Haematoma
- Reaction to the sedative used during the procedure

Specific risks (particular to this procedure)

- Thrombosis or embolization, potentially leading to loss of the limb
- Perforation of the artery, requiring further surgical intervention
- Aneurysm or pseudo-aneurysm of the artery at the site of dilatation and stenting or at the puncture site
- Reaction to the contrast dye used in the angiography

What are the main types of dressings for ulcers?

- **Low-adherence dressings:** useful only if there is little exudate that needs soaking up because they have little adherence, but they can often be left in place for 7 days.
- **Hydrogel dressings:** as the name implies, they are useful for hydrating dry ulcers (e.g. arterial) and for encouraging debridement of dead tissue (e.g. diabetic neuropathic ulcers).
- **Alginate dressings:** like the dry algae they are based on, they mop up water and are thus useful for wet ulcers (e.g. venous ulcers, fungating ulcers) that need drying.
- **Antibacterial dressings:** these prevent growth of bacteria by incorporating silver, honey, iodine, or metronidazole. There is little evidence base other than for iodine.

 For a range of Single Best Answer questions related to the topic of this chapter go to www.oxfordtextbooks.co.uk/orc/OCMS/

29

Index

Index of cases